SEVENTH EDITION

HAIRDRESSING AND BARBERING

THE FOUNDATIONS

The Official Guide to Hairdressing and Barbering NVQ at Level 2

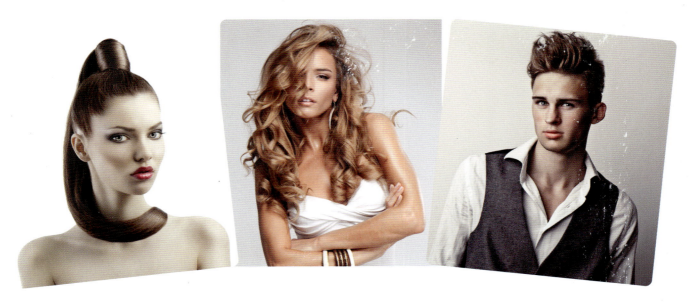

MARTIN GREEN

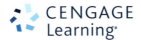

CENGAGE
Learning®

Australia • Brazil • Japan • Korea • Mexico • Singapore • Spain • United Kingdom • United States

HABIA SERIES LIST

Hairdressing

Student textbooks

Hairdressing and Barbering The Foundations: The Official Guide to Hairdressing and Barbering NVQ at Level 2 7e *Martin Green*

Begin Hairdressing: The Official Guide to Level 1 REVISED 2e *Martin Green*

Hairdressing and Barbering The Foundations: The Official Guide to Hairdressing and Barbering VRQ at Level 2 1e *Martin Green*

Professional Hairdressing: The Official Guide to Level 3 REVISED 6e *Martin Green and Leo Palladino*

The Pocket Guide to Key Terms for Hairdressing *Martin Green*

The Official Guide to the City & Guilds Certificate in Salon Service 1e *John Armstrong with Anita Crosland, Martin Green and Lorraine Nordmann*

The Colour Book: The Official Guide to Colour for NVQ Levels 2 & 3 1e *Tracey Lloyd with Christine McMillan-Bodell*

eXtensions: The Official Guide to Hair Extensions 1e *Theresa Bullock*

Salon Management *Martin Green*

Men's Hairdressing: Traditional and Modern Barbering 2e *Maurice Lister*

African-Caribbean Hairdressing 2e *Sandra Gittens*

The World of Hair Colour 1e *John Gray*

The Cutting Book: The Official Guide to Cutting at S/NVQ Levels 2 and 3 *Jane Goldsbro and Elaine White*

Professional Hairdressing titles

Trevor Sorbie: The Bridal Hair Book 1e *Trevor Sorbie and Jacki Wadeson*

The Art of Dressing Long Hair 1e *Guy Kremer and Jacki Wadeson*

Patrick Cameron: Dressing Long Hair 1e *Patrick Cameron and Jacki Wadeson*

Patrick Cameron: Dressing Long Hair 2 1e *Patrick Cameron and Jacki Wadeson*

Bridal Hair 1e *Pat Dixon and Jacki Wadeson*

Professional Men's Hairdressing: The Art of Cutting and Styling 1e *Guy Kremer and Jacki Wadeson*

Essensuals, the Next Generation Toni and Guy: Step by Step 1e *Sacha Mascolo, Christian Mascolo and Stuart Wesson*

Mahogany Hairdressing: Step to Cutting, Colouring and Finishing Hair 1e *Martin Gannon and Richard Thompson*

Mahogany Hairdressing: Advanced Looks 1e *Martin Gannon and Richard Thompson*

The Total Look: The Style Guide for Hair and Make-up Professional 1e *Ian Mistlin*

Trevor Sorbie: Visions in Hair 1e *Trevor Sorbie, Kris Sorbie and Jacki Wadeson*

The Art of Hair Colouring 1e *David Adams and Jacki Wadeson*

Beauty therapy

Beauty Basics: The Official Guide to Level 1 3e *Lorraine Nordmann*

Beauty Therapy – The Foundations: The Official Guide to Level 2 VRQ 5e *Lorraine Nordmann*

Beauty Therapy – The Foundations: The Official Guide to Level 2 5e *Lorraine Nordmann*

Professional Beauty Therapy – The Official Guide to Level 3 4e *Lorraine Nordmann*

The Pocket Guide to Key Terms for Beauty Therapy *Lorraine Nordmann and Marian Newman*

The Official Guide to the City & Guilds Certificate in Salon Services 1e *John Armstrong with Anita Crosland, Martin Green and Lorraine Nordmann*

The Complete Guide to Make-Up 1e *Suzanne Le Quesne*

The Encyclopedia of Nails 1e *Jacqui Jefford and Anne Swain*

The Art of Nails: A Comprehensive Style Guide to Nail Treatments and Nail Art 1e *Jacqui Jefford*

Nail Artistry 1e *Jacqui Jefford*

The Complete Nail Technician 3e *Marian Newman*

Manicure, Pedicure and Advanced Nail Techniques 1e *Elaine Almond*

The Official Guide to Body Massage 2e *Adele O'Keefe*

An Holistic Guide to Massage 1e *Tina Parsons*

Indian Head Massage 2e *Muriel Burnham-Airey and Adele O'Keefe*

Aromatherapy for the Beauty Therapist 1e *Valerie Worwood*

An Holistic Guide to Reflexology 1e *Tina Parsons*

An Holistic Guide to Anatomy and Physiology 1e *Tina Parsons*

The Essential Guide to Holistic and Complementary Therapy 1e *Helen Beckmann and Suzanne Le Quesne*

The Spa Book 1e *Jane Crebbin-Bailey, Dr John Harcup, and John Harrington*

SPA: The Official Guide to Spa Therapy at Levels 2 and 3, *Joan Scott and Andrea Harrison*

Nutrition: A Practical Approach 1e *Suzanne Le Quesne*

Hands on Sports Therapy 1e *Keith Ward*

Encyclopedia of Hair Removal: A Complete Reference to Methods, Techniques and Career Opportunities, *Gill Morris and Janice Brown*

The Anatomy and Physiology Workbook: For Beauty and Holistic Therapies Levels 1–3. *Tina Parsons*

The Anatomy and Physiology CD-Rom

Beautiful Selling: The Complete Guide to Sales Success in the Salon *Rath Langley*

The Official Guide to the Diploma in Hair and Beauty Studies at Foundation Level 1e *Jane Goldsbro and Elaine White*

The Official Guide to the Diploma in Hair and Beauty Studies at Higher Level 1e *Jane Goldsbro and Elaine White*

The Official Guide to Foundation Learning in Hair and Beauty 1e *Jane Goldsbro and Elaine White*

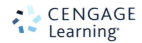

**Hairdressing and Barbering: The Foundations —
The Official Guide to Hairdressing and Barbering
NVQ at Level 2**
Martin Green

Publishing Director: Linden Harris
Commissioning Editor: Lucy Mills
Development Editor: Claire Napoli
Editorial Assistant: Lauren Darby
Production Editor: Alison Cooke
Production Controller: Eyvett Davis
Typesetter: MPS Limited
Cover design: HCT Creative
Text design: Design Deluxe

For product information and technology assistance,
contact **emea.info@cengage.com.**

For permission to use material from this text or product,
and for permission queries,
email **emea.permissions@cengage.com.**

British Library Cataloguing-in-Publication Data
A catalogue record for this book is available from the British Library.

ISBN: 978-1-4080-7110-6

Cengage Learning EMEA
Cheriton House, North Way, Andover, Hampshire, SP10 5BE United Kingdom

Cengage Learning products are represented in Canada by Nelson Education Ltd.

For your lifelong learning solutions, visit **www.cengage.co.uk**

Purchase your next print book, e-book or e-chapter at **www.cengagebrain.com**

Printed in China by RR Donnelley
2 3 4 5 6 7 8 9 10 – 16 15 14

Dedication to Leo Palladino [B.A.]

This edition is dedicated to the memory of Leo Palladino whose original chapters, on the science of hairdressing, formed the basis of the Official Guides to Hairdressing as they are known today. Leo's knowledge and understanding of this subject contributed to his success in becoming the best-selling author in the United Kingdom and beyond, on practical and theoretical hairdressing. His books have become and continue to be the industry standard for this subject.

During his successful career in hairdressing, trichology and education Leo lectured at college level progressing to Head of Science at Gloucestershire College of Arts and Technology. He served on the Hairdressing Council as an advisor and toured the country with companies such as Wella. As Chief Examiner for City & Guilds he had the ultimate responsibility for setting Syllabi and marking examination papers, and as a board member of Habia, setting the standards as we know them in the United Kingdom today.

Throughout life Leo's dedication to both his family and his industry was second to none.

His legacy will live on through his lifetime's contribution to the Hairdressing industry.

Contents

PART ONE Generic salon skills

PART TWO Technical services

Foreword

When Habia first began to promote the NVQ Level 2 qualification in hairdressing back in 1989, no one envisaged the phenomenal success that would be achieved. Within five years the NVQ established itself as the accepted qualification throughout the hairdressing industry. Fundamental to this achievement was the success of the first edition of this book.

Ever since 1989 when the first edition of this book was published, Habia and the standards it creates have been an integral part of Hairdressing and Barbering, The Foundations.

It seems incredible we are now on the 7th edition, and still managing to find ways to keep the content original and informative whilst providing learners with the key knowledge they need to progress in their studies.

Rob Young, Habia MD

Acknowledgements

The author and publisher would like to thank the following:

For providing the cover image:

Habia

For providing images for this book:

Prof Andrew Wright

Andy Lynch (**www.andylynch.co.uk**)

BaByliss PRO

Balmain

Beauty Express

Denman

E A Ellisons & Co LTD

The Glove Club **www.gloveclub.co.uk**

Goldwell UK

Habia

HairTools Ltd (**www.hairtools.co.uk**)

HSE

IT&LY

Dr John Gray

King Research, Inc

L'Oréal Professionnel

Majestic Towels

Mediscan

Paul Falltrick for Matrix

Redken

REM UK LTD

Saks (**www.saks.co.uk**)

WAHL UK

Wella

Wellcome Images

The publisher would like to thank the many copyright holders who have kindly granted us permission to reproduce material throughout this text. Every effort has been made to contact all rights holders but in the unlikely event that anything has been overlooked please contact the publisher directly and we will happily make the necessary arrangements at the earliest opportunity.

For their help with the photo shoot:

The author and Cengage Learning wish to extend a huge thanks to the Hairdressing Department at Abingdon and Witney College and in particular, all the students and staff who played a key part in the organization, direction and production of photographic content for this book. Particular thanks go to:

Sarah Barnardt – Team leader, technical supervision and coordination for colouring

Hayley Dunbar

Leanne Collins

Natalie Timms – Team leader, technical supervision and coordination for styling and long hair effects

Laura Clark

Bianca Clanfield

Carloyn Nutley

Charlotte (Charlie) Donaldson – Team leader, technical supervision and coordination for cutting and barbering

Kathy Selby

Katie Jones

Sophie Day

And a special thanks to our stylists:

Ashleigh Farmer

Keri Stowe

Emma Sykes

Sarah Scott

Sam Ruddock

Tash Wingfield

Katie Arnold

Hayley Allen

Le-Ann Proto

Lottie Smith

Harley Askew

Shaun Fitzgibbon

Katie Glynn

Jo Walker

Karen Goddard

About the author

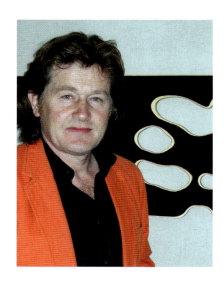

Martin Green is an experienced hairdresser and college lecturer with 40 years in the industry. During that time, he has been a consultant to Habia, where he was part of the original team that created the first NOS. He has worked for awarding organizations such as City and Guilds of London Institute (C&G) where he was a Regional Verifier for the South West, and at the Vocational Training Charitable Trust (VTCT) writing assessment materials.

Martin writes the *Official Guides to Hairdressing*. These include *Begin Hairdressing NVQ Level 1, Hairdressing and Barbering the Foundations VRQ Level 2 and Professional Hairdressing NVQ Level 3*.

Martin's energy and passion for the craft is not only demonstrated through being a practitioner, teacher and author, his enthusiasm has been unyielding, and he has keen interests in the development of e-learning and online resources too. More recently, he won a national award at *Advanced Level for Widening Participation* in education through e-learning, awarded by JISC RSC.

Level 2 NVQ (QCF) Diploma in Hairdressing or Barbering

In order to reach our customers' ever-increasing expectations, the standards of what we do must rise too. In a changing world the industry needs staff that are flexible, highly self-motivated and most importantly, very well trained. But in order for this to happen, other things need to change too and this book has been updated to reflect these changes within training and education.

The NVQ is the only type of qualification that provides the learner with a 'job ready' job recognized qualification. This means that for those who want to be trained as apprentices in a salon, they will reach Junior Stylist status by the end of their Level 2 training. Similarly, those students who have chosen to do an NVQ at college can expect that at least part of the course will be spent out on placement in a commercial salon too.

NVQ Diploma (QCF) – An Introduction

HABIA, The Hair and Beauty Industry Authority, is the representative organization responsible for defining the standards for our hair and beauty industry. The National Occupational Standards (NOS) that they produce are then taken and used by awarding organizations to create the qualifications that you take part in. So in simple terms HABIA produce the standards that you work towards and awarding organizations define the conditions and specifications against which you are assessed.

All NOS have a common structure and design. That is to say, they all follow a particular format for all vocational sectors. Each vocational qualification is structured in the same way and is made up from a number of grouped components.

Each grouping or **unit** addresses a specific task or area of working, e.g. reception. So when a staff member is asked to 'do reception' the work involves many different tasks such as handling payments, making appointments, receiving clients and restocking products and stationery materials. These individual learning objectives are referred to in NVQ terms as the 'main outcomes'.

Level 2 NVQ Diploma in Hairdressing

Structure of units

Candidates must complete all **eight mandatory units** and gain a **minimum of six optional credits** to achieve the qualification.

The mandatory units are:

Unit title	Credit value	Chapter
G20 Make sure your own actions reduce risks to health and safety (ENTO HSS 1)	4 credits	1
G17 Give clients a positive impression of yourself and your organization (ICS Unit 9)	5 credits	3
G7 Advise and consult with clients	4 credits	6
GH8 Shampoo, condition and treat the hair and scalp	4 credits	7
GH9 Change hair colour	11 credits	16
GH10 Style and finish hair	6 credits	8
GH11 Set and dress hair	6 credits	10
GH12 Cut hair using basic techniques	8 credits	12

(All of these must be completed.)

Plus a unit (or units) that add up to **minimum of six optional credits** from the list below:

Unit title	Credit value	Chapter
G4 Fulfill salon reception duties	3 credits	4
G18 Promote additional services or products to clients (ICS Unit10)	6 credits	5
G8 Develop and maintain your effectiveness at work	3 credits	2
GH13 Plait and twist hair	4 credits	10
GH14 Perm and neutralize hair	8 credits	17
GH15 Attach hair to enhance a style	3 credits	11

A minimum of 54 credits must be achieved in order to gain the full Level 2 NVQ Diploma in Hairdressing (QCF).

Level 2 NVQ Diploma in Barbering (QCF)

Structure of Units

Candidates must complete the **six mandatory units** and a **minimum of nine optional credits** with **one** unit to be taken from **each** of the following optional groups:

The mandatory units are:

Unit title	Credit value	Chapter
G20 Make sure your own actions reduce risks to health and safety ENTO (HSS 1)	4 credits	1
G7 Advise and consult with clients	4 credits	6
GH8 Shampoo, condition and treat the hair and scalp	4 credits	7
GB3 Cut hair using basic barbering techniques	8 credits	13
GB4 Cut facial hair to shape using basic techniques	4 credits	14
GB5 Dry and finish men's hair	4 credits	9

(All of these must be completed.)

Plus one of the following optional units from this group:

Unit title	Credit value	Chapter
AH21 Create basic patterns in hair	4 credits	15
GH14 Perm and neutralize hair	8 credits	17
GB2 Change men's hair colour	11 credits	16

Plus one of the following optional units from this group:

Unit title	Credit value	Chapter
G4 Fulfil salon reception duties	3 credits	4
G8 Develop and maintain your effectiveness at work	3 credits	2
G17 Give clients a positive impression of yourself and your organization (ICS Unit 9)	5 credits	3
G18 Promote additional services or products to clients (ICS Unit10)	6 credits	5

A minimum of 37 credits must be achieved in order to gain the full Level 2 Diploma in Barbering

Units and learning outcomes

The individual units listed on the previous page denote the smallest components of the NVQ that can be awarded by certificate. Each unit comprises a unit title and one or more learning outcomes and these are the smallest meaningful components within an NVQ.

Unit title and learning outcomes (example from: Health and safety unit)

Unit title	Learning outcomes
G20 Make sure your own actions reduce risks to health and safety	G20.1 Identify the hazards and evaluate the risks in your workplace G20.2 Reduce the risks to health and safety in your workplace

The learning outcomes

Learning outcomes are brief statements that outline the tasks that need to be done. Their titles are always expressed in a 'do this' language, e.g. 'Identify the hazards and evaluate the risks in your workplace'. However, while giving you an idea of what needs to be done, it doesn't say how it's to be done.

The NOS cover this in greater detail. They specify how each task is to be performed by listing the **performance criteria**; they also cover the circumstances, conditions or situations in which these actions must be done, which is called the **range**.

Performance criteria

The performance criteria are a list of the essential actions. Although these may not be necessarily in the order in which they should be done, they do provide a definitive checklist of what needs to be done. During assessment, these performance criteria form the specification of how a task must be done.

Example of performance criteria showing how the task must be done:

Learning outcome	Performance criteria
GH8.1 Maintain effective and safe methods of working when shampooing, conditioning and treating the hair and scalp	1 Ensuring your client's clothing is effectively protected throughout the service 2 Wearing personal protective equipment, if required 3 Positioning your client to meet the needs of the service without causing them discomfort 4 Ensuring your own posture and position whilst working minimizes fatigue and the risk of injury

Range

The range statements provide a number of conditions or applications in which the learning outcomes must be performed. Quite simply, they state under what particular circumstances, and on what occasions, or in which special situations, the activity must take place.

Example of range statements identifying which situations or circumstances need to be included when doing the task:

Learning outcome	Range
GH8.1 Maintain effective and safe methods of working when shampooing, conditioning and treating the hair and scalp	**Look to identify any contra-indications such as:** skin and scalp disorders and diseases **Look to identify any contra-indications such as:** cuts and abrasions **Ask questions to identify any contra-indications such as:** product allergies

Essential knowledge and understanding

NVQs are not just about doing though; when you do your work properly, you need to know what you are doing and why you are doing it. The terms 'theory', 'learning' and 'principles' generally refer to essential knowledge and understanding, in other words, what you must know.

Learning outcome	What you must know (EKU)
GH8.1 Maintain effective and safe methods of working when shampooing, conditioning and treating the hair and scalp	**You should know:** when and how to complete client records **You should know:** the range of protective clothing that should be available for clients **You should know:** why it is important to use personal protective equipment

At the point where a task's performance criteria and range have been covered and knowledge has been learnt and understood, the task is carried out competently and a skill has been acquired.

Shared knowledge

Units and learning outcomes often share similar components, i.e. some of the performance criteria used within a main outcome from one task is often similar to that used within another.

Example

GH12.1 Maintain effective and safe methods of working when cutting hair, and GH10.1 Maintain effective and safe methods of working when styling and finishing hair.

Similarly, the knowledge that is essential underpinning one learning outcome, will often occur in another. This duplication may at first seem unnecessary, but it happens because of the modular, stand-alone design of NVQ units. (Remember, each individual unit can be awarded on a certificate.)

This can be useful in terms of speeding up the learning process as sometimes knowledge or skills learnt in one activity are then directly applicable to other tasks. This is also useful when it comes to recording these learnt experiences, because the knowledge learnt in one situation can be quickly cross-referenced to other similar activities in your portfolio.

Under assessment

Your competence, your ability to carry out a task to a standard, is measured during assessment. Your ability to carry out the task, 'performance evidence', will be observed and checked against the performance criteria. Therefore your assessor will be watching to see how you carry out your work.

Sometimes it is not possible to cover all the situations that might crop up in one performance. So, in that situation, your assessor might ask you questions about what you have done and how you might apply that in different circumstances. To help you get used to this, the activities that appear throughout the book contain lots of the types of questions that you might be asked.

Your understanding and background knowledge of work tasks is also measured through questions asked by your assessor. Sometimes you might be asked to give a personal account of what you have learned. This could take the form of writing a sequence of events that need to be done to complete the task satisfactorily. Other questions may ask you specifically about particular tasks; more often than not, these types of questions take the form of short-answer, or multiple-choice questions. Again, the activities covered within this book give plenty of examples and practice.

About this book

The common structure and design that exist within National Occupational Standards (NOS) are mirrored in many ways within this text. For the first time in the hairdressing NVQ/SVQ official series, revisions and updates have been totally reworked to provide:

A) the fastest possible navigation to the things that you want to find out about

B) a book that covers all the aspects of the NVQ Diploma for both hairdressing and barbering standards

C) a chapter structure that now mirrors the NVQ Diploma standards in unit as well as outcome format.

D) a large glossary and index to help you understand and find key information

All of these features and illustrations have been redesigned and reorganized in order to help you accelerate through your Level 2 programme.

How to use this book

You can use this book in a number of differing ways:

1 You can use the revised chapter structure to cover complete units as you get to them within your training.

2 You can use the book as a quick guide and overview to the things that you will be doing and the things that you will learn.

3 You can use it as your standalone course guide covering the A–Z of hairdressing at NVQ Diploma Level 2.

The new format will help you to use and read this book more easily. Each chapter opens with a simple quick look at what you need to do, and what you will need to know, and then extends further by covering each aspect in a comprehensive way.

Throughout this textbook you will find many colourful text boxes designed to aid your learning and understanding as well as highlight key points. Here are examples and descriptions of each:

BEST PRACTICE

Suggests good working practice and help you develop your skills and awareness during your training.

HEALTH & SAFETY

Draws your attention to related health and safety information essential for each technical skill.

ACTIVITY BOX

Feature within all chapters and provide additional tasks for you to further your understanding.

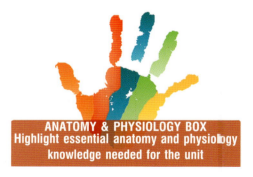

Directional arrows point you to other parts of the book that explore similar topics, in order for you to expand your learning.

CourseMate video boxes highlight some techniques which are available to view online

ANATOMY & PHYSIOLOGY BOX
Highlight essential anatomy and physiology knowledge needed for the unit

TOP TIP

share the author's experience and provide positive suggestions to improve knowledge and skills for each unit.

Knowledge Check

These boxes are designed to check your knowledge of the subject being discussed on the page. These will often include information about the current laws surrounding a topic.

SUMMARY

Summary boxes can be found at the end of each chapter and are designed to:

1 Provide a final reflection on what you have covered in the chapter.

2 Provide a clearer picture of all the essential aspects of the topic, including the tools and equipment you should be using.

3 Ensuring you have a basic understanding of the key principles.

ASSESSMENT OF KNOWLEDGE AND UNDERSTANDING

Are provided at the end of all core chapters. You can use the questions to prepare for oral and written assessments and help test your own knowledge throughout. Seek guidance from your supervisor/assessor if there are areas you are unsure of.

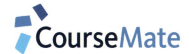

About the website

Use Hairdressing and Barbering Level 2 NVQ CourseMate alongside *The Official Guide to Hairdressing and Barbering Level 2 NVQ 7e* textbook for a complete blended learning solution!

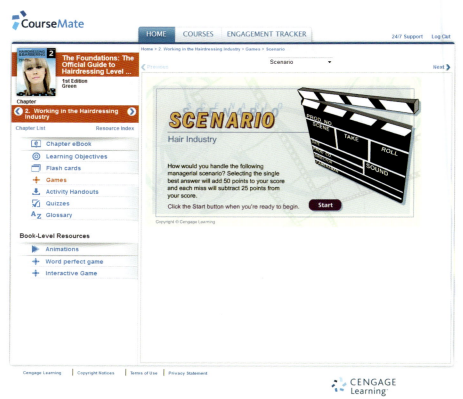

This highly interactive resource brings course concepts to life and is designed to support lecturers and students through the range of online resources which can be perfectly integrated in to the classroom to cover the guided learning hours for each unit.

For Students:

- Searchable eBook
- Step by step videos
- Interactive multiple choice quizzes
- Interactive activities and games

For Lecturers:

- Lessons plans
- PowerPoint slides
- Activity handouts
- 'Engagement Tracker' tools so students' progression and comprehension can be fully monitored

For more information please email emea.fesales@cengage.com

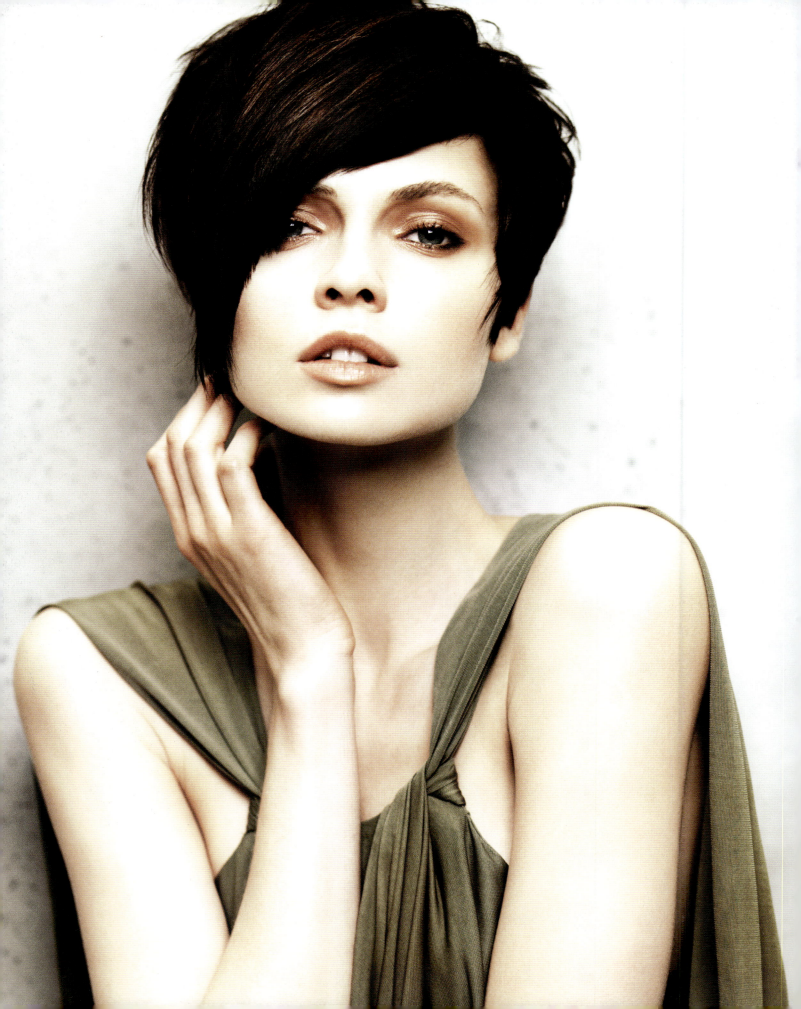

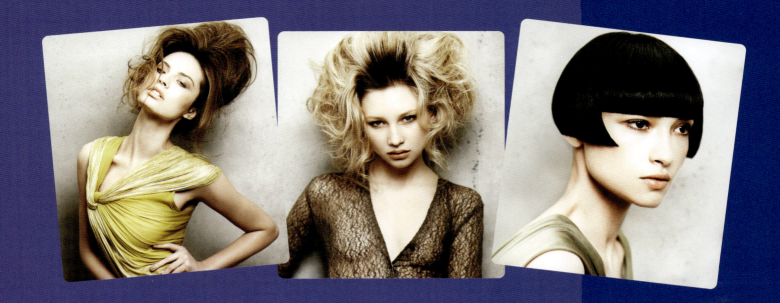

PART ONE

Generic salon skills

This section of the book looks at the range of non-technical services that play an essential supporting role in the delivery of the commercial services to salon clients.

1 Health and safety

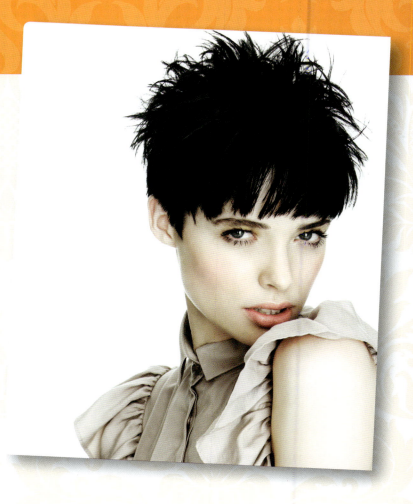

LEARNING OBJECTIVES

◆ Be able to identify any potential hazards within your salon

◆ Be able to reduce the risks to health and safety within your salon

◆ Know how to take action to eliminate potential hazards

◆ Know who you should report health and safety issues to, in situations that are beyond your normal work remit

KEY TERMS

assessments
body language
colouring products
communications
cross-infection
dermatitis
evacuation procedures

hazard
Health and Safety at Work
    Act 1974
limits of your own authority
Permanent colours
perming
perm solution

personal presentation
personal protective equipment
portfolio
project
risk
scalp
sharps box

G20 Make sure your own actions reduce risks to health and safety

Information covered in this chapter

- Hazards and risks
- Good salon hygiene and preventing infection
- Safe, hygienic use of salon tools and equipment
- Dealing with emergencies
- Health and safety regulations

INTRODUCTION

The ways in which you and your colleagues go about daily duties has a direct effect upon the general health and safety of everyone within the workplace. Poor hygiene, careless preparation, not thinking for others or not clearing up properly and not noticing potential hazards – can all have a disastrous impact on the safety and well-being of others.

At Level 2 you should be able to identify and reduce risks within the working environment, so this chapter looks at the types of hazard that you might find in your workplace, and also how you should go about reducing or eliminating risks to health and safety.

If you would like to find out more about hairdressing health and safety, or the relevant legislation covered in the Health and Safety at Work Act 1974 (HASWA), there is more information in Appendices 1 and 2 at the back of this book. Alternatively go online to the Health and Safety Executive website – www.hse.gov.uk/hairdressing/ – to find out more about these issues.

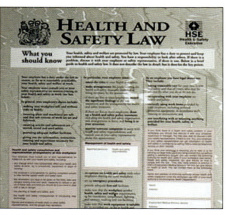

Health and safety law

HMSO

The Health and Safety at Work Act 1974 is continually being reviewed and updated, it covers many smaller component regulations. See if you can match the individual legal regulations on the left with the appropriate health and safety issues on the right. (Tip: look at the regulation wording to work out its appropriate link.)

Workplace (Health, Safety and Welfare) Regulations 1992	Always wear gloves and aprons when handling chemical compounds
Manual Handling Operations Regulations 1992	Correct and safe operation of salon equipment
Provision and Use of Work Equipment Regulations 1992	Salon chemical products must be stored and be kept safely at all times
Personal Protective Equipment at Work Regulations 1992	**Dermatitis** a notifiable skin condition that results from sensitivity to chemicals
Control of Substances Hazardous to Health Regulations 2002 (COSHH)	Monitoring and maintenance of workplace hygiene and cleanliness
Electricity at Work Regulations 1989	Always keep well stocked, just in case of accidents occurring at work
Reporting of Injuries, Diseases and Dangerous Occurrences Regulations 1995	Manufacturer information relating to the use of chemical products
Cosmetic Products (Safety) Regulations 1989	The movement and handling of objects needs to be done safely and properly
Health and Safety (First Aid) Regulations 1981	Items of salon electrical equipment must be checked and tested each year

HEALTH & SAFETY

Health and safety laws are being continually reviewed and updated. Make sure you are aware of the latest information and look at the health and safety posters within your salon.

HEALTH & SAFETY

Employers have a responsibility to ensure the health, safety and welfare of the people within the workplace.

All people at work have a duty and responsibility not to harm themselves or others through the work they do.

Identify hazards and evaluate the risks in your workplace

Hazard and risk

Almost anything may be a **hazard**, but may or may not become a **risk**. For example:

◆ A trailing electric cable from a piece of equipment is a hazard if it is trailing across a passageway as there is a high risk of someone tripping over it, but if it lies along a wall out of the way, the risk is much less.

◆ Poisonous or flammable chemicals are hazards and may present a high risk. However, if they are kept in a properly designed secure store and handled by properly trained and equipped people, the risk is much less than if they are left about for anyone to use.

◆ A failed light bulb is a hazard. If it is just one of many in a room it presents very little risk, but if it is the only light on a stairwell, it is a very high risk. Changing the bulb may be a high risk, if it is up high, or if the power has been left on, or a low risk if it is in a table lamp which has been unplugged.

◆ A box of heavy items is a hazard. It presents a higher risk to someone who lifts it incorrectly, rather than someone who uses the correct manual handling techniques.

You share a responsibility with your work colleagues for the safety of all the people within the salon (clients, visitors and staff) so you need to be aware of the types of hazards that could exist. You need to be aware of:

1 Hazards within the working environment, such as:

- ◆ wet or slippery floors
- ◆ cluttered passageways or corridors
- ◆ hair clippings left on the salon floor
- ◆ trailing electrical flexes.

2 Hazards to do with equipment and materials, such as:

- ◆ worn-out or faulty electrical equipment
- ◆ incorrectly labelled materials
- ◆ inaccurate measurement of chemical products.

3 Hazards connected with people, such as:

- ◆ bad posture
- ◆ handling and moving stock
- ◆ poor health, **cross-infection**, disease.

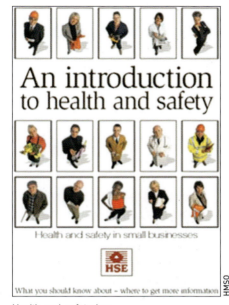

An introduction to health and safety

Health and safety in small businesses

HSE

What you should know about – where to get more information

HMSO

Health and safety law

Simply being aware of potential hazards is not enough. You have a responsibility to contribute to a safe working environment, so you must take steps to check and deal with any sources of risk to people's health and safety.

You could do this in two ways:

1 You could deal with the hazard yourself. This will probably apply to obvious hazards such as:

- ◆ trailing flexes – roll them up and store them safely
- ◆ cluttered doorways and corridors – remove objects and store them safely or dispose of them appropriately
- ◆ sweep the floor to remove loose hair clippings.

2 You tell a responsible person, e.g. your manager or supervisor. This applies to hazards which are beyond your responsibility to deal with, such as:

- ◆ faulty equipment, such as dryers, tongs, straightening irons, kettles, computers, etc.
- ◆ worn floor coverings or broken tiles
- ◆ loose or damaged fittings, such as mirrors, shelves or backwashes
- ◆ obstructions too heavy for you to move safely
- ◆ fire – follow the correct procedures to raise the alarm and help with the salon's **evacuation procedures**.

ACTIVITY

Hazards at work

◆ Your ability to spot potential hazards helps to prevent accidents within the salon environment.

◆ Complete this activity by identifying the things that you need to check for.

Hazards	Things to check for
Floors and flooring	
Corridors	
Chemicals	
Electrical equipment	
Basins and sinks	

HEALTH & SAFETY

Being aware of potential hazards is not enough: you can minimize risks by taking prompt action.

ACTIVITY

Find out the following information from your place of work, then complete the details in the space provided.

Q1. Who has overall responsibility for health and safety at your salon?
A1. Name

Q2. What is their job role in the workplace?
A2. Job role

Q3. If you found something at work that you felt was not safe, whom would you report to?
A3. Name

Q4. What sort of potential hazards do you think you might find? (List as many as you can.)
A4.

Q5. In relation to product use, why are manufacturers' instructions important?
A5.

Q6. What is your salon's policy in respect to maintaining a healthy and safe work environment?
A6.

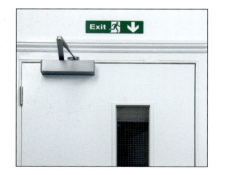

A safe working environment

Being a responsible person The word 'responsible' is used many times and in many ways at work. It may be something that you are already used to and it may be something that you welcome. However, as we all have a role to play at work, the role of self-responsibility – shouldering the weight of our actions and the impact that it has on others – really comes into play. You play an important part in spotting potential hazards and preventing accidents and therefore helping your salon and colleagues to avoid any emergency situations arising.

So how can I make a difference?

Suppose, for example, that someone had carelessly blocked a fire door with recently delivered stock. You could take the initiative and move the stock items to a safe and secure location.

However, there are occasions where being responsible requires that you make a quick judgement of what you have found and tell someone else about it. When you notice a potential hazard that you cannot easily rectify yourself, tell your supervisor immediately.

Imagine, for instance, that the lower cutting blade on a pair of clippers became loose. If this was unnoticed by one of the stylists they might pick the clippers up and use them on a client and cut their neck!

In this situation your swift action might save a client from a serious injury. You see the hazard and understand the risk, but the essential readjustment of the blades should only be undertaken by a suitably trained person.

Salon/workplace policy
Salons will vary in size, layout and organizational structure and because of this each salon has its own set of rules relating to safe and healthy practices, processes and procedures. This information is made available to you at the point of joining an organization, usually within an induction process.

The induction training sets out the basic rules of your employment: what's expected of you and what you can expect from the company. During your induction you may be given a number of documents that you should keep for future information and later use. Amongst these (typically) will be the salon's policy in relation to the following health and safety issues:

◆ fire and emergency evacuation procedures

◆ people to whom you should report in the event of emergency or significant risk to people's safety

◆ the things that you *may* undertake yourself to control risks to the health, safety and welfare of others

◆ the things that you *may not* undertake yourself to control risks to the health, safety and welfare of others

◆ health and safety training information.

In addition to the above, you will find the following prominently placed health and safety notices/records available on display:

◆ health and safety information poster

◆ COSHH information booklet

◆ salon risk **assessments**

◆ Public Liability Insurance certificate

◆ fire safety evacuation procedures

◆ accident book (records of injuries and treatments provided)

◆ written health and safety policy.

HEALTH & SAFETY

Always read the manufacturers' instructions before using their equipment or products.

ACTIVITY

Salon layout

Draw a floor plan of your salon. Within your sketch you need to show where the following can be found:

1. Fire extinguisher(s)
2. Storage for products/equipment
3. Disposal of waste and sharps
4. Sterilizing equipment
5. Personal protective equipment
6. Accident book
7. Fire exit(s)
8. First-aid box/kit
9. Health and safety information

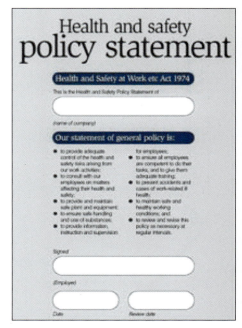

An example health and safety policy statement

Reduce the risks to health and safety in your workplace

People are exposed to all kinds of hazardous substances at work. These can include chemicals that people make or work with directly, and also dust, fumes and bacteria which can be present in the workplace. Exposure can happen by inhalation, (i.e. breathing them in), making contact with the skin, splashing them into the eyes or ingestion (i.e. swallowing them).

If exposure is not prevented or properly controlled, it can cause serious illness, including cancer, asthma and dermatitis, and sometimes even death.

The health and safety laws are designed to protect you, the clients and your fellow staff members. So your personal health and safety and safe methods of work are absolutely essential. This chapter will explain how you can help reduce risks to health and safety within the working environment for everyone's benefit.

The **Health and Safety at Work Act 1974** is the main, overarching legislation, made by parliament, relating to business premises, under which all other regulations exist. Although the Act contains many individual regulations the responsibility for maintaining these falls upon you and your employer. In short: *employers have a legal duty under the HASAWA (1974) to ensure that:*

◆ the premises are safe to work within

◆ all equipment and salon systems are safe to use

◆ employees have access to personal protective equipment

◆ contractors and self-employed staff working on the premises benefit from the same health and safety policy

◆ health and safety procedures are appropriately reviewed and updated

Employees have duties too. They should:

◆ follow appropriate working methods laid down for their safety

◆ make proper use of equipment provided for their safety

◆ cooperate with their employer on health and safety matters

◆ inform the employer if they identify hazardous activities/situations

◆ take care to ensure that their activities do not put others at risk

Both employers and employees have a joint responsibility for:

◆ the safety of the working environment

◆ taking reasonable care of themselves or others who may be affected by their working practices and must support their employer in fulfilling their obligations in the compliance of current health and safety requirements.

For more specific information on the health and safety regulations see Appendix 1, pages 440–444.

Obstructions

Passageways and corridors are dangerous, regardless of whether the obstruction is in a doorway or a corridor, on stairs or in a fire exit. In an emergency, people might have to leave the salon in a hurry – perhaps even in the dark if the electricity has gone off. It could be disastrous if someone injured themselves or fell. So:

◆ always be on the lookout for any obstruction in these areas

◆ if you see something that could present a risk, tell your work supervisor.

Spillage and breakages

You do need to act quickly in the event of a spillage or breakage, but stop and think before doing anything.

◆ First of all, what has been spilled or dropped, do you know what it is?

◆ Is this something that needs special care and attention when handling?

◆ Should you report the situation to someone else, or can you handle the situation yourself?

◆ If you can, should you be wearing gloves?

◆ What else do you need to get to rectify the situation safely without creating another hazard?

ACTIVITY

Find out your salon's policy in respect of the following procedures and write your responses in your **portfolio.**

Briefly describe what safe working practices are.

How should hazardous substances be stored, dispensed and used?

What are the salon's rules regarding smoking, consuming food and drink on the premises and policy in respect to alcohol and other drugs?

What is the salon's policy in the event of an emergency occurring?

What are the salon's expectations in respect to **personal presentation** and hygiene?

Disposal of waste

General salon waste General salon waste should be placed in appropriate waste recycling bins. When these are full they can be put ready for weekly recycling collection. Where a swing bin becomes contaminated by spilt waste materials, make sure that you wash out the inside of the bin with hot water and detergent.

Being environmentally aware requires us to be more responsible in the ways in which we dispose of our waste items. Take particular care in following the salon's procedures for the safe disposal of:

◆ aluminium foil and cans, glass bottles and plastic waste, packaging, etc.

◆ paper, cardboard and other biodegradables

◆ chemical hairdressing products (not down drains and sinks)

◆ aerosols such as hairspray cans and other pressurized items.

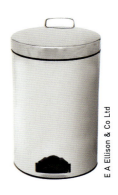

E A Ellison & Co Ltd

ACTIVITY

Use the Internet to find out what the policy for recycling is in your local area:

Go to your local authority's website and find out how different items are recycled or are safely disposed of.

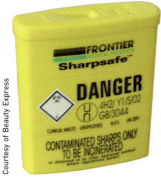

Sharps box

Disposal of sharp items Used razor blades and similar items should be placed into a **sharps box**. When the container is full it can be disposed of safely in accordance with your local authority's policy. Look on your local authority's website (Environmental Health Department) for more information.

Lifting and handling

(A list of health and safety regulations can be found in the appendices section of this book.)

As manual handling is an everyday part of salon processes, it is also covered here, as a range of skeletal and muscular disorders can occur if safe lifting procedures are not observed.

Bad posture resulting from the incorrect handling of large and/or heavy items can result in lower back pain/problems, repetitive strain injuries and strain disorders.

Think about the situations that can occur in a salon environment:

◆ moving stock into storage

◆ unpacking heavy or awkward items

◆ lifting equipment and moving salon furniture

◆ working heights – chairs, trolleys, dryers etc.

The health and safety regulations require employers to:

◆ *avoid* the need for hazardous manual handling

◆ *assess* the risk of injury from any hazardous manual handling that can't be avoided; and

◆ *reduce* the risk of injury from hazardous manual handling, (so far as is reasonably practicable).

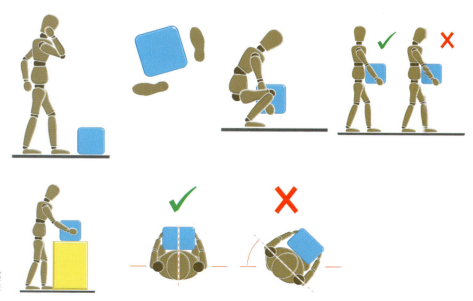

HMSO

ACTIVITY

Risks in the salon environment

From the list below tick the risks that could apply to you within the salon and then make brief notes on how they can be avoided.

1. Inhaling fumes from chemicals
2. Chemical burns
3. Cutting yourself
4. Tripping over boxes of stock
5. Slipping on hair clippings
6. Falling down the stairs
7. Developing dermatitis
8. Injury due to unsafe practices
9. Electric shock from equipment
10. Food poisoning
11. Slipping on wet floor

Avoiding dermatitis

Stop dermatitis now! Up to **70 per cent** of hairdressers have to give up hairdressing because of this common occupational health hazard (Source: Health and Safety Executive, see www.hse.gov). You can avoid this condition by making sure that you always use disposable (nitrile or polyvinyl) gloves. Always dry your hands thoroughly after washing and moisturize them to keep them healthy.

Five steps to prevent dermatitis

Step 1. Wear disposable nitrile or polyvinyl gloves when shampooing, conditioning, colouring, lightening or using any chemical substances.

Step 2. Dry your hands thoroughly with a soft cotton or paper towel.

Step 3. Moisturize after washing your hands, as well as at the start and end of each day. It's easy to miss fingertips, in-between fingers and wrists.

Step 4. Change gloves between clients. Make sure you don't contaminate your hands when you take them off.

Step 5. Check your skin regularly for early signs of dermatitis.

What do you do if you think you have it?
If you think you are suffering from dermatitis, then you should visit your doctor for advice and treatment. If you believe it has been caused or made worse by your work as a hairdresser, then you should mention this to your doctor and you must also tell your employer.

Handling chemicals

Many of the hairdressing services involve some contact with chemicals and salons have safe ways of dealing with this. Employers have a legal obligation to control the exposure of hazardous substances in the workplace and you are protected by the Control Of Substances Hazardous to Health Regulations 2002 (COSHH). The vast majority of hairdressing chemicals are safe and only pose a risk to health at the point when they are handled and used.

TOP TIP

Up to 70 per cent of hairdressers suffer from skin damage. Keep your hands healthy and wave goodbye to bad hand days.

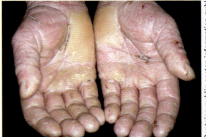

Contains public sector information published by the Health and Safety Executive and licensed under the Open Government Licence v1.0

COSHH precautions Risk assessments made by your employer will indicate the types of chemicals available within the salon and the safe ways in which they may be handled or used. These chemical products will vary from cleaning items – such as washing materials, bleach and polish – to the more typical salon specific items such as **colouring products**, lighteners, hydrogen peroxide and general styling materials.

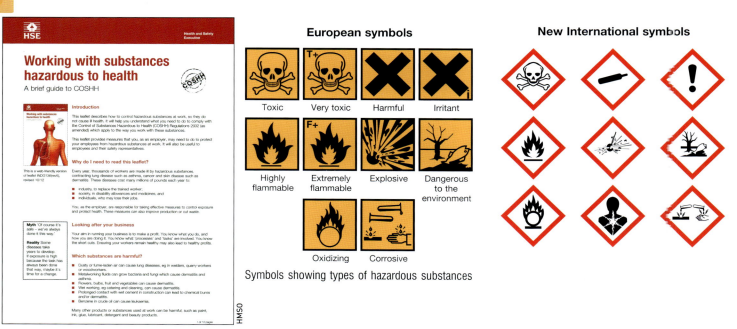

COSHH leaflet

European symbols

Toxic | Very toxic | Harmful | Irritant

Highly flammable | Extremely flammable | Explosive | Dangerous to the environment

Oxidizing | Corrosive

Symbols showing types of hazardous substances

New International symbols

Make sure that you use the lists provided by your employer, these will indicate the level of risk that each of the chemical products presents to you. They will give a hazard rating and details on how they can be handled safely with the personal protective equipment provided by your employer.

For more information see Personal Protective Equipment at Work Regulations 1992 in Appendix 1 page 442.

Keep floors clear and swept

The most common causes of injuries at work are slips and trips. Resulting falls can be serious and a busy salon means lots of people: the more clients there are, the more hair clippings there will be. Loose clippings left on the salon floor present a hazard to staff and clients alike.

Both wet and dry hair clippings are easily slipped on, so make sure that you sweep the working areas regularly. Don't wait for stylists to finish; get rid of clippings before they build up. Clear them away from areas where people are working or walking and then brush them into a dustpan and put them into the waste bin.

Working with computers

Using a computer for long periods of time can give rise to back problems, repetitive strain injury or other musculoskeletal disorders. These health problems may become serious if no action is taken. They can be caused by poor design of workstations (and associated equipment such as chairs), insufficient space, lack of training or not taking breaks from display screen work.

Work with a screen does not cause eye damage, but many users experience temporary eye strain or stress. This can lead to reduced work efficiency or taking time off work.

Working with electricity

Electricity can kill. Although deaths from electric shocks are very rare in hairdressing salons, even a non-fatal shock can cause severe or permanent injury. An electric shock from faulty or damaged electrical equipment may lead to a fall (e.g. down a stairwell).

Those using electricity may not be the only ones at risk. Illegal DIY electrical installations and faulty appliances can lead to fires which can also result in death or injury to others.

Get into the habit of looking for loose cables and plugs on tongs, straighteners and hand dryers *before* plugging them in for use. If you think that a piece of electrical equipment is faulty or damaged, tell your supervisor immediately. Remove it from the salon area and label it clearly, making sure that no one else tries to use it.

For more information see Electricity at Work Regulations 1989 in Appendix 1 page 444.

BEST PRACTICE

Hazards	Check for
Floors	✓ Are they slippery or wet?
Doorways	✓ Are they clear of obstacles?
Electrical flexes	✓ Are they loose or trailing?
Chemicals	✓ Are they labelled and stored correctly?
Equipment	✓ Is it worn or in need of attention?

Stress at work

Many people argue about the definition and sometimes even the existence of 'stress'. However, research has shown that whatever you choose to call it, there is a clear link between poor work organization and subsequent ill health. HSE has chosen to use the word stress and define it as:

> *the adverse reaction people have to excessive pressure or other types of demand placed on them.*

Stress at work can be tackled in the same way as any other risk to health. Hazards can include:

◆ lack of control over the way you do your work, work overload (or underload)

◆ lack of support from your managers/supervisors

◆ conflicting or ambiguous roles

◆ poor relationships with colleagues (including bullying) or

◆ poor management of organizational change.

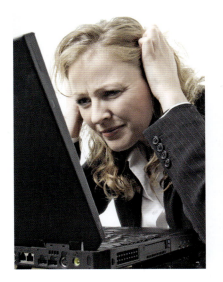

TOP TIP

HSE-related information
Stress website: www.hse.gov/uk/stress

ACTIVITY

1. List the things that the staff use within the salon that could be potentially unsafe if they are not used the right way.

2. Find out what sorts of things could be a danger in the staff room.

3. What sorts of waste are generated during normal daily routines in the salon?

Did you know?

◆ All employers and self-employed people have to assess risks at work?

◆ Employers with five or more employees should have a written health and safety policy?

◆ Employers with five or more employees have to record the significant findings of their risk assessment?

◆ Employers have a duty to involve their employees or their employees' safety representatives on health and safety matters?

◆ Employers have to provide free health and safety training or protective equipment for employees where needed?

Personal health and hygiene

Hairdressing, beauty therapy and nail craft are all personal services, and as such are very different to trades such as retail, joinery or engineering in the way that practitioners communicate with and handle their clients. Salon staff and their clients can have quite a close relationship, which has both advantages and disadvantages. Your clients will judge your personal and professional standards by your personal presentation, the way in which you present yourself. Remember, hairdressing is an image-conscious industry. We aim to provide a high-quality service that gives clients well-cut, well-styled and well-groomed hair, so that they feel pleased and confident and have greater self- esteem. Would you give clients confidence if you turned up for appointments with stained overalls, unkempt hair and dirty hands and nails?

Hands and nails   Your hands should always be perfectly clean. Dirt on your hands and under your nails harbours harmful bacteria, and by spreading germs you could infect other people. Your hands need washing not only before going to work, but several times throughout the day. When you are shampooing and conditioning, your hands could lose moisture and become dry and cracked. Broken skin allows germs to enter and infection may follow. To prevent this from happening, you should always wear disposable nitrile or polyvinyl gloves.

HEALTH & SAFETY

Don't attempt to carry out any type of electrical repairs at work!

Only those qualified with the technical knowledge are allowed to do this.

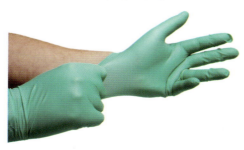 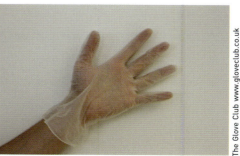

The Glove Club www.gloveclub.co.uk

ACTIVITY

General salon hygiene

Complete this table by listing how you would maintain a clean, hygienic salon.

Jobs to do:	How is this cleaned and maintained?
Work surfaces	
Floors	
Salon tools and equipment	
Towels and gowns	
Salon seating	

HEALTH & SAFETY

Always wear disposable vinyl gloves.
When? On any occasion where you come into contact with chemicals.
Why? Because gloves are a protective barrier against infection.
Always wash your hands.
When? Before work, after eating, after using the toilet and after coughing, sneezing or blowing your nose.
Why? Because your hands are one of the main sources for spreading infection.
Always wear protective clothing/equipment.
When? Always wear a plastic apron for any salon procedure involving chemicals.
Why? This will prevent spillages onto your clothes, particularly when colouring and **perming**.

Your body Human skin contains sweat glands that secrete waste in the form of sweat. Skin in areas such as the armpits, feet and genitals have more sweat glands than elsewhere and the warm, moist conditions provide an ideal breeding ground for bacteria.

Decaying bacteria causes body odour (BO), so it is essential to take a shower/bath on a daily basis to remove the build-up of sweat, dead skin cells and surface bacteria.

Mouth Frequent tooth-brushing will help to eliminate bad breath and maintains good, personal oral hygiene by removing the particles of food from between the teeth that can cause a build-up of plaque and even start tooth decay!

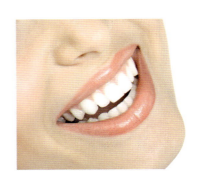

Safe posture It is important that you adopt the correct posture whilst working, as bad posture can lead to clinical fatigue – symptoms include impaired coordination – aches, pains, an accident or even longer-term skeletal injury. An incorrect standing position will put undue strain on your back, shoulders and neck muscles.

Professional posture is derived from standing correctly. Professionals' shoulders are level, their head upright and their body weight distributed evenly over their legs with their feet slightly apart. Any other standing position – dropped shoulder, hip pushed forwards or sideways – looks unprofessional. Slouching is not only uncomfortable; it is dangerous and is an example of poor **body language**: it communicates to customers and colleagues an uncaring attitude.

Personal behaviour Work should be enjoyable but knowing the difference between general friendly banter between colleagues and taking things too far is vitally important. Treat your fellow workers with respect. Courtesy amongst staff s just as important as it is with client **communications**. Behave sensibly at all times within the salon; it's one thing acting quickly to avert mishaps, such as spillages or breakages, but rushing about the salon could cause an accident.

Always use the equipment in the way it was intended. If you're not sure how something works or is handled, ask first! Remember, always use the manufacturer's instructions: that is what they are there for.

ACTIVITY

Match the information on the left with the relevant statements on the right.

Regular washing	Occurs when food particles are left between teeth
Bad breath (halitosis)	Catch on the client's **scalp** and hair
Personal cleanliness and a smart appearance	Can lead to fatigue or longer-term injury
Bracelets, necklaces and rings	Will prevent build-up of sweat and BO
Bad posture	Reflects your pride in your work

Good salon hygiene

It is important you develop an awareness of health and safety risks and that you are always aware of any risks in any situation. Quite simply, a tidy salon is easier to clean so get into the habit of clearing up your work as you go.

ACTIVITY

Now find out what the expected standards at your place of work are in relation to the following aspects.

Aspect to consider: **Salon's expected standards:**

Your personal hygiene

Your jewellery

Your work shoes

Your work clothing

What is your company's policy if you fail to meet these standards?

Floors and seating Floors should be kept clean at all times. This means that they will need regular mopping, sweeping or vacuuming. When working areas are damp-mopped during normal working hours, make sure that adequate warning signs are provided close to the wet areas. The salon's seating will be made of material that is easily cleaned. It should be washed regularly with hot water and detergent. After they have dried, the seats can be made hygienically clean by wiping over with disinfectant or an antiseptic lotion.

Working surfaces All surfaces within the salon, including the reception, staff and stock preparation areas, should be washed down at least once each day. Most salons now use easily maintained wipe-clean surfaces, usually some form of plastic laminate. They can be cleaned with hot water and detergent, and after the surfaces are dry they can be wiped over with a hygienic, antiseptic spray. Don't use rough, gritty scourers as these will scratch plastic surfaces. If a surface becomes scratched, it will look dull and unattractive and will contain minute crevices in which bacteria will develop.

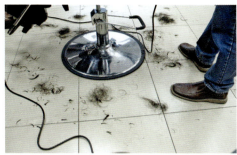

Floors need sweeping regularly

Mirrors Glass mirrors should be cleaned every morning before clients arrive. Never try to style a client's hair while they sit in front of a murky, dusty or smeary mirror. Glass surfaces should be cleaned and polished using a glass-cleaning spray that evaporates quickly without smearing.

HEALTH & SAFETY

Take all precautions to avoid occupational contact dermatitis – always use protective disposable nitrile or polyvinyl gloves.

Towels and gowns Each client must have a fresh, clean towel and gown. These should be washed on a suitable (washing machine) wash programme at 60°C to remove any soiling or staining and to prevent the spread of infection by killing any bacteria. Fabric conditioners may be used to provide a luxurious softness and freshness.

HEALTH & SAFETY

You have a duty to your work colleagues and clients to minimize the possible spread of infection or disease. Hairdressers are, by the nature of their work, in constant close contact with their customers and therefore need to pay particular attention to healthy, hygienic and safe working practices.

ACTIVITY

See if you can answer these questions in your portfolio

Q1a What type of container is liquid or crème hydrogen peroxide kept in?

Q1b Why is hydrogen peroxide hazardous to health?

Q2a Permanent colours (hair dyes) are packaged in what sort of container?

Q2b What chemicals are found in permanent hair colours?

Q3a How should hair lightening powder be stored?

Q3b Why is hair lightening powder hazardous to health?

Q4a How are shampoos and conditioners stored ready for use at the backwash?

Q4b How are they dispensed when they are used on clients?

Q5a What type of container is perm solution kept in?

Q5b What hazard to health does perm solution present?

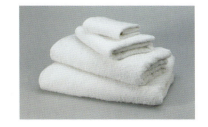

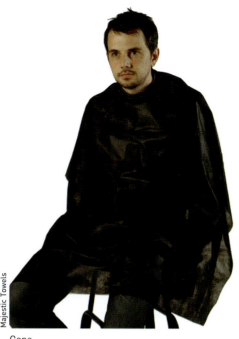

Majestic Towels

Cape

Styling tools Most pieces of salon equipment, such as combs, brushes and curlers, are made from plastics. These materials are relatively easy to keep hygienically safe, if they are used and cleaned properly.

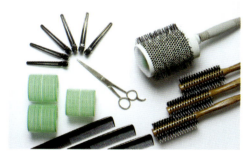

Combs should be washed daily. When not in use they should be immersed into an antibacterial solution like Barbicide™. When they are then needed they can be rinsed and dried and are then ready for use.

If any styling tools are accidentally dropped on to the floor, do not use them until they have been adequately cleaned. Don't put contaminated items on to work surfaces as they could spread infection and disease.

Handle non-plastic items, such as scissors and clipper blades, with care. When they need cleaning, the flat edges can be wiped over after spraying with a disinfectant then wiped over carefully with cotton wool. Although most of these items are made of special steels, don't immerse them in the Barbicide™ jar. These fluids contain chemicals that will corrode the precision-made surfaces of the blades.

(More information relating to sterilizing hairdressing equipment can be found in Unit GH12 Cut hair using basic techniques, ultraviolet and chemical methods, page 270)

Regularly used clippers in the hairdressing salon will require frequent routine checks for both safety and efficiency. Hair will get trapped between the blades; this reduces cutting performance and constant vibration may loosen the cutting edges. The tiny, cut fragments of hair between the blades will increase friction between the cutting surfaces and reduce the amount of movement of the upper, cutting edge. This will need routine checking and lubrication.

ACTIVITY

General health and safety checklist

	Yes	No
Do you know who is in charge of health and safety in your salon?		
Has your salon got a written health and safety policy?		
Has your salon done risk assessments?		
Do you know what COSHH means?		
Do you know where the first-aid kit is?		
Do you know where the accident book is?		
Do you know the salon's emergency procedures?		

ACTIVITY

Personal protective equipment

The column on the left lists items of personal protective equipment (PPE) that your salon provides for staff and client safety. Complete the information in the space provided.

PPE	When is it used	Why it is used
Disposable (nitrile or polyvinyl) gloves		
Gowns and towels		
Stylists' waterproof apron		
Barrier cream		
Cotton 'neck' wool		

SUMMARY

Remember to:

- ✓ work safely and hygienically in the salon at all times
- ✓ prepare and protect the clients correctly at the start of a technical service
- ✓ always wear personal protective wear for technical services
- ✓ look out for potential hazards and take action to eliminate any risks
- ✓ keep the work areas clean, hygienic and free from hazards
- ✓ clean and sterilize the tools and equipment before they are used
- ✓ dispose of waste items safely and be ECC friendly
- ✓ be aware of the salon's first-aid procedures
- ✓ always work within the **limits of your own authority**

Knowledge Check

Project

For this **project** you will need to use the information from the salon's risk assessments and the COSHH salon information booklet.

For each of the following:

- ◆ one cold wave perming lotion
- ◆ one tube of permanent colour
- ◆ one powder lightening product

Find out:

- ◆ the chemical composition
- ◆ how it is used safely
- ◆ how it should be stored safely
- ◆ how it is handled
- ◆ any other special conditions that apply to it.

A selection of different types of questions to check your health and safety knowledge. (Also see Appendix 2.)

ASSESSMENT OF KNOWLEDGE AND UNDERSTANDING

Q1   A _____ is something with potential to cause harm.   Fill in the blank

Q2   Risk assessment is a process of evaluation to develop safe working practices.   True or false

Q3   Which of the following are environmental hazards? (Select all that apply)   Multi selection

Boxes of stock left in the reception area   ☐ 1

Stock upon shelves in the store room   ☐ 2

Wet or slippery floors   ☐ 3

Shampoo backwash positions   ☐ 4

Salon work stations   ☐ 5

Trailing flexes from electrical equipment   ☐ 6

Q4   First-aid boxes should contain paracetamol tablets.   True or false

Q5   Which of the following regulations relates to the safe handling of chemicals?   Multi choice

PPE   ○ a

RIDDOR   ○ b

COSHH   ○ c

OSRPA   ○ d

Q6   All salons must have a written health and safety policy.   True or false

Q7   Which of the following records must a salon keep up to date by law?   Multi selection

Telephone book   ☐ 1

Accident book   ☐ 2

Appointment book   ☐ 3

Electrical equipment annual test records   ☐ 4

Health and safety at work checklist   ☐ 5

Fire drill records   ☐ 6

Q8   The _____ regulations require employers to provide adequate equipment and facilities in case of an accident occurring.   Fill in the blank

Q9   What colour is the label on a dry powder-filled fire extinguisher?   Multi choice

Red   ○ a

Cream   ○ b

Black   ○ c

Blue   ○ d

Q10   A dry powder-filled fire extinguisher can be used on all classes of fire.   True or false

2 Professional development

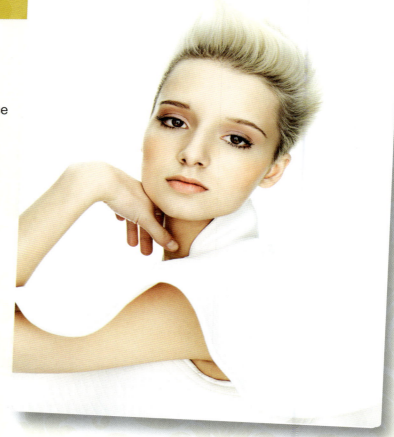

LEARNING OBJECTIVES

- ◆ Be able to improve your personal performance at work

- ◆ Be able to work effectively as part of a team

- ◆ Understand your job role and the work processes involved

- ◆ Understand how you can improve your performance and achieve targets

- ◆ Understand how to work as part of a team

KEY TERMS

appraisal

client care

client consultation

disciplinary procedures

layering

grievance

gross misconduct

Habia

National Occupational
  Standards

personal targets

salon services

SWOT analysis

Unit title

G8 Develop and maintain your effectiveness at work

Information covered in this chapter

- ◆ Identifying personal strengths and weaknesses
- ◆ Job roles and descriptions
- ◆ Performance reviews, appraisals and targets
- ◆ Effective teamwork

INTRODUCTION

This unit is about you taking the responsibility at work to improve your performance, achieve **personal targets** and get along with your colleagues. Doing well in your job really makes a difference to the whole team, as the staff in any salon situation are an integral part of the formula for success. Salons cannot afford to carry dead weight; everyone needs to shoulder their responsibilities, do their job and achieve the targets that have been set for them.

Working towards known targets is the baseline or benchmark in the world of work; without them we wouldn't know if we got things right. Targets are set by management and are a condition of your employment, therefore it is your job to work hard and achieve. The feeling that you get from reaching those goals will transform you. You will feel more confident in what you are doing, gain more respect from the people you work with and begin to take on the role of a true professional.

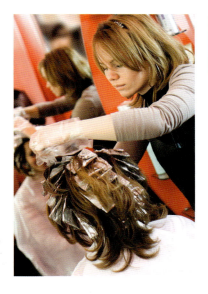

TOP TIP

The **National Occupational Standards** (NOS) can be obtained from the Hairdressing and Beauty Therapy Industry Authority (**Habia**).

BEST PRACTICE

'Continuing professional development' (CPD) is the term used by people in professional roles who have to continually update their skills. Your CPD could involve attending courses or seminars, going to trade shows and exhibitions, or even taking part in competitions.

Improve your personal performance at work

You should have a clear understanding of what you should be doing and what you are aiming to achieve at work. If you don't know this how can you tell whether you are getting it right?

The tried and tested system for looking at personal effectiveness is the appraisal process. It is conducted on a once or twice yearly basis with your manager, to review your progress, agree suitable courses for action and to set targets for the next few months. The way in which you work and the impact that has on the team and salon is vital to the success of the business as a whole. What you do and say affects others; the positive and helpful way that you assist colleagues in their work and the way in which you relate to them is called teamwork.

Your ability to meet the expected standards at work is referred to as 'personal effectiveness' and this is the result of care, interest, respect and ongoing training.

You should be able to:

◆ make use of opportunities to learn

◆ work towards the industry-recognized National Occupational Standards (NOS)

◆ identify your own strengths and weaknesses

◆ work to achievable, mutually agreed personal and salon targets

◆ review your progress towards targets.

Make use of opportunities to learn

In order to make use of opportunities to learn you have to be able to recognize those opportunities as they arise. So what sort of things are learning opportunities?

Everything that you do in the salon provides a learning opportunity. Each task that you haven't been able to carry out yourself before, provides you with a target for the future. It's never a case of: 'I'll never be able to do that' or 'It's OK for you; you've been doing it for ages'. It's also about continual improvement. In order to learn something, it has to be practised and that means several times in different situations before it can be done correctly, every time.

Watch how the senior staff tackle difficult or complex tasks. Stand by them and offer your help, you can learn a lot more if you are able to see closely how procedures are completed. Ask questions, sometimes things are far more complex than they seem.

If you are wandering around aimlessly at work it is probably because you don't know what you should be doing. Just think how your colleagues will see this; they might view you as lazy or deliberately trying to avoid working as a team player. If you are unclear about what you should be doing at work, ask.

Working towards the industry-recognized National Occupational Standards (NOS)

The standards set down by Habia provide the minimum requirements for anyone working competently. At Diploma Level 2, the NOS encompass all the jobs that you will be doing as a junior stylist in work. As you work through the programme you will find that some tasks are easier than others, but you shouldn't be worried as there can be many reasons for that. Everyone is different and, in training, people have different learning styles.

Some trainees handle visual tasks easier than others, they watch closely looking at details and methods. Others find that practise makes perfect; the continual repetition of practical processes is the only way that they can master the skill. Yet others can be told something once and it is etched into their minds.

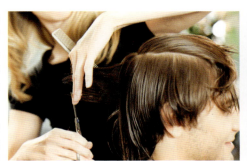

When a trainee or apprentice starts work in a salon, much of what goes on seems quite alien. This can seem overwhelming; the large majority of people who come into the craft wanting to be hairdressers are shocked by the amount of things that they need to learn. The NOS comprise of many units and each one can have several component parts. When the units are broken down into smaller, more manageable bits, they don't seem quite so bad. In fact much of what is learned in one unit can be applied to others as well.

The NOS provide a specification, a template, for the correct methods of working. They highlight the techniques that you need to use when working and the order or sequence in which hairdressing tasks are done. If you don't follow these pre-set procedures and try to do things your own way, these things will happen:

1 The result of what you are attempting to do will be wrong.

2 You will not only be letting yourself down, but all your other colleagues with whom you work too.

3 You will find yourself in the manager's office explaining why you thought your way was a better idea.

But there is always more than one way to achieve the desired result, and this provides flexibility and alternatives in what you do. But like most other things in life, there is an easy route and a hard one. The choice is yours, and this is one of the reasons why the National Occupational Standards exist: they provide you with the simplest, correct ways of doing things so that you can be assured that you are getting it right.

Identifying your own strengths and weaknesses

The process of evaluating and reviewing progress is called 'appraisal' and this can be undertaken in two ways: either by yourself, that is self-appraisal (where you measure your own strengths and weaknesses against set standards) or, in conjunction with your manager on a more formal basis.

Being able to spot your own mistakes is a starting point. We all know that if we do things the right way, we gain the personal satisfaction of getting it right. On the other hand, if we keep making mistakes and get it wrong more times than right, we lose confidence and it affects everything else that we do. This low self-esteem needs to be avoided; it is negative and starts a downward spiral, which is hard to get out of.

The important aspect of self-appraisal is being honest in what you can do. Try the activity below as an example of how you could do this for yourself.

ACTIVITY

Fill in the middle column with the letters A, B, C, etc. for the statements that best apply to you (here is an example):

Level of ability	Employee fills in this column	Supervisor fills in this column
Example: I can do this very well	A, G, H, P	
I can do this very well		
I can do this OK		
I think I'm getting there		
I find this a bit tricky		
I can't do this at all		

A. *I can highlight on both short and medium-length hair*

B. *I can apply colour to longer hair*

C. *I handle payments by cards at reception*

D. *I make appointments for all services*

E. *I help, assist and communicate with clients on a routine basis*

F. *I can prepare the chemical products for the stylists*

G. *I recommend products to clients which encourages them to buy*

H. *I recommend treatments to clients, encouraging them to buy*

I. *I deal with client enquiries over the phone*

J. *I blow-dry clients' hair to help out the stylists*

K. *I apply colour for stylists*

L. *I am always punctual for work*

M. *I am particular about my appearance*

N. *I thoroughly clean and prepare the working surfaces*

O. *I monitor the usage of stock and materials*

P. *I notice when things need doing*

Q. *I recognize situations where there may be a potential hazard*

After you have completed the activity of putting the letters A–Q in the appropriate box, you may have other additional statements that you want to add to your list. Does your manager agree with your responses? Hand this to your manager and ask to have your responses checked. Finally, your manager can fill in the last column in the same way. Now see if both columns match.

Work to achievable, mutually agreed personal and salon targets

In many work settings you will be asked to complete some form of self-evaluation before the performance appraisal. The self-evaluation will provide a discussion document which can be used to *shape* the appraisal process and identify the areas where you now meet expectations or alternatively, have further room for improvements.

The appraisal process At the beginning of the appraisal period, the manager and the employee jointly discuss, develop and mutually agree the objectives and performance measures (targets) for that period. An individual development plan will then be drafted, outlining the expected outcomes over the next review period.

If there are any significant changes in performance, these will be discussed and any amendments will be added in to the overall plan.

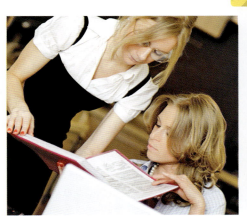

At the end of the appraisal period, the results are discussed by the employee and the manager, and both manager and employee sign the appraisal. A copy is prepared for the employee and the original is kept on file.

An appraisal of performance will contain the following information:

- ◆ appraisee's name
- ◆ appraisal period
- ◆ appraiser's name and title
- ◆ performance objectives
- ◆ job title
- ◆ work location
- ◆ results achieved
- ◆ identified areas of strengths and weaknesses
- ◆ an ongoing action plan (individual learning plan)
- ◆ an (optional) overall performance grading.

TOP TIP

The appraisal is a positive and forward-looking process, including:

- ◆ positive feedback for the things that are going well
- ◆ constructive and fair criticism where there are weaknesses
- ◆ positive suggestions
- ◆ setting of specific targets
- ◆ follow-up after appraisal.

ACTIVITY

Self Appraisal Name ....

This self-appraisal is designed to help you reflect on your job performance. After completion this will be used as a discussion document within your appraisal

1. In what aspects of your job do you feel that you have performed well?

2. In what aspects of your job do you think that you could do better?

3. What aspects of your job do you particularly like?

4. What aspects of your job do you dislike?

5. What things have you encountered within your work that you have found difficult?

ACTIVITY

Getting ready for the appraisal meeting – use the appraisal form to focus your attention on the issues.

◆ Think of examples of how you do your job well.

◆ Gather information and evidence about what you have achieved in your job.

◆ Think about what you would like to develop or improve in the future.

TOP TIP

Preparing for appraisal

◆ Think about each statement on the form.

◆ Think about the things you are good at.

◆ Think about any issues you have.

◆ Write some notes to remind you what you want to talk about during the meeting. These may include things that are not covered by the form. (Don't forget to take your notes with you to the meeting.)

For you, the appraisal is a good way to air any problems in the workplace and to make points about training needs and the future. For your supervisor or manager, it is a good way to identify possible problems in the workplace, training needs and to contribute towards effective management.

At the meeting   Refer to your appraisal form and your notes to remind yourself of what you want to say.

◆ Be positive, express yourself clearly.

◆ Ask questions.

◆ Discuss and agree your next steps with your manager.

◆ Make sure the appraisal form is filled in with details of what is agreed.

After the meeting

◆ Remind your manager about how he or she agreed to help you.

◆ Make sure you keep to the agreements you made.

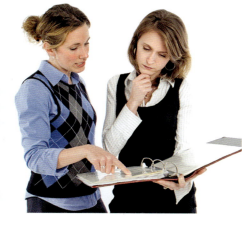

Review your progress towards targets The joint review process of appraisal would fulfil no purpose at all unless it looks at your current situation, your feelings and work performances. It should then measure that against the mutually agreed targets and then finally, create an ongoing development plan/individual learning plan, which can be reviewed at a future date.

Ask for help However, you should not wait for a formal review or appraisal. If you are having problems with any aspect of your training or your job you should ask for support or assistance from a senior stylist, your trainer or manager. If you have completed the objectives set out in your training or appraisal before the due target date, ask for more objectives to be set. This will help to keep you more motivated by completing your training earlier and increasing your knowledge of the job, enabling you to do higher-skilled work.

An appraisal form

Performance appraisal	
Name:	*Kira Kortova*
Job title:	*Trainee stylist*
Date of previous appraisal:	*N/A*
Review of prior targets and objectives:	*New employee (started 5/1/2014)*
Date of this appraisal:	*5/6/2014*
Objectives:	*To obtain competence within:* ◆ *cutting hair **layering** techniques across the range.* ◆ *blow-drying hair on a variety of hair types and lengths.*
Notes on achievement:	*Competence has been achieved across the range for all the cutting requirements.*
	Competence has been achieved for most blow-drying range requirements.
Training requirements:	*Further training and practise is needed within the area of blow-drying longer length effects.*
Any other comments on performance by appraiser:	*Kira is working towards commercially accepted standards as defined in the NOS*
Any comments on the appraisal by the staff member appraised:	*I feel that this has been a fair appraisal of my progress although I did not achieve all of my performance targets. K.Kortova*
Action plan:	*To achieve occupational competence across the range for blow-drying (i.e. longer length hair).*
	To undergo training and practise in perming methods and techniques.
	To take assessment for perming.
Date of next appraisal:	*10/12/2014*

Get SMART Smart objectives are used a lot in education and even if you haven't heard of them before, they will crop up in the future. Quite simply, SMART objectives are a way of setting targets in a well-defined and uniform format. The letters within the word SMART are an acronym or abbreviation, as these letters stand for:

◆ **Specific** – Any targets should be clearly defined as objectives.

◆ **Measurable** – The objectives need to be set in measureable units, i.e achieve 100 per cent attendance or reach £200 worth of retail sales.

◆ **Achievable** – The objectives must reflect the person's abilities.

◆ **Realistic** – The objectives must be appropriate to the person.

◆ **Timed** – The objectives must be time-bound, i.e. By December 31 the employee should have attained. ....

ACTIVITY

Strengths and weaknesses chart

This activity provides a way for you to study and assess your strengths and weaknesses at work.

When you have filled in the table below ask your trainer to check your responses.

Personal skill	My strengths	My weaknesses
Dealing with clients		
Communicating with work colleagues		
Organizing my own work		
Helping others in their work		
Sorting out things myself		

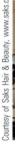

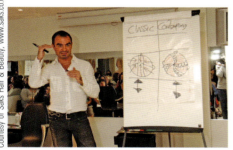

Measuring effectiveness

To be able to measure progress towards training targets as well as overall work contributions, there needs to be clear, stated expectations of the performance required of you. For both training and work activities, this is the standard to which you will need to demonstrate competence.

In training situations, your personal development plan will state the:

◆ training activities that will take place

◆ tasks which need to be performed

◆ standards and the levels of performance expected

◆ types of assessment that should be expected

◆ review of your progress towards these agreed targets and when it is to take place.

In normal work situations, performance appraisal will be based on the following factors:

◆ results achieved against set objectives and job requirements

◆ any additional accomplishments and contributions

◆ contributions made by the individual as compared with those of other staff members.

The job requirements will be outlined in your employee's job description. A job description is a list of the functions and roles expected within the job. The job description should include details of the following:

◆ the job title

◆ the work location(s)

◆ responsibility (to whom and for what)

◆ the job purpose

◆ main functions (listed)

◆ standards expected

◆ any other special conditions.

The standards expected from the job holder will often be produced in the staff handbook. They would normally include:

◆ standards of behaviour and appearance

◆ the salon's code of conduct

Job description – Stylist	
Location:	Based at salon as advised
Main purpose of job:	To ensure customer care is provided at all times
	To maintain a good standard of technical and **client care**, ensuring that up-to-date methods and techniques are used following the salon training practices and procedures
Responsible to:	Salon manager
Requirements:	To maintain the company's standards in respect of hairdressing/beauty services
	To ensure that all clients receive service of the best possible quality
	To advise clients on services and treatments
	To advise clients on products and after care
	To achieve designated performance targets
	To participate in self-development or to assist with the development of others
	To maintain company policy in respect of: ◆ personal standards of health/hygiene ◆ personal standards of appearance/conduct ◆ operating safely whilst at work ◆ timekeeping and service provision ◆ brand image and public promotion
	as laid out in employee handbook
	To carry out **client consultation** in accordance with company policy
	To maintain company security practices and procedures
	To assist your manager in the provision of **salon services**
	To undertake additional tasks and duties required by your manager from time to time.

TOP TIP

Whether it is called appraisal, evaluation, assessment or review, a meeting or interview with your manager can help you to think about:

◆ how you feel about your job

◆ how your training is going

◆ what you would like to do in the future.

◆ job description

◆ the grievance procedure

◆ employee legal entitlements and responsibilities

◆ health and safety requirements.

When these are clearly defined at the beginning, then the employee knows what is expected. If you do not have a job description ask your employer or manager if you can have one, so that you know precisely what is expected of you and how your job role fits into or alongside those of your colleagues. You will have a clear guide on your limits of authority. Some large salons will have a staff structure chart that explains everyone's role in the salon and the reporting structure.

ACTIVITY

Look at the statements on the left and match them up with the corresponding statement on the right.

Relationships at work are based upon	personal preferences and choice
Friendships outside work are based upon	effective communication takes place
Customer care is built on	mutual respect and teamwork
Good customer relations occur when	professionalism and personal service
Teamwork takes place when	making the best of personal strengths and working to improve weaknesses
Self-development in the job role means	all the staff do their jobs efficiently

Work effectively as part of a team

Creating and maintaining good working relationships with your fellow staff members is essential. Only a harmonious working team can be productive and effective. The relationships that are built at work are very different to those that exist outside of that environment. A hairdressing business relies upon providing a repeated service to its customers at a price that is profitable and that they can afford.

The formula may seem simple: unfortunately it isn't. There are so many factors that affect this delicate balance. Unlike other businesses, personal services rely solely upon people and the communication between them.

Hairdressing is not just about selling. Why is that? Well, when a product is sold, more often than not, the purchaser has made a conscious decision to buy. The standard or quality is defined by the product's component parts. The only factors affecting the sale are competing products and their price, availability, features and benefits.

TOP TIP

There is a huge difference between the friendships that you build out of choice and the others that you have to accept and work with in the professional world.

Being an effective team member

When you work in a salon, regardless of whether it is a large company chain or a small independent salon, you will be an important part of their team. You will be working with other people whom you don't know, yet you will have to get on with them. As a team member you will need to know:

◆ the other members of the team

◆ who is responsible for different things

◆ to whom you need to go if you need any help.

Teamwork is about making an active contribution, seeking to assist others even if it is only holding brushes whilst the stylist is blowdrying. Don't expect to be asked to do things all the time; think ahead and see if you can anticipate what others will need.

Anticipating the needs of others is a follow-on from providing support by cleaning and preparing the work areas ready for use, locating and preparing products as and when they are required.

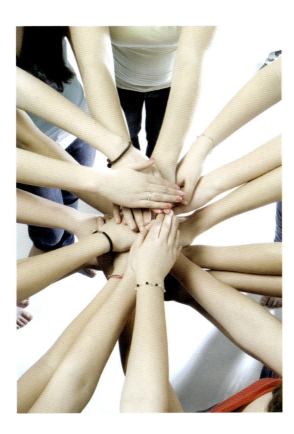

Respond to requests willingly

Cooperate with your colleagues. Make a positive contribution to your team. When a colleague asks you for help you should respond willingly and politely to the request. Remember, working in a public place is like being on show all the time. Clients will see, hear and *feel* any tension within the salon. How others see you in your work role will have a huge impact on your professionalism: you would rather be thought of as a willing, helpful trainee than a quiet, moody one!

Maintain harmony and always try to minimize conflicts. Most good working relationships develop easily; others, however, will need to be worked at. People at work are different, so in order for you to work as a team player you must develop a mutual respect for others, even if they would *never* get on your personal friends list.

Make effective use of your working day

Always make good use of your time. In a busy salon there is always something that needs doing, so sometimes you will have to juggle between two or three things at the same time!

◆ Keep a list of the different tasks you have been asked to do (that way you won't get into trouble for trying to remember them all).

◆ Find out which ones take priority. Some jobs are more important or urgent and they will need to be done first.

◆ If you don't understand what has been asked of you, ask someone before it's too late!

◆ Remember, if you do have to leave something halfway through, make sure that you get back to complete it at the earliest convenient moment.

ACTIVITY

Show how you are an effective team member
Complete the table below by filling in the empty column with actions that demonstrate being an effective team member.

Work aspect:	I do this by:
Being an effective team member	
Making good use of your time at work	
Responding to others' requests for help	

Report problems to relevant people

Within any organizational structure there is a hierarchy and this is important for you to know to whom you should go if you need any help or have any grievances.

ACTIVITY

Organizational chart

Look at the following organizational diagram and first of all answer the questions. Then, in the space provided complete the structure for your own workplace environment.

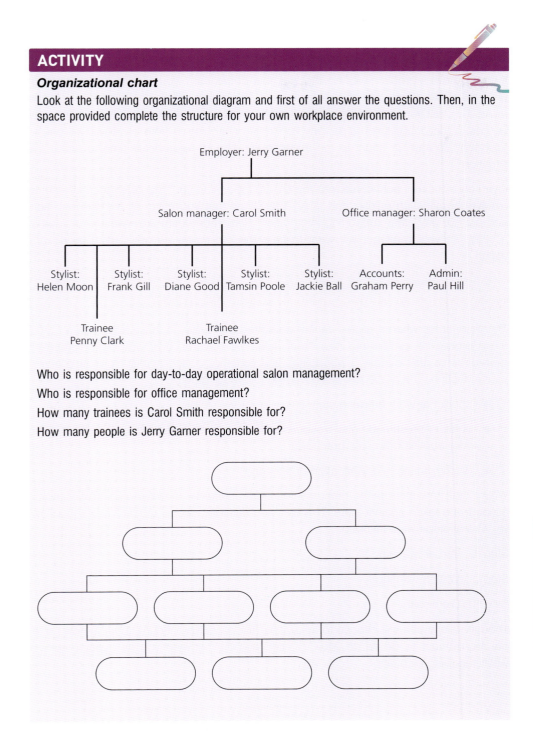

Who is responsible for day-to-day operational salon management?

Who is responsible for office management?

How many trainees is Carol Smith responsible for?

How many people is Jerry Garner responsible for?

As you can see from the example above, different people do different jobs. For example, you would need to know whom to contact if you were ill and couldn't get into work. Conversely, if you had a query about your wages you might need to contact somebody else.

In another situation, imagine that a client has returned to the salon with a complaint about her hair and she is demanding her money back. You won't have the authority to deal with this; you will have to get someone to handle the complaint.

Resolving problems with other members of the team

If you do have a problem with another member of the team, you need to approach them privately about it first. You should think carefully about what you are going to say and make sure that your time and place is suitable. It is highly unprofessional to air your grievances in the public salon area; any backchat or arguing in front of clients will not be tolerated. So save it, count to ten and choose a more appropriate time to tackle the situation.

If you cannot sort it out yourselves, you should report it to your manager who will want to resolve the situation quickly and fairly. Make sure that you cover all the relevant facts and provide any other supporting information. Remember there are always two sides to a story, so your manager will want to hear the other side as well before taking any action.

Grievance and disciplinary procedures

There are times when disputes cannot be sorted out easily. In these situations a formal salon procedure comes into play. Your salon will have its own way of implementing **grievance** or **disciplinary procedures**, and you should receive this information during your induction. The procedure will cover the following issues:

◆ conflict at work between staff

◆ unfair or presumed unfair treatment at work (e.g. being asked to do tasks beyond your abilities or unsafe practices)

◆ discrimination in any situation or scenario.

Where staff members fail to meet the required standards, they can expect disciplinary action to be taken against them. This can vary between salons. Up until now the following formal steps were involved:

Step 1   Verbal warning

Step 2   Written warning

Step 3   Dismissal

Though salons can still choose to follow this disciplinary procedure, there is now no legal requirement to do so, to allow greater flexibility between you and your employer when resolving disputes.

Acts of gross misconduct/gross incompetence

Your salon will have its own standards and expectations relating to conduct and behaviour and the team are happier in their work if they know what is expected of them.

The following list provides examples of acts of **gross misconduct**:

◆ carrying or taking illicit drugs on the work premises

◆ thieving from the salon or fellow staff members

◆ drinking alcohol on the premises

◆ wilfully damaging company property

◆ endangering yourself, fellow staff members or salon clients and visitors

◆ disclosing private company information and data.

Acts of gross incompetence will have the same summary dismissal as gross misconduct. These actions of negligence can occur during normal work activities and will put the salon's good name and reputation in jeopardy. Typical examples of this would be:

◆ careless or improper use of chemicals on clients, e.g. spillages causing bodily harm incurring hospitalization

◆ careless timing of chemical treatments, e.g. causing scalp burns, hair damage or loss

◆ careless or improper use of equipment, e.g. tampering with electrical items causing harm to others, incorrect timings of processes causing harm or damage.

TOP TIP

If you are unsure of what constitutes an act of gross misconduct or an act of gross incompetence/negligence, ask your supervisor.

ACTIVITY

SWOT analysis

After completing your SWOT analysis (from page 30), you can refocus again upon the positive and negative aspects.

Choosing the positive aspects first, how can you develop these attributes further?

Now select the negative aspects. What do you need to do in order to change these into positives too?

This exercise will help you form the basis of your next action plan: discuss your SWOT analysis and your suggested routes for further development with your trainer.

Keep copies of all the information for use in your portfolio.

SUMMARY

Remember to:

✓ communicate positively and effectively in the salon at all times

✓ develop yourself in those activities that provide further progress in your career

✓ work together harmoniously with others as a team player

✓ recognize the occasions when others need assistance

✓ work at maintaining professional relationships with fellow staff members

✓ use your time efficiently and effectively

✓ work towards personal targets and know why they should be achieved.

Knowledge Check

For this project you will need to gather information from other people with whom you work.

There is a simple tried-and-tested method for self-assessing one's own current position: the SWOT analysis. This helps you think through your:

◆ strengths

◆ weaknesses

◆ opportunities

◆ threats

in relation to where you are now and where you need to be.

For each of the titles – strengths, weaknesses, opportunities and threats – write a small summary of your attributes, and then show this to your supervisor to see if they agree.

The completed SWOT analysis can be recorded in your portfolio and will provide a basis for your future action plan.

ASSESSMENT OF KNOWLEDGE AND UNDERSTANDING

A selection of different types of questions to check your personal effectiveness knowledge.

Q1 Working in _____ minimizes conflict between staff members. — Fill in the blank

Q2 Relationships at work are different to those outside of work. — True or false

Q3 Which of the following are examples of good teamwork? — Multi selection

Sitting in the staff room exchanging jokes	☐ 1
Preparing trolleys with curlers	☐ 2
Sitting at the reception desk	☐ 3
Recognizing the needs of others	☐ 4
Collecting cakes at break time	☐ 5
Passing up materials to the stylists	☐ 6

Q4 Personal development is about getting your own way. — True or false

Q5 Which of the following is part of SWOT analysis? — Multi choice

Diluting peroxide strengths	○ a
Identifying personal opportunities	○ b
Threatening others	○ c
Feeling weak	○ d

Q6 Talking and listening to your seniors is an important part of good team communications. — True or false

Q7   What takes place in an appraisal?   Multi selection

                                A review of your aspirations   ☐ 1

                           A review of your current position   ☐ 2

                             A review of your future conduct   ☐ 3

                               A review of your past conduct   ☐ 4

                      A review of clients' treatment history   ☐ 5

                      An informal chat about your fellow staff   ☐ 6

Q8   Your non-verbal communication will say more about what you are _____   Fill in the blank
           than your mouth.

Q9   Which of the following is contained in a job description?   Multi choice

                                    Records of your conduct   O a

                        Terms and conditions of employment   O b

                                  Roles and responsibilities   O c

                                   Records of your training   O d

Q10   Your effectiveness at work is also linked to your efficiency.   True or false

3 Professional client care

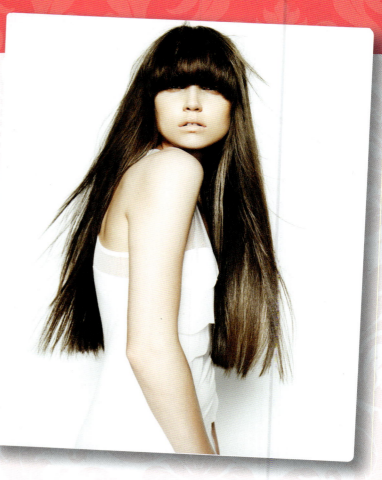

LEARNING OBJECTIVES

◆ Be able to establish a rapport with clients

◆ Be able to respond appropriately to clients

◆ Be able to communicate effectively with clients

◆ Understand how to give clients a positive impression of you and the business

KEY TERMS

body language

closed questions

confidential information

Consumer Protection Act

Data Protection Act

good customer service

non-verbal communication

open questions

professional standards

role play

G17 Give clients a positive impression of yourself and your organization

Information covered in this chapter

- ◆ Personal appearance and behaviour
- ◆ **Good customer service**
- ◆ Client communication
- ◆ Verbal and written communications
- ◆ **Non-verbal communication** (recognizing body language, gestures and mannerisms)

INTRODUCTION

If there were a motto that you needed to learn for this chapter it is this one.

You don't get a second chance to make a good first impression.

Good customer communication is an essential part of any successful business. Get it right and many positive aspects are conveyed to the client; professionalism, good service, respect, care, consideration and loyalty. All these things are indicators of a quality service. Whereas poor customer communication is none of these!

All of us enjoy the experience of good service if we feel that the person serving us really wants to create the right impression, i.e. by responding to our needs and giving us useful, accurate information. So as hairdressers and barbers we are always on show, every detail of our behaviour when we deal with clients is plain to see. How we conduct ourselves affects the impression that the clients form of the service they receive. Excellent client service can only be provided by people who are good with people and the key word here is communication, in particular professional communication.

Establish a rapport with clients

Presenting yourself

The introduction to this section referred to creating a positive impression as being the first part of good customer communication. Unfortunately, it is human nature to be judge mental and that means that we all tend to try to quantify and make assumptions of everything that we come into contact with. We observe it and our minds quickly give it a label. In other words, we see something and we quickly search through our memories to see if it resembles something or a situation that we have already encountered. If we have, we 'pigeonhole' it and give it a label with that reference. The whole catalogue process takes moments!

Lazy, reticent, moody, eager, pushy, professional, scary, attractive

There are a few labels that we attach to others. So how do you want to be viewed?

Personal standards

BEST PRACTICE

A good hairdresser considers others, adapts to situations and is respectful to clients at all times.

Appearance Your personal appearance is as important as your personal cleanliness. The effort you put into getting ready for work reflects your pride in the job. Your own individual look is OK as long as you appreciate and accept that there are professional standards of dress and appearance that must be followed.

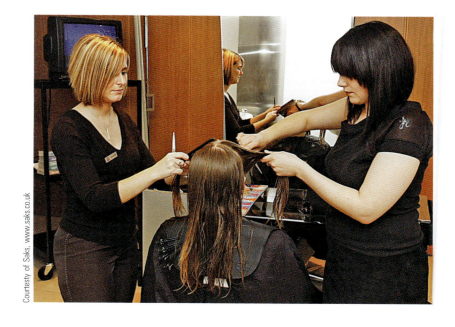

Courtesty of Saks, www.saks.co.uk

Clothes It's far easier to wear a uniform at work than your own clothes. Uniforms are created specifically with work in mind; they are an easy option for cleaning, and they form part of your PPE. (See Health & Safety – Personal Protective Equipment)

Whatever clothes you wear, they should be clean, well ironed and made from fabrics that are suitable not only for your intended work, but also for the time of year. Remember, clothes revealing too much of your body will be considered unprofessional and possibly provocative!

Shoes Hairdressing involves a lot of standing and your feet can get tired, hot, sweaty and even sore, so wear shoes with low heels and make sure the shoe will protect your feet from any falling objects.

It is also better to wear shoes that allow your feet to 'breathe', as ventilated feet remain cool and comfortable throughout the working day. Many modern materials can combine comfort with contemporary style. Trainers are great but check that your workplace permits them before turning up at work in them.

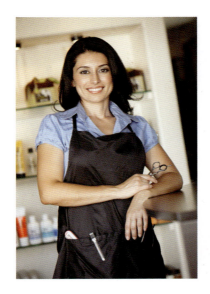

Your hair When working in a salon, it is important to maintain a professional appearance and your hair needs to be clean and well presented. Long hair should be kept away from your face to allow eye contact with clients and display positive body language.

Jewellery It is better not to wear too much jewellery because it harbours germs. Rings, bracelets and long necklaces can get in the way of everyday tasks and get tangled in services such as washing hair. Moisture and shampooing products may get trapped under rings and this can cause dermatitis.

Meeting and greeting clients – with a professional etiquette

Your greeting of the client is the next way, beyond the first impression, in which you will be judged. Get this right and any previous invisible barriers or uncertainties will disappear.

New customers entering into the salon need to be made to feel welcome. Don't forget; they are walking into an alien environment. They don't know what to expect and may not know anyone who works within the salon. Similarly, a regular client needs to feel part of the business too, they expect the familiar faces whom they see on a regular basis to recognize them and to welcome them too.

This is the difference between being a customer at a shop and a valued client in a salon. We can show people that we remember them by the way that we greet them.

- ◆ Stop what you are doing.
- ◆ Make eye to eye contact.
- ◆ Say 'Good morning (or afternoon) Mrs XXXX'.
- ◆ 'My name is XXXXXX, how can I help you?'

BEST PRACTICE

There are three main reasons for talking to clients and colleagues:

1. to welcome people
2. pass on information and
3. get information.

Respond appropriately to clients

What is good customer service?

Good customer service means making the client your number one priority. Quite simply, it is looking after their individual needs and making sure that their visit to the salon is both a pleasurable and enjoyable experience. This begins from the point that the client makes contact with or enters into the salon, and continues until they leave. Helping the client to manage their own hair between visits extends the service they receive from you further. Initially, aftercare advice is provided by the stylist, but you can help too. If you have any tips or have found that certain equipment or accessories work well, tell them how they can get the results they are looking for.

How can I respond appropriately to clients?

✓ Be respectful and polite in the way that you speak to them.

✓ Listen and *hear* what they have to say when they make their requests.

✓ Identify their needs and understand their requests.

✓ Find out things quickly and provide accurate, honest information.

✓ Remember that some clients need more time, be patient, understand their needs.

TOP TIP

Good customer relationships are built to L.A.S.T.

L = Listen

◆ Concentrate on what the client is saying.

◆ Show the client that you are listening properly through open body language.

◆ Ask for further information or for details to be repeated, if required.

◆ Check the information – repeat details back to the client.

A = Apologize

◆ Empathize with the client.

◆ Always remain calm, polite and professional.

◆ Use appropriate language, tone and body language.

◆ Don't make excuses or blame others.

S = Solve

◆ Follow company guidelines or procedures.

◆ Deal with problems as quickly as possible.

◆ Tell the client what you are going to do and by when.

◆ Follow up any problems you passed on to someone else.

T = Thank

◆ Thank the client for bringing the problem to your attention.

◆ Use a sincere tone of voice.

ACTIVITY

Customer care and communication

Complete this table by writing in the space on the right the sorts of things that you could do that would demonstrate good customer care in relation to the word(s) on the left.

Items:	How could you demonstrate good customer care?
Magazines	
Tea or coffee	
Towel and gown	
Products and services	

Being respectful

We are familiar with being told that you can't demand respect you have to earn it, but it's different for customers: they can expect it – **because they're paying for it!**

For more information on listening and hearing see the section on communication (page 47).

Listening and hearing

Identify the client's needs The simplest way of finding out what somebody wants is to ask them.

Questioning If we don't ask, we won't know; we want the client to feel valued and properly served during their visit. We can't just assume the needs of others, guessing what they want; in nine cases out of ten we would be wrong. Good customer service is finding out what the client wants by questioning and then doing something about it with a prompt, accurate and respectful response.

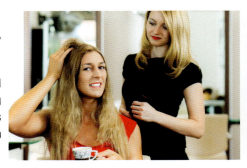

Avoid gossip! Generally speaking, people like to talk and the hairdressing salon is one of those places where conversation is not only expected, but good fun too. However, beware: you must be a professional at all times. Be careful what you say and who you are saying it to!

Never get drawn into conversations that lead to gossip. It's OK to talk about TV programmes, music interests, celebrities and the reported things that they have done, but it's quite another to discuss stories about people that you or the client knows!

There are other taboos too: keep away from politics and religion. It's OK for you to have your opinions, as long as you don't end up *haranguing* other people about them. Remember, what you believe in is personal and important to you, but you can't and must not expect everyone else to hold the same views.

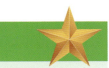

BEST PRACTICE

When talking to clients
What you believe in is personal and important to you, but you can't and mustn't expect everyone else to hold the same views.

Keep clients informed Many of the salon's services and treatments involve lengthy processes and procedures, and that can mean plenty of waiting around. Well, that's how it can seem to a client when they are waiting for a perm or treatment to develop.

For example: if a client is waiting in reception, tell them what is happening and why they haven't been attended to yet. Similarly, if a client has had a colouring service, then the colour needs a certain amount of time to develop. Explain what is happening and give an indication of how long it will take. (And if you don't know, find out from the stylist first.)

Good service checklist

The client's trust and goodwill are enhanced by clear communication and in the ways that you communicate with them. Poor explanations and miscommunication can undermine a great deal of hard work. So, while you are working, make sure that you:

- Tell the client the reasons for any delays or disruptions in services. Give them reassurance in what is taking place, particularly if it involves a new service or a different look.

- Learn to recognize the needs of your clients. Everyone is different with differing requirements.

- Remember your clients and things about them; even the simplest of things can make all the difference – whether a client prefers coffee to tea, or if they take sugar in hot drinks. Little things like this show that you have listened and learned and, what's more, you have taken an interest in them.

- Tell your client about the services that your salon provides, the special techniques and promotions that are currently on offer.

- Get help from your team. If there is something that you are not sure about or something unexpected is happening, get a senior's opinion and avoid something going wrong.

ACTIVITY

In your own words, write down what these words mean to you:

Goodwill

Client care

Professional etiquette

Positive communication

Miscommunication

Body language

Good service

BEST PRACTICE

The language you use depends on to whom you are talking, why you are talking and where you are.

With colleagues
Your language may be quite informal (but not in front of clients). You may also use some technical terms.

With clients
Your language will generally be more formal but you will need to simplify or explain technical terms.

TOP TIP

Can you hear me yet?!!!

A loud voice is often thought of as aggressive or overbearing.

A quiet or soft voice is often thought of as timid or polite.

ACTIVITY

Barriers to communication

Certain situations like those listed below can get in the way of effective communication. Discuss ways in which these potential barriers can be overcome.

1. Physical barriers

2. Time constraints

3. Assumptions

4. Moods and attitudes

5. Language barriers

6. Personality clashes

7. Background noise

Communicate information to clients

Positive communication

Good communicators use a mixture of skills in their daily routines. They have:

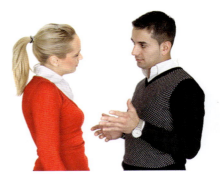

◆ *Excellent listening skills* – This is the ability to hear and understand what the client is saying. This can be particularly useful as sometimes the person prompting the change may not be the client in the chair, but sitting at home with their feet up! Remember, other people can have a strong influence on our clients, so you need to find out if the proposed changes are realistic, suitable, practical or even possible.

◆ *Good speaking skills* – Long silences can often be uncomfortable, but filling in gaps in conversation with nervous chatter makes you look foolish. Knowing when it is right to speak or when to keep quiet is an invaluable interpersonal skill.

◆ In day-to-day, routine communication with a client the balance can change. More often than not, the client will have plenty to say, particularly when you ask them about what has happened since their last visit.

◆ *'Reading' skills* – The ability to read situations, to understand what has been said or not said, is particularly useful. There are times when your client will take on a certain facial expression, or say something that makes you think. In these situations, your ability to read the situation, your perceptiveness in picking this up and responding appropriately may have a crucial impact on your long-term business relationship.

TOP TIP

It's not what you say it's how you say it

Vocal (voice)

Volume (how loud or quiet)

Pace (how fast or slow)

Pitch (how high or low)

Tone (the manner of speaking)

Feedback sounds ('mmm', 'ah-ha', 'errr').

ACTIVITY

Communication

Good communication with clients is essential. Without it, a stylist will not make the right decisions or take the correct courses of action.

Write down what you think are the advantages or disadvantages for the following communication techniques.

Communication technique	Advantages	Disadvantages
Example: Hand gestures	Helps to direct people – shows them the way	Can appear rude if it isn't backed up with helpful advice
Other body language		
Oral communication		
Written communication		

TOP TIP

Tone of voice

You can often tell what mood someone is in from the tone they use.

We communicate to one another in the following ways:

◆ verbal communication

◆ non-verbal communication

◆ written communication.

Verbal communication

Verbal communication is what you say and what others hear, it should always be:

◆ clear to the listener

◆ brief and to the point

◆ uncomplicated – easy to understand, avoiding the use of technical terms

◆ friendly and courteous.

Speech is used to pass on information and to ask questions. We have already covered the professional ways of passing on information to clients and staff. But we also need to gain information from others too, and that's done by questioning:

◆ *Closed questions* – Closed questions lead the client to give only simple yes or no responses and yield very little information. Examples are: 'Have you washed your hair with anything different lately?' 'Do you find the colour application at home is easy?' 'Have you always had a centre parting?' 'Did you have your highlights done recently?'

◆ *Open questions* – These are a better type of question to use when you want the client to give you information, particularly during consultation. Examples are: 'What products do you use when you wash your hair at home?' 'How do you apply the colour when you do it at home?' 'Which way do you style the front of your hair?' 'When was the last time that you had a whole head of highlights?' You will have informal conversations chatting with your client during the service and more formal, structured conversations greeting your client and in a consultation situation.

Talking and listening to your client is one of the most important parts of the hairdressing service. It will enable you to find out what the client wants and if they have any problems with their hair. You need to listen closely to what they are saying and ask questions to clarify any areas you are not sure about. You also need to ask open questions about their hair to ensure that you get enough information to make a choice, explore ideas and give opinions, such as:

◆ Would you like to change anything about your hairstyle?

◆ What products do you use on your hair?

◆ How much time do you have to style your hair?

ACTIVITY

How would you change the wording of these closed questions to turn them into open questions and find out more about the client's hair?

Is this a permanent colour on your hair?

Would you consider a different hairstyle?

Did you find that the new conditioner helped you manage your hair?

Do you like styling products on your hair?

Non-verbal communication

Non-verbal communication is commonly referred to as 'body language' and this type of communication is an effective way of letting others know what we really mean.

We express ourselves with **body language** through our:

◆ posture

◆ gestures

◆ facial expressions.

Body language As well as using words we show our interest, attitude and feelings by bodily expressions. Non-verbal communication (NVC), or body language to put it more simply, is especially important. It can truly show what we are feeling, even if our mouths are saying something quite different!

In the animal world the main form of communication and interaction from one creature to another is through body language. The cat that is alarmed when it is confronted by a dog on the street turns sideways on and hunches up. This makes him look larger than he actually is. Size means everything. When the dog is pulled away sharply he sulks; he gets right in your view and turns his back to you. Animals' positioning, posturing and mannerisms all mean something; they all convey a very clear and strong message.

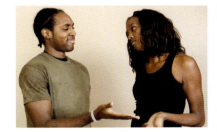

We too (like animals), express our interest and attitudes via non-verbal communication through eye contact, posture and general body positioning. So it is very important that we send the right message, particularly when dealing with clients and potential customers as they will be making their mind up about you!

Eye contact The first rule of good communication is always maintaining eye contact when talking to the client. Where possible, maintain eye level as well. For example, if you are carrying out a consultation, sit down with your client; never stand over them or talk to them through the mirror. Standing over or above your client and looking down conveys a feeling of authority, as if you were trying to assert control.

Body zones – space invaders! People have a comfort zone. This is the space around the body within which they feel at ease. Obviously the extent of this space varies from person to person. Within a close, intimate relationship, shared proximity may be welcome, but an uninvited invasion of this space is at best, very uncomfortable, and at worst, menacing or threatening!

Physical contact Most people are embarrassed by physical contact from someone they do not know well, and knowing when to be *tactile* is almost a science in itself. For example, touching a client's shoulder with the palm of the hand, whilst they are waiting, and asking if they are OK, or if they need anything, is fine. It shows that you are taking an interest in them and your genuine concern.

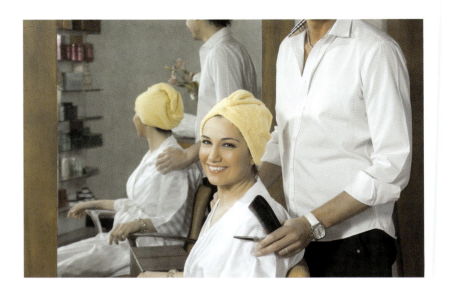

Posture, body position and gestures

Much has been written on the subject of body language and the psychological effects that it has on those reading it. It is far too complex a subject to address in a few simple paragraphs, but there are a few simple rules:

◆ Slouching in the salon or at reception looks very unprofessional.

◆ Folded arms and the crossing of arms on the chest is a protective gesture that portrays a closed mind or shows defensiveness.

◆ Open palms, as a gesture supporting explanation or information, with hands at waist height and palms upward, indicates openness or honesty.

BEST PRACTICE

Body zones – proxemics

Do not crowd or appear over-familiar with your client. Imagine how you would feel if someone came up to you and got a little too close. What do you do? Immediately back off and go onto the defensive.

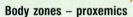

Good Posture

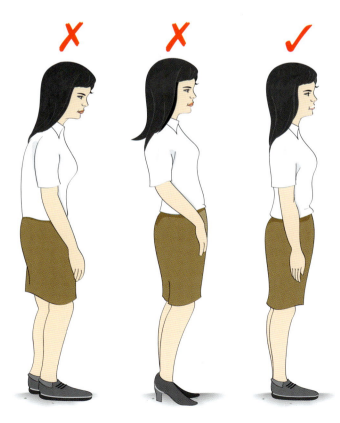

◆ Inspecting fingernails or looking at a watch is rude, it's a plain and simple indication of boredom or vanity.

◆ Talking with your hand in front your mouth may lead the listener to believe you are not being honest. You're hiding yourself by your gestures.

◆ Shifting from foot to foot shows that you're worrying about getting found out! It also says that you would rather be somewhere else; to get away so that no guilty expressions are spotted.

These forms of communication are only an indication of feelings and emotions. In isolation they may not mean anything at all. However, taken together they can convey a very clear message. Make sure that you send the appropriate signals and look interested, keen, ready to help and positive. Above all show that you can listen.

You're a liar!

◆ sweating

◆ excessive hand movements

◆ biting of fingernails

◆ chewing of the inside of the mouth

◆ drying up of the mouth, and

◆ lack of eye contact.

The list above provides a general indication that shows we are telling 'porky pies'. Some people are very good at masking these indicators, but in most cases they are obvious and a plain indication that someone is not telling the truth.

ACTIVITY

Which of the examples of non-verbal communication below would be considered to be positive expressions of communication when listening to a client explaining what she wants?

Non-verbal communication	Tick which ones ✓
Yawning	
Looking at the ceiling	
Shaking the head	
Sitting with arms and legs crossed	
Making eye contact	
Nodding	
Putting your arm around the client	
Frowning	
Smiling	

Written communication

Most day-to-day communication between staff or clients is spoken. However, there are times when information has to be recorded. Client records, taking messages and stock procedures are typical examples of this.

Client records can be manual or computerized; in either event they will contain similar information:

◆ client name and title

◆ address and contact information

◆ previous service, treatment, tests and product information

◆ date, costs and timings of previous visits

◆ stylist/operator details and any other additional memos.

The client record is normally used during consultation; this will give you detailed background information relating to their previous visits and allows you a more informed basis for planning a suitable course of action. The information needn't be too long; as long as you have covered the essential aspects that will do.

Taking messages – write it down! A quick memo is an easy way of recording information rather than trying to remember and pass on messages later. In most cases we don't remember or if we do it's too late to do anything about it.

An effective memo is clear and includes the following:

✓ for whom it is intended

✓ who took the message

✓ the date and time

✓ its purpose

✓ clear details or instructions.

Handling confidential information

Throughout all of your dealings with your clients you must remain professional. This is particularly true when it comes to handling **confidential information**. There are more clients lost by stylists through careless talk than through poor hairdressing!

◆ Make sure that your discussions with clients remain discreet. Private information should remain private.

◆ You should never repeat to another person what has been said to you in confidence. Even if it is true!

◆ Recorded or documented information is personal to the clients. The **Data Protection Act** protects you and your clients from unlawful disclosure of information to others.

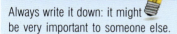
BEST PRACTICE
Always make sure that your written records are accurate. Incorrect or incomplete client information could result in a future disaster.

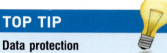
TOP TIP
Always write it down: it might be very important to someone else.

TOP TIP
Data protection

The Data Protection Act 1998 protects peoples' personal information held on file. The law ensures that personal information is not mishandled, mismanaged or used inappropriately.

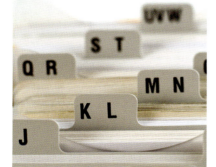

Handling clients in different situations

As discussed on the previous page, good communication is vital. It will help you deal with many situations. However, not all clients are easy to get along with or to extract information from. Some clients may be angry because they have been made to wait or may be unhappy with the finished effect. Some clients may find it difficult to explain what they want or may not understand what you are asking. As a stylist it is your job to remain calm and deal with the situation in a supportive, concerned and caring way.

Angry clients Stay calm, listen to the client and let them explain why they are angry. Use open, friendly body language and maintain eye contact. Keep your speech clear and low when asking questions or giving information to clarify the situation. If you are not in a position to deal with the problem make sure that you get someone who can – this may be a senior stylist or the manager. Never ignore the client; they are angry for a reason and usually the situation can be easily rectified.

Confused clients Not all clients know what they want when they book for an appointment or what you are suggesting for their hairstyle. Make sure that you give the client time to talk and ask questions. Listen to them again, maintain eye contact, use open body language and gestures such as nodding your head or open palms to confirm your honesty in listening and being ready to support your client. Use simple explanations and questions to extract information. Use visual aids such as style books or colour charts to confirm the requirements.

Dealing with complaints A client has every right to expect the service that was agreed and paid for and when an unexpected result occurs the client has every right to complain. Dealing with a dissatisfied client is not easy and should therefore be referred to a senior member of staff.

If a client approaches you with a complaint you should:

- move your client away to a quieter area of the salon
- seek assistance from a senior member of staff.

The complaint may then be resolved by the senior who will:

- find out exactly what the problem is
- assess the validity of the complaint
- mutually agree on a suitable course of action
- carry out/organize any corrective work
- make a record of the complaint for future use.

Special note

If the complaint is serious – such as hair breakage or discolouration – it may be difficult to rectify. The client has a legal right to pursue acts of gross negligence and recently this has proved a popular route to gaining compensation. If a client does follow this course of action the salon's insurers will need to be notified sooner rather than later.

> **TOP TIP**
>
> Don't be in a hurry to solve a problem, you might make it worse. Always remain calm and give careful consideration to the problem, making sure the client understands and agrees to any course of corrective action.

ACTIVITY

Preparing for the unexpected is always difficult, but one way of doing this is through a **role play**. Role play is a way of 'acting out' the different things that could happen during different client situations.

Simple misunderstandings do occur during consultation and this can be due to many different reasons. Unfortunately, the final hair effect that results from poor consultation can be quite different to what the client wanted.

Take it in turns to play client and stylist to see if you can improve your consultation skills before it happens to you!

ACTIVITY

Expressions

What do each of these emotions express? Match up the 4 emotions below with the corresponding picture.

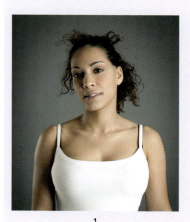

1

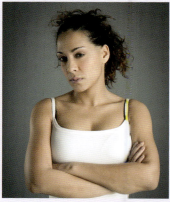

2

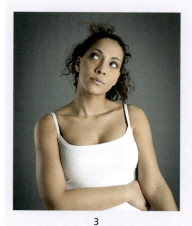

3

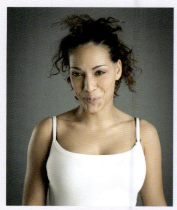

4

Angry =

Fed up =

Happily surprised =

Content =

ACTIVITY

Getting the right information

I've got to pick my children up from school at 3.30.

I've been sitting here waiting for 25 minutes now.

My appointment was for two o'clock! Is there any chance I might be seen within the next five minutes?

First of all, which of the following repeats the main points of the client's complaint?

A. The client's appointment is for 3.30 and they're sitting here and waiting for it.

B. The client's appointment was at two o'clock and they've been waiting for 25 minutes.

C. The client needs to be seen in the next five minutes because they have to pick their children up at 3.30. The appointment was at two o'clock and they've been waiting for 25 minutes.

D. The client has to leave now to pick up their children up from school.

What would be the best thing to say to this client?

A. You'd better go now to be sure you'll be at the school in time.

B. I'm sorry we have kept you waiting so long. Would you like to make another appointment?

C. We're really short-staffed at the moment. Everybody is having to wait. Twenty-five minutes is nothing. *She's* been here an hour already.

D. I'm sorry you've had such a long wait. Will you accept this sample product with our compliments? Perhaps I can make you another appointment at a time to suit you?

ACTIVITY

What is the appropriate thing to say to a client who has been kept waiting for their appointment?

A. 'Sorry to keep you waiting. We're always very busy this time of year.'

B. 'I'm afraid Sue will be about another fifteen minutes. Can I get you a coffee or some magazines?'

C. 'Not long to wait now, Mrs Portman.'

D. 'Sue's running late again, Mrs Portman. Here are some magazines while you wait.'

E. 'Sorry for the delay, Mrs Portman. Sue will be free in about a quarter of an hour. If you prefer, Mike can cut your hair instead.'

SUMMARY

Remember to:

✓   communicate positively and effectively in the salon at all times

✓   be polite, but confident in carrying out communications with clients

✓   maintain confidentiality and the consequences of failing to keep things private

✓   listen to clients and show them that you care

✓   use positive body language and the reasons why it plays such an important part in good customer service

Knowledge Check

For this project you will need to gather information from a variety of sources.

For the following legislation find out how:

1   the Disability and Discrimination Act

2   the **Consumer Protection Act**

affects or has an impact on the services that can be provided to clients.

In your project pay particular attention to the aspects that would have impact on a business and the implications if this legislation were not considered.

ASSESSMENT OF KNOWLEDGE AND UNDERSTANDING

A selection of different types of questions to check your customer communication knowledge.

Q1   Good personal _____ is essential in a personal service industry.   Fill in the blank

Q2   Poor posture leads to clinical fatigue.   True or false

Q3   Which of the following are essential PPE for the clients?   Multi selection

Towels	☐ 1
Barrier creams	☐ 2
Aprons	☐ 3
Gowns	☐ 4
Plastic capes	☐ 5
Latex gloves	☐ 6

Q4	Poor quality combs are uncomfortable and can scratch the client's scalp.	True or false
Q5	Which of the following is an example of poor customer service?	Multi choice
	Checking that the towels and gowns are clean	O a
	Cleaning the work surfaces	O b
	Sweeping up loose hair clippings	O c
	Forgetting to offer the client a drink	O d
Q6	Talking and listening to your client is one of the most important parts of good communication.	True or false
Q7	What information should you remember to get when taking messages?	Multi selection
	Address of contact	☐ 1
	Time and place of call	☐ 2
	Purpose of call	☐ 3
	Details and instructions	☐ 4
	Client treatment history	☐ 5
	Client service details	☐ 6
Q8	Non-verbal communication is another name for _____ language.	Fill in the blank
Q9	Which of the following is poor body language?	Multi choice
	Maintaining eye contact with the client	O a
	Moving into someone's personal space	O b
	Smiling when you greet someone	O c
	Maintaining the same eye level as the client	O d
Q10	Hands at waist height, with palms upward, indicate that the person has nothing to hide.	True or false

4 Reception

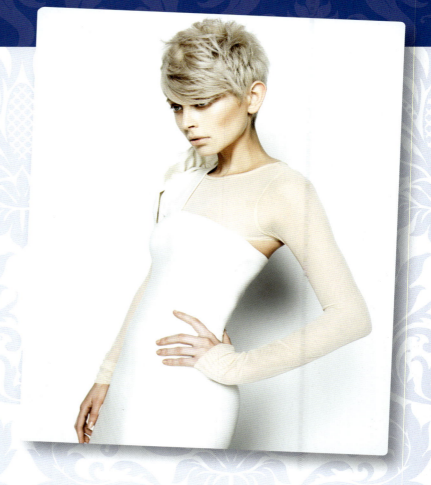

LEARNING OBJECTIVES

◆ Be able to maintain the reception and retail areas

◆ Be able to attend to enquiries

◆ Be able to make appointments

◆ Be able to calculate bills and handle payments

◆ Understand your client's legal rights in relation to consumer, and data protection

◆ Know your salon's range of products and services

KEY TERMS

appointment system	double booking	stock control
confidential information	overbooking	x readings
Data Protection Act (1998)	resources	z reading
database	restyle	

G4 Fulfil salon reception duties

Information covered in this chapter:

◆ Reception duties and maintenance

◆ Good customer service

◆ Manual and electronic payment systems

◆ Appointment systems

◆ Legislation – confidential information – consumer protection

INTRODUCTION

The reception is the most important area of the salon, as it is here that the client makes their first contact with the business. With clients and visitors arriving, incoming telephone calls, stock deliveries, appointments and payments being made, it's a busy place.

Because of all these daily duties that they perform, the receptionist needs a variety of skills: good communication, good organizational abilities, accuracy and above all attention to detail.

Apart from the receptionist's tasks, the reception area is equally important for creating the overall, professional impression. The waiting area, retail displays and reception desk should always be clean, organized and welcoming. It is the job of reception staff to maintain the area throughout the day as things are constantly changing. Stationery items, till rolls, pens and pencils can all run out, retail displays need restocking, magazines and cups and saucers all need attention.

BEST PRACTICE

Meet your clients' expectations by offering a prompt, welcoming and efficient service with the minimum of delay.

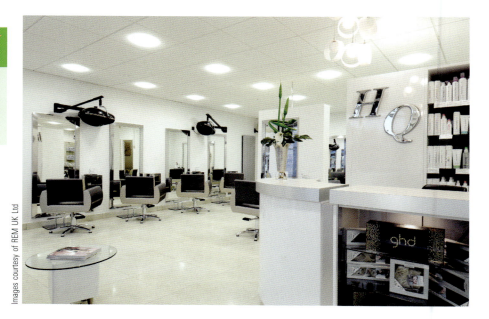

Images courtesy of REM UK Ltd

A professional salon reception

Customer service is at the heart of the hairdressing industry and it is good customer service that brings the clients back again and again. Clients want to feel that their custom is valued and that you and the rest of the staff will respond to their needs and problems with efficiency and empathy.

This chapter covers a range of skills required for reception work. It includes:

- making clients welcome and dealing with enquiries face to face
- making appointments
- using the phone
- handling money, in both cash and non-cash transactions
- balancing the till
- **stock control**
- working within the law.

A receptionist receives the clients and makes them feel welcome. They must greet them properly, respond to their needs and deal with their enquiries in a professional and friendly way.

If you are going to help in reception you will need good communication skills as you will have to deal with a wide range of people who expect the best from you. You will also need to know about the services and products that are available so that you can explain these to clients and promote your business.

You may also be responsible for making sure that there is enough stock and for accepting payments from clients and giving change. In addition, you may have to check that the money in the till is correct at the end of the day.

All this has to be done within the law, so you need to know which laws apply to you when you are handling clients' personal information and selling salon products.

Maintain the reception area

First impressions

Hairdressing is a personal service industry and if we are going to keep our clients happy, we have to provide a complete and professional service. This service is not just focused around the stylist's abilities – cutting, styling, perming or colouring – though, it has to be right from the point of entry to the exit from the salon. It's the first and the last impression of the salon.

The reception area is the hub of the salon; clients arrive, calls are received, visitors arrive, bills are paid and appointments are made. As part of your duties as the receptionist you will be responsible for making sure that the client waiting area is kept clean and tidy; that magazines are regularly checked for condition and currency and that the style books are replaced after use. A client who has had to wait will feel less angry if they have been attended to, offered something to drink or at least had something at hand to pass the time.

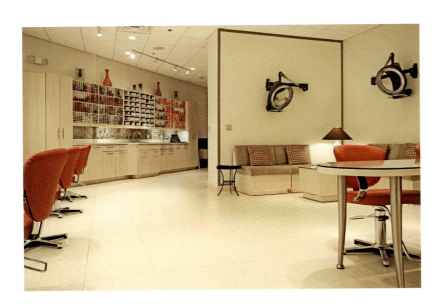

ACTIVITY

What is your salon's policy in respect to dealing with clients and enquiries?

What is the procedure for receiving clients? (Write your answers in the space below.)

ACTIVITY

Match the following operations to the tasks. We have already done the first one for you.

Retail products should be dusted daily	because handling information correctly is so important
Hairstyle books and magazines are useful	because people don't buy or handle dirty items
Offer clients a drink or magazines	because we must convey a professional image and service
Appointment books are essential	because they help people describe a new look
Good communication is essential	because sometimes they have to wait for a while
Messages should always be passed on to the right person	because they organize the stylist's day

Make sure that the retail displays are regularly cleaned and refilled, that retail products are checked for condition and that price labels are clearly visible. The retail products must look attractive: we want the clients to be encouraged to draw closer, pick them up and handle them.

The reception area is always busy with clients arriving or wanting to pay their bill, the telephone is often ringing with clients wanting to make appointments. Therefore the desk must be well organized. Stationery, such as memo pads, pens and payment-processing items, should be checked each morning before the salon opens, and you should make sure that there is enough to last throughout the day. The receptionist is also responsible for the till; there should also be enough change and card-processing materials to last all day.

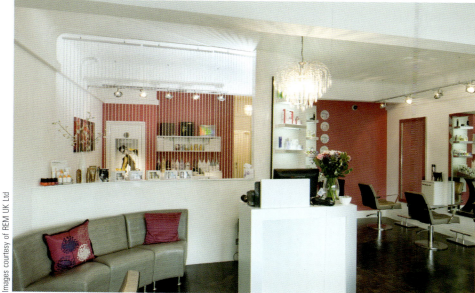

Images courtesy of REM UK Ltd

Maintaining reception – checklist Salon tidiness is essential and maintenance in reception is equally important. Make sure that each of these is done every day:

- ✓ Dust and polish shelves and surfaces in reception before clients arrive
- ✓ Appointment diary must be ready for use
- ✓ Card-payment receipt rolls and till rolls replenished and spares available
- ✓ Stationery items; pens, pencils, note paper, till rolls and clips, etc. ready at hand
- ✓ Damaged or faulty product packaging removed and reported to the manager
- ✓ Products rearranged and gaps in product lines removed from displays
- ✓ Product information, price lists and brochures ready for distribution
- ✓ Product promotions clearly displayed and stock items ready to sell

BEST PRACTICE

Clients' expectations of service are high. Always offer a prompt, welcoming, efficient service, be attentive and be helpful.

Being organized

All salons use some form of booking system for scheduling appointments and allocating work. Some prefer to use a manual appointment system; others prefer to use computer based applications. In either event the **appointment system** is the most important business process within the salon as it provides:

- ◆ a snapshot of expected levels of business
- ◆ a detailed action plan of work for staff
- ◆ a minute-by-minute schedule of business activities
- ◆ a record of client visits, creating a pattern of repeat business.

From this information you can:

- ◆ plan the salon **resources**, e.g. people, time, stock and equipment
- ◆ organize client records, contact details and treatment history
- ◆ prepare the till and electronic payment processes.

From this it is easy to see that the appointment system is the centre of an efficiently run business. The information it contains must be clear, accurate and up to date. However, maintaining the appointment system doesn't always guarantee the smooth running of the salon. You will always need to be prepared for the unexpected, such as late arrivals, walk-ins and clients turning up on the wrong day.

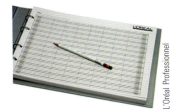

Typical appointment page/book

Attend to clients and enquiries

Good client care at reception

Good customer service and client care are essential to creating a thriving repeat business model. Without returning clients there would be no future for the salon or the people that work within it! So be hospitable, treat the clients well, greet each one with a smile and make sure that your body language (see Unit G17 page 51) is positive.

See Unit G17 page 51 for information on body language.

Five Steps to client care at reception

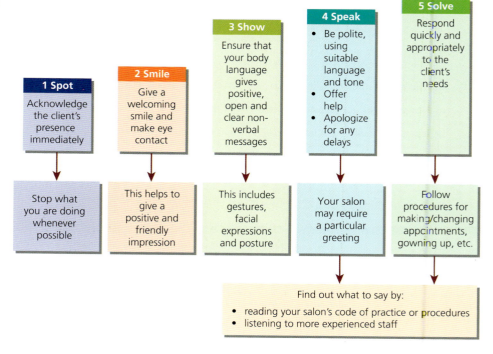

1 Spot	2 Smile	3 Show	4 Speak	5 Solve
Acknowledge the client's presence immediately	Give a welcoming smile and make eye contact	Ensure that your body language gives positive, open and clear non-verbal messages	• Be polite, using suitable language and tone • Offer help • Apologize for any delays	Respond quickly and appropriately to the client's needs
Stop what you are doing whenever possible	This helps to give a positive and friendly impression	This includes gestures, facial expressions and posture	Your salon may require a particular greeting	Follow procedures for making/changing appointments, gowning up, etc.

Find out what to say by:
• reading your salon's code of practice or procedures
• listening to more experienced staff

Handling enquiries

We want visitors to become clients and there are ways to make this happen. An important part of this process and one that affects the conscious decisions people make about us is communication. We want people to see us as professional communicators.

Effective communication takes place in the following ways:

◆ *speech* – what we say to others and the way in which we say it

◆ *listening* – hearing the requests of others properly

◆ *writing* – recording information accurately and clearly

◆ *body language* – the way we communicate our feelings and attitude to situations by posture, expression and mannerisms.

Enquiries made by a client either in person (i.e. face to face) or on the telephone should be handled in the same way. In both instances, we need to respond promptly and politely. If you don't know the answer to a question, ask someone who does: accurate information is essential. So stop! Listen to what is being said, hear the request and act on the information.

Misinterpreting what has been said will lead to giving or recording the wrong information.

On the telephone Good telephone skills are important to give a good impression and deal with clients effectively. You will be judged by what you say, so you should be polite, cheerful and helpful from the moment you pick up the telephone receiver to the moment you replace it.

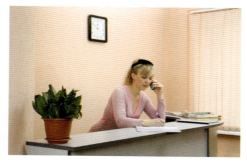

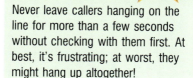

BEST PRACTICE

Never leave callers hanging on the line for more than a few seconds without checking with them first. At best, it's frustrating; at worst, they might hang up altogether!

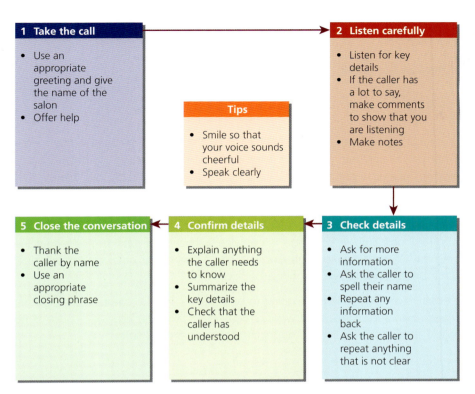

Five steps to handling calls

1 Take the call
- Use an appropriate greeting and give the name of the salon
- Offer help

Tips
- Smile so that your voice sounds cheerful
- Speak clearly

2 Listen carefully
- Listen for key details
- If the caller has a lot to say, make comments to show that you are listening
- Make notes

5 Close the conversation
- Thank the caller by name
- Use an appropriate closing phrase

4 Confirm details
- Explain anything the caller needs to know
- Summarize the key details
- Check that the caller has understood

3 Check details
- Ask for more information
- Ask the caller to spell their name
- Repeat any information back
- Ask the caller to repeat anything that is not clear

Memorandum

TO: John
FROM: Linda
DATE: 1/10
SUBJECT: Staff absence

Jayne will not be in for the rest of the week as she has a virus. Please could you reschedule her appointments, and advise all clients accordingly. Thanks.

Smile when you answer the telephone: people will 'hear' the friendliness in your voice. At the same time speak clearly so that the caller can understand everything you say. After listening to the caller's request, confirm the main points back to them. This summarizes the information and ensures that all details are correct. Keep in mind the length of the call: calls cost money and waste valuable salon time.

Face to face When clients arrive in person, they should be attended to promptly, their appointment and time should be checked before they are directed to a seat. Always make a point of making them feel welcome; perhaps offer a magazine or a drink before informing the stylist that their client has arrived. This is important as it will avoid any unnecessary waiting or possible embarrassment when the stylist realizes (perhaps much later) that their client has actually arrived.

There will be occasions when you need to seek assistance or advice from others. Being able to recognize situations where you are unable to help is not a failure, it is all part of professional communication. There will be situations that require the attention of someone else, perhaps when the window cleaner arrives and says 'Shall I just get on with it?' or when stock arrives and the signature of a person responsible for taking delivery and accepting condition of goods is required.

The visual impressions made from a person's body language are equally important.

Confidentiality Certain circumstances need special care and attention, and probably the most important aspect of professional communication is confidentiality. During our day-to-day work it is possible that we come into contact with information that others consider private. It is important that you recognize these situations and handle them accordingly. This **confidential information** will be disclosed in numerous ways: during

See **Chapter 3** Unit G17 on giving clients a positive impression of you and your organization.

See page 79 for information on the Data Protection Act (1998)

routine conversation between staff or clients and from business contacts and enquirers. Whatever the source, it is vitally important that you do not divulge personal or potentially sensitive information to anyone. Failure to maintain client confidentiality is not only a breach of professionalism and customer loyalty; it could in some cases (under the Data Protection Act (1998)) be against the law!

Late arrivals

Hardly a day will go by when there isn't someone who is late for their appointment. People are not deliberately late, it's just one of those things put down to modern living, transportation hold-ups, last-minute duties and trying to fit too much into a busy day. All have an impact on time. Unfortunately, it's not your time they are using: in most cases it's the next client's! In a situation where the client has arrived late you do need to be sympathetic and understanding. The first thing to do is be sympathetic, find out if there is still enough time to complete the service without over running throughout the rest of the day. If there isn't enough time left, see if one of the other stylists can help out: often a bit of 'juggling' will put things back on track.

Will the client have to wait? Is there going to be a delay? Tell the client immediately, let them choose between staying and waiting, coming back a little later or, if there is no other option, re-booking for another appointment at some other time.

Unscheduled arrivals and 'walk-ins'

The client who arrives without an appointment should always be accommodated if at all possible. If you think about the situation from their point of view, they have made the decision to come into your salon. Why? Is it because they have been recommended by someone else? Did they like the look of the salon from the outside? Or did they just happen to be in the area at the time? Whatever the reason, it's all good business.

Double booked!

Overbooking, or double booking, does occur, but shouldn't do too often. It is usually the result of either a staff member or the client making a mistake, or through poor communication. Don't try to beat the appointment system; you may upset clients, colleagues or both. Providing a high-quality service includes making sure people know the expected time scales and duration of services and if there will be any waiting.

Changes to booked services

There will often be occasions where a client has booked for one service, but by the time they reach the salon they have changed their mind and want something else totally different. People change their minds all the time. Don't worry, this could be good business – a client may come in expecting a restyle, cut and finish, and go out with highlights too. In fact many salons set incentives around this very activity; for example, staff performances and commissions may be based on 'upselling' or 'client conversion'.

Staff absences

Staff sickness will always stretch the salon's resources to its limits but every salon needs to plan for the unexpected:

When someone is off ill:

◆ check to see if another member of staff can 'step in' to provide the service

◆ rearrange the appointments – by calling the clients to let them know before they set out.

ACTIVITY

Typical assessment questions and model answers: when clients arrive at the salon…

Q1 What's the first thing you should do when a client arrives?

A1 Check the client's name, appointment time, what they are having done and who it is with.

Q2 What should you do next?

A2 Take their coat and any shopping etc. and put them away carefully and safely.

Q3 The stylist is not quite ready for the client. What should you do next?

A3 Ask the client to take a seat and offer them a drink and a magazine to look at for the time being.

BEST PRACTICE

Never bill a client for an amount that was not agreed.

TOP TIP

First impressions are lasting impressions

The human brain can take in a wide variety of information from different channels at the same time. How is that? We are aware of our surroundings by using any number of the five senses: sight, hearing, smell, touch and taste. These senses analyze and interpret the information we receive, helping us to create an overall impression, whether right or wrong! We all process the information so quickly that we are trying to create a judgement or understanding for what we see. Generally speaking our first and lasting impression is created in fewer than ten seconds! Hence, 'You don't get a second chance to create a good first impression'.

ACTIVITY

Explain why taking messages and passing them on to the correct person is so important.

Making appointments

Know your salon's services

The appointment system is the very centre, the 'hub' of the whole salon operation. Without an appointment system the business would stop! So it is essential that appointments are made accurately and promptly, every time, whether a client makes an appointment over the telephone or in person.

Before you can schedule appointments you must know the services available. Each salon provides a unique 'menu' of services. Different stylists will have different abilities and skills, and so might be available for certain services at certain levels. You need to know the variety of services available, their timings and relevant costs.

Making appointments needn't be difficult. It's about matching client requests with the time available. We want to help the customer make the booking, while bearing in mind the time that it will take and who will be providing the service. When clients are contacting the salon by telephone you should always speak first saying, 'Good morning/afternoon, this is Head Masters hair salon. This is Clare speaking, how may I help you?' This friendly and positive approach will immediately give a professional image of both the salon and yourself.

Appointment entries

Make sure when the booking is made that you record the information accurately and clearly and that you have considered all the following:

- date and time
- service required
- stylist required
- the client's name
- client's contact details (at least a telephone number).

Record the client's name clearly in the appointment system, alongside the service, and check that it is scheduled for the correct day and time with the appropriate stylist. As a matter of good customer service it is also useful to give the client an approximate idea of service cost and length of appointment time. At the end, summarize all the information back to the client, thus ensuring that all the details are correct.

Checklist for making appointments

- ✓ You need to know the different service abbreviations
- ✓ Ask the correct questions to get the right information
- ✓ Be patient with people, listen to their needs
- ✓ Know the prices of the different retail products and services
- ✓ Check the staff rotas – see who's in at the beginning of the day
- ✓ Check the spellings of people's names
- ✓ Check the stationery at the beginning of the day

When in doubt ask!

There may be situations where you are not sure. It is always better to ask someone else than to make mistakes such as:

- making incorrect or inaccurate bookings
- providing inaccurate information, e.g. incorrect costings of services or products.

When unsure always ask someone for help. There is nothing worse than a stylist who is running late, particularly if this is the result of someone else's booking error. The situation will be stressful for the stylist but, more importantly, we do not want any clients waiting longer than absolutely necessary, whatever the reason.

BEST PRACTICE

Always introduce yourself when handling calls. People like to speak to people with whom they can associate, not strangers or machines!

Service abbreviations	
Cut and blow-dry	CBD
Blow-dry	BD
Shampoo and set	S/S
Ladies' wet cut	WC
Gents' wet cut	G W/C
Gents' cut and blow-dry	G CBD
Highlights T section	H/L T
Highlights full head	H/L fh
Highlights half head	H/L½
Retouch colour	Col rt
Full head colour	Col fh
Permanent wave	PW
Chemical straightening	Strght

ACTIVITY

In this exercise you need to read the following service information and then complete the blank appointment sheet accordingly with the appropriate abbreviations.

A salon employs three experienced hairstylists:

Jane: A stylist who works part-time 1 pm to 5.30 pm

Samantha: A stylist who works full-time 9 am to 5.30 pm and has an hour for lunch

Tina: A colourist who works mornings only 9 am to 12 noon

Service		Duration
Cut and blow-dry	(CBD)	45 mins
Blow-dry	(BD)	30 mins
Wet cut only	(WC)	30 mins
Dry trim	(DT)	15 mins
Highlights T section	(HLT)	30 mins (plus 30 mins' development)
Highlights full head	(HL fh)	45 mins (plus 30 mins' development)
Retouch colour	(Col rt)	30 mins (plus 45 mins' development)

Add the name of each stylist at the top of the appropriate column. Now read the following service information and complete the blank appointment page.

Miss Cooper and her daughter would like full head highlights at the same time as each other with a cut and blow-dry back with Samantha later.

Mrs Ford wants the earliest appointment available with Jane for a cut and blow-dry and would like to bring her two children for dry trims with whoever is available at the same time.

Miss Jones would like a mid-morning cut and blow-dry appointment with Samantha.

A Miss Collins telephones to ask if there is an appointment for retouch colour and then a cut and blow-dry back with Samantha after 10.30 am. Mark out time for Samantha's lunch.

Two college girls, Miss Green and Miss Dorkin, call in and ask if there are any appointments for cut and blow-dry after lectures and as near to 2.00 pm as possible. They don't mind who they have, but they would like their appointments at the same time.

Someone telephones at 1.00 pm and asks for their children, Paula and Cheryl Tombs, to have a wet cut and a dry trim respectively, before 3.00 pm. Where can they be fitted in?

Appointment sheet			
Date:			
Time			
9.00			
9.15			
9.30			
9.45			
10.00			
10.15			
10.30			
10.45			
11.00			
11.15			
11.30			
11.45			
12.00			
12.15			
12.30			
12.45			
1.00			
1.15			
1.30			
1.45			
2.00			
2.15			
2.30			
2.45			
3.00			
3.15			
3.30			
3.45			
4.00			
4.15			
4.30			
4.45			
5.00			

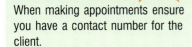

BEST PRACTICE

When making appointments ensure you have a contact number for the client.

Handle payments from clients

Different types of payment

When the hairdressing services have been completed and the client is satisfied with the result, the last thing that takes place before leaving the salon is the payment. The payment is made and kept in either an electronic or computerized till.

Both types of till can be programmed to perform a number of functions. Each person may be given a department key code which identifies their takings; this code can be used to calculate commission payments. On an automated till, a turnkey system can display X and Z totals. These readings when printed out are used to check the amounts registered against the actual amount in the till.

- ◆ **X readings** may be used to provide subtotals throughout the day: this is particularly useful in larger companies where it may be helpful to check takings when the cashier or receptionist leaves the till, removes cash, etc. from the till, or leaves the reception for break or for lunch.

- ◆ The **Z reading** is a figure taken at the close of business at the end of day. This provides a breakdown of the payment types, the times that payments were made and the allocations of sales against individuals.

The computerized till has advantages over the electronic till as it has the ability to provide a better analysis of salon sales. As well as keeping a central point of access to all the clients' records and treatment history it will monitor individual client sales, client repeat patterns, products sold or used within the salon, marketing information and also provides a wide range of management reports.

TOP TIP

If the change in the till is getting low tell a relevant person immediately. Running out of change will disrupt service and give a poor impression of salon organization.

BEST PRACTICE

Any tips given by clients should always be kept separately from the money in the till.

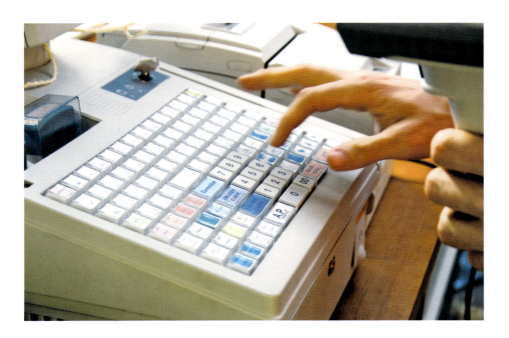

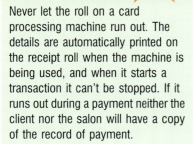

BEST PRACTICE

Never let the roll on a card processing machine run out. The details are automatically printed on the receipt roll when the machine is being used, and when it starts a transaction it can't be stopped. If it runs out during a payment neither the client nor the salon will have a copy of the record of payment.

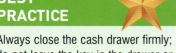

BEST PRACTICE

Always close the cash drawer firmly; do not leave the key in the drawer or the till open.

TOP TIP

Fraud is happening all the time! Find out what your salon's policy is in relation to fraudulent or attempted fraudulent transactions.

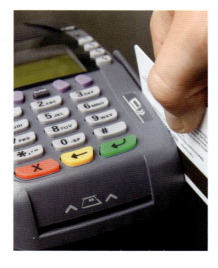

Sales-related equipment

- *Calculator* – Always a useful and necessary item to be kept somewhere handy on the desk for totalling large bills or during end-of-day summaries.

- *Till rolls and spare rolls for card-processing machines* – These provide records of sales and provide the client with a receipt for payment. Always keep spares handy just in case they run out in daily use. As the rolls get close to running out you will notice a red continuous marking, indicating that the roll must be changed at the earliest possible moment.

- *Credit card equipment* – the electronic terminal processes payments automatically, using 'Chip and Pin'. The machine is loaded with a receipt roll and the details of the sale are automatically printed onto the receipt.

- *Cash float* – At the start of the day a small sum of money in low-denomination notes and smaller coins is put in the till in order to provide change to clients paying in cash. This float is removed at the end of the day before any of the rest of the money is tallied. (A typical float, say £50.00, would be made up of the following: one × ten-pound note, two × five-pound notes, five × two-pound coins, ten × one-pound coins, ten × fifty-pence coins, ten × twenty-pence coins, 20 × ten-pence coins, 20 × five-pence coins.)

Methods of payment

Cash When taking cash from clients make sure that you follow these simple steps:

1 Take care to 'ring up' all the services and products provided to the client into the till and press 'subtotal'.

2 Inform the client of the amount to be paid.

3 Look carefully but not suspiciously to make sure that the money offered is legal tender (you should check that the notes are still valid, and not counterfeit).

4 Place the money tendered to you on the ledge at the top of the till drawer, so that it can be seen by the client too.

5 Press the numeric keys of the till to equal the amount tendered by the client.

6 Press the total button. The till will automatically show the amount of change to be given and the till drawer will open.

7 Take out and count back this amount into the client's hand.

8 Tear off the till receipt and don't forget to thank them as well as asking, 'Would you like to make your next appointment now?'

9 If the amount given back to the client is disputed, ask how much is missing. It is quite simple to make a genuine mistake, but if you are in any doubt call for a senior member of staff to assist. (If there is any dispute the till will need to be cashed up there and then to check for discrepancies.)

BEST PRACTICE

Checking the validity of notes

Hold the note in front of you with the Queen's head uppermost and on the right. You are looking for:

◆ a clear, detailed watermark of the Queen (facing to the right) in the lower centre of any denomination note

◆ a continuous metal strip through the note

◆ a hologram decal in the mid-left section of the note.

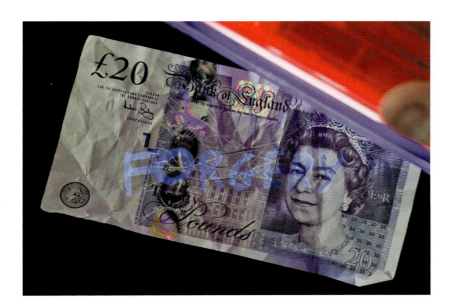

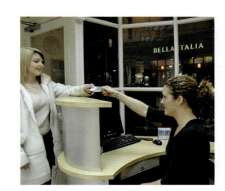

Cheques Cheques are no longer a popular form of payment and not accepted in most retail environments. Check to see your salon's policy.

Payments by card Payment by card is the most popular form of payment and there are a number of reasons why clients prefer to use this type of payment:

◆ *Cash availability* – Most people are paid directly into their bank accounts, therefore it is easier to draw down on these funds by debit card than to queue at an ATM (automated teller machine) to get cash out.

◆ *Cost of drawing out cash* – Many competing banking organizations will charge for withdrawing cash. If you can't find a branch of the bank with which you have an account, you could be charged for withdrawing from another bank's ATM.

◆ *Easier to account for expenditure* – It is simpler to keep a tally on the bank account as each amount drawn will be itemized on a monthly statement.

◆ *Different types of card* – There are many different types of card, so people can make choices on how they pay. Therefore people can manage their money easier by opting to pay by debit card, credit card or charge card.

◆ *Easier to use than cheques* – Cheques are no longer popular for secure tender for goods and services, although they are still used as a method of postal payments.

BEST PRACTICE

A post-dated cheque, i.e. a cheque made out for a date later than the current day's date, is not a valid form of payment.

Card types There are three basic types of card:

◆ debit card

◆ credit card

◆ charge card.

◆ *Debit cards* – VISA DEBIT is the most popular way of drawing down funds directly from your bank account at the time that the transaction is made. The card-processing company will apply a small nominal fee for each card transaction made.

◆ *Credit cards* – These are accepted as a method of payment at the discretion of the salon. When a card has been accepted as the method of payment, a fixed percentage of the total bill is charged by the card-processing company for the use of this facility. A list of cards that are accepted by the salon for payment should be clearly displayed on the door or front window as well as the reception desk.

◆ *Charge cards* – These provide another payment alternative. Many businesses now accept charge-card payments too – American Express is the main operator in this field. Charge-card payments are made in a similar way to credit or debit cards and therefore can be treated the same way. The difference is more for the card holder. The cards are often used as business cards, for travel, accommodation and business expenses. Each month the card holder receives a statement for the purchases made on the card over the period. This statement is a request for settlement and the bill must be paid.

ACTIVITY

Make a list of all the different card types that may be used for payment in your salon, and the differences between them.

Processing payments Before you accept a card payment you should make sure that the card is genuine and valid. Within the salon information pack you will find a card recognition guide for each card that is permitted. The guide provides the following information:

1 *Card symbol* – This is a logo (Visa, MasterCard) which will appear at the front lower right corner of the card. On charge cards, i.e. American Express, the Centurion head is printed across the centre of the card.

2 *Card hologram* – The card hologram service mark is in the centre right-hand edge of the card. This service mark is etched on to a foil decal which is superimposed on the card's printed background. The service mark on the holographic service mark (e.g. Visa, which appears as a dove ascending) is visible when angled in the light. The hologram changes according to the angle from which it is viewed.

3 *Card member number* – The card member's number will be embossed on to the surface and across the width of the card.

4 *Card validity dates* – The card will show a 'valid from' date as well as an 'expires end' date. If the card is not in date it can not be accepted.

5 *Card holder's name* – Check that the name on the card and the title of the card member, if it is embossed, match the person presenting it.

Chip and pin payments

1 Check that the terminal is in sale ready mode.

2 Insert the card into the chip reader.

3   Enter the amount by using the key pad (if you make a mistake you can clear the figures using the 'clear' button).

4   Press 'enter', which will connect the terminal to the card-processing company.

5   The customer details are automatically accessed and after a few moments, a message will prompt for 'Enter customer pin'. The customer can enter their four-digit pin on the customer keypad and press enter. The payment is authorized or declined automatically.

6   Separate the receipts. Pass the bottom copy back to the client and retain the top copy for the till.

Gift vouchers   These may be sold by the salon for payment against hairdressing and beauty services or retail sales. When the salon is operating as a concession, gift vouchers may be available for purchase from the host company. You in turn will require reimbursement from the source of the voucher. Company policy should outline procedures for issuing and receiving gift vouchers.

Discrepancies

Inconsistencies, disagreements or differences – invalid currencies being tendered, out-of-date cheque cards or unsigned cheques – should be dealt with as soon as possible. Where a payment card is being fraudulently used or there is a payment dispute, such as a bill totalling more than was previously agreed, then a senior member of staff should be referred to. Should an illegal transaction or even one suspected of being illegal be attempted, it may be decided to refer the matter to the police. This decision should always be made by the manager alone; however, in these circumstances you must act discreetly as serious allegations must be backed up with a formal statement and/or evidence.

Discrepancies within the till where the sales don't balance with the money in the till could be a genuine mistake or, alternatively, indicate dishonesty. The till should be neither up nor down at the end of the day and your salon will have a procedure for looking into 'unders' or 'overs' more closely.

Theft   Theft is a crime. If someone is caught in the act of theft or if it is proven that a previous theft has taken place, then it should be reported to the police.

Police strongly urge businesses to prosecute staff who have stolen from the business. Theft is an act of gross misconduct and any person found guilty of it will be dismissed immediately without any justifiable recourse.

Computers   There is a salon application suitable for any size of business. The benefits that they bring to a business in helping it to run more effectively are really compelling as they provide a wide variety of management information that couldn't be collected in any other way.

Most of these **database** applications provide a very comprehensive package and have features that address the following business aspects:

◆ *appointment booking system*

◆ *client records*: patterns of repeat business and history, as well as contact information, product usage, stock control and retail sales

◆ *staff details*: sales, commissions, hours of work, sickness, holidays, etc.

BEST PRACTICE

All information regarding clients should be handled in strict confidence. This safeguards all concerned and helps to reduce the possibility of embarrassment and loss of clients.

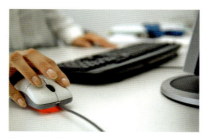

Online booking systems

◆ *sales functions*: sales audits, tracking and VAT, as well as normal till operation

◆ *management information*: reports, accounting, financial breakdowns, trading patterns.

As more clients do their business, accounts and shopping online, a growing number of salons communicate to their customer base either through their website or by email.

It's just as easy to make an appointment online as it is on the telephone, so there will be a big take-up over the next few years in hairdressing and beauty therapy online booking systems.

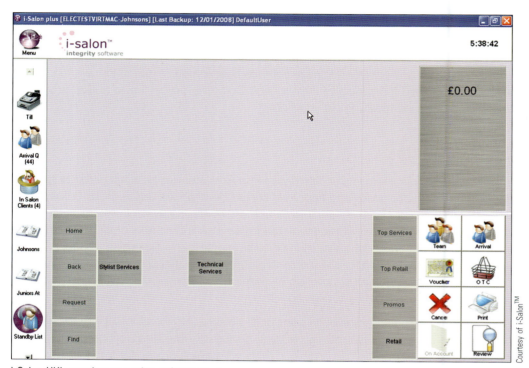

i-Salon UK's number one salon software system

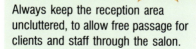

BEST PRACTICE

Always keep the reception area uncluttered, to allow free passage for clients and staff through the salon.

ACTIVITY

Collect information about the different types of computer-based systems available. When you have information on say two or three, make a comparison between them. See what features and benefits each one has to offer.

Reception security

The reception is the first part of the salon that people walk into off the street so this area must maintain a high level of security. All monies must be kept safely locked away and products should be monitored so that they are not maliciously removed. Records relating to the business, client details, accounts books, etc. should never be left unattended. If a client were to see these things left around that would be bad enough but if an unknown viewed them, then the salon's security measures would have been breached and personal information disclosed. In order to avoid these situations:

◆ the salon reception should be manned at all times

◆ money is not kept on the premises when the salon is shut and keep cash in the till during working hours to an absolute minimum

◆ never leave the till drawer open when it is not in use

◆ check all notes that have been handed over in payment to avoid counterfeits

◆ always leave the cash drawer, or at least the chassis that it fits into, open over-night: this discourages forced entries

◆ money should be regularly transferred to the company safe or banked

◆ never make regular visits to the bank at the same times

◆ receipts should be given for all payments

◆ never use the cash in the till for petty cash purchases

◆ any other money removed for whatever reason must always be recorded

◆ follow the salon's safety and security procedures at all times.

Laws affecting the salon's clients: consumer rights, discrimination and data protection

Data Protection Act (1998) Any organization that records information about staff or clients, whether on a card index system or a computer, must register with the Data Protection Registrar. This information must be kept accurate and up-to-date and be available to the person whose information it is to see on their request. In salons, this means that information about clients must be kept confidential, as must any information held about the staff. All staff have a responsibility to maintain this confidentiality at all times.

Data Protection Act 1998

The Data Protection Act (DPA) applies to any business that uses computers or paper-based systems for storing personal information about its clients and staff.

It places obligations on the person holding the information (data controller) to deal with it properly.

It gives the person that the information concerns (data subject) rights regarding the data held about them.

The duties of the data controller

There are eight principles put in place by the DPA to make sure that data is handled correctly. By law, the data controller must keep to these principles. The principles say that the data must be:

1. fairly and lawfully processed
2. processed for limited purposes
3. adequate, relevant and not excessive
4. accurate
5. not kept for longer than is necessary
6. processed in line with your rights
7. secure
8. not transferred to other countries without adequate protection.

ACTIVITY

What is your salon's policy in respect to your personal safety in aspects of salon security? Find out and put this information in your portfolio.

BEST PRACTICE

Clients may have the legal right to take action against you if you reveal information about them to anybody else.

ACTIVITY

It is important to know about the laws and legislation that affect your work in the salon. Your knowledge of the law can affect what you do every day.

A client or visitor asks you about the contact details of a friend who is also a client at the salon. Which of the following responses would be the correct way to handle confidential information?

> Good morning Mrs Green you want Mrs Peel's phone number? Yes, it's 01234 567890.

> I'm sorry Mrs Green, I can't provide you with that information as our records are kept private.

> Yes, Mrs Green, we do keep the record cards on the desk so that anybody can get to the information easily.

The Sale of Goods Act (1979) and Sale and Supply of Goods Act (1994)

The Sale of Goods Act 1979 and the later Sale and Supply of Goods Act 1994 are the main legal instruments helping buyers to obtain redress when their purchases go wrong. It is in the interest of anyone who sells goods or services to understand the implications of these Acts and the responsibilities they have under them. Essentially, these Acts state that what you sell must fit its description, be fit for its purpose and be of satisfactory quality. If not, you – as the supplier – are obliged to sort out the problem.

Briefly these Acts require the vendor:

◆ To make sure that goods *conform to contract*. This means that they must be as you describe them, e.g. highlight shampoo stops your highlights from fading.

◆ The goods must also be of *satisfactory quality*, meaning they should be safe, work properly and have no defects.

◆ You must also ensure the goods are *fit for purpose.* This means they should be capable of doing what they're meant for. For example, a brush shouldn't fall apart when it is first used.

The Consumer Protection Act (1987)

This Act follows European laws to protect the buyer in the following areas:

◆ *product liability* – a customer may claim compensation for a product that doesn't reach general standards of safety

◆ *general safety requirements* – it is a criminal offence to sell goods that are unsafe; traders that breach this conduct may face fines or even imprisonment

◆ *misleading prices* – misleading consumers with wrongly displayed prices is also an offence.

The Act is designed to help safeguard the consumer from products that do not reach reasonable levels of safety. Your salon will take adequate precautions in procuring, using and supplying reputable products and maintaining them so that they remain in good condition.

The Prices Act (1974) The price of products has to be displayed in order to prevent a false impression to the buyer.

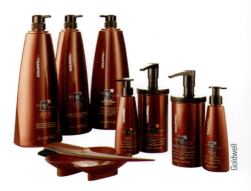

The Trades Descriptions Act (1968 and 1972) Products must not be falsely or misleadingly described in relation to their quality, fitness, price or purpose, by advertisements, orally, displays or descriptions. And since 1972 it has also been a requirement to label a product clearly, so that the buyer can see where the product was made.

Briefly, a retailer cannot:

- mislead consumers by making false statements about products
- offer sale products at half price unless they have been offered at the actual price for a reasonable period.

The Resale Prices Act (1964 and 1976) The manufacturers can supply a recommended price (MRRP or manufacturers' recommended retail price), but the seller is not obliged to sell at the recommended price.

Disability Discrimination Act 2005 (DDA 2005) The Act makes it unlawful to discriminate against disabled persons in connection with employment, the provision of goods, facilities and services or the disposal or management of premises; to make provision about the employment of disabled persons; and to establish a National Disability Council.

The Act protects the rights of disabled people and new revisions in 2005 have particular relevance to the business proprietor. For more information on this or accessibility issues visit **www.disability.gov.uk/legislation**.

Equality Act (2010)

Now covers all the following aspects

What is the Equality Act?

There are nine main pieces of legislation that have merged:

- ✓ the Equal Pay Act 1970
- ✓ the Sex Discrimination Act 1975
- ✓ the Race Relations Act 1976
- ✓ the Disability Discrimination Act 1995
- ✓ the Employment Equality (Religion or Belief) Regulations 2003
- ✓ the Employment Equality (Sexual Orientation) Regulations 2003

✓ the Employment Equality (Age) Regulations 2006

✓ the Equality Act 2006, Part 2

✓ the Equality Act (Sexual Orientation) Regulations 2007

http://www.equalityhumanrights.com

ACTIVITY

It is important to know about the laws and legislation that affect your work in the salon. Your knowledge of the law can affect what you do every day.

1. How many days must a product have been on sale before you can advertise it as a sale item at a reduced price?

    A. 14 days?

    B. 28 days?

    C. 90 days?

2. Who is responsible for the state of the products sold in a salon?

    A. the person who made it?

    B. the person who sold it?

    C. the person who bought it?

3. A client buys a hairbrush from the salon and returns the next day saying, 'This hairbrush you sold me is plastic. It says on the box it has natural bristles.' Which of these is the correct response that you should give?

    A. 'I'm sorry. The boxes must have got muddled up. I'll find you a real bristle brush.'

    B. 'Plastic bristles would be best for your hair.'

    C. 'I'm sorry. There's a muddle in the stock room. Somebody needs to sort t out.'

SUMMARY

Remember to:

✓ promote the range of services available in the salon and know what they cost

✓ promote the range of products available in the salon and know what they cost

✓ keep the reception area clean and tidy at all times

✓ keep stationery stocks handy at reception and know where to find replacements

✓ cover all the salon's payment types and methods

✓ always make appointments correctly, according to the salon's policy

✓ take messages and pass them on to the right person promptly

✓ give the right change when payment is made by cash

✓ recognize the current and valid forms of payment that the salon accepts

✓ keep the reception area and the till secure at all times.

Knowledge Check

With two of your colleagues you can practise and document the different scenarios that occur in a hairdressing salon.

Let one person take the place of the client and another, the receptionist. The third acts as an observer and takes notes for the others. Take it in turns to cover the following salon situations:

1   An angry client who is not happy with their hair.

2   A client who needs assistance with buying retail products.

3   A client who wants to make several bookings for her daughter's wedding.

In your notes you need to cover how the client was handled, how, if at all, the service could be improved and what information needs to be recorded in each of the different scenarios.

Case study

A client has asked for an appointment with a stylist who no longer works at the salon. Describe your salon procedures for:

◆   what you say to the client

◆   the questions you would ask

◆   the alternatives that you would offer the client

◆   what you would do if you could not deal with the situation.

ASSESSMENT OF KNOWLEDGE AND UNDERSTANDING

A selection of different types of questions to check your reception knowledge.

Q1   Visa and MasterCard are both forms of _____ card.   Fill in the blank

Q2   A charge card is the same as a debit card.   True or false

Q3   Which of the following card types are debit cards?   Multi selection

Loyalty card	☐	1
Switch card	☐	2
American Express card	☐	3
MasterCard	☐	4
Maestro card	☐	5
Store card	☐	6

Q4   A float in the till contains one × £10.00 note, two ×£5.00 notes, £20.00 in £1 coins and £5.00 in 50p coins. How much is in the float?   Multi choice

£40.00	O	a
£45.00	O	b
£45.50	O	c
£46.00	O	d

Q5   You should always take a contact number when making appointments.   True or false

Q6 Which of the following are examples of ineffective use of resources?   Multi selection

Explaining services and costs to clients on the telephone   ☐ 1

Discarding excess product after application   ☐ 2

Overrunning on appointments   ☐ 3

Turning the lights off in corridors and staff areas   ☐ 4

Washing up in the dispensary   ☐ 5

Ordering stock over the telephone   ☐ 6

Q7 _____ retail products are for maintaining hair between visits.   Fill in the blank

Q8 Which of the following procedures monitors the usage of products within salons?   Multi choice

Stock control   ○ a

Monitoring wastage   ○ b

Retail product and display cleaning   ○ c

Stock rotation   ○ d

Q9 A job description is a document containing the employee's terms and conditions of employment.   True or false

5 Promote services and products

LEARNING OBJECTIVES

◆ Be able to identify additional services or products that are available

◆ Be able to inform clients about services or products

◆ Be able to promote additional services or products

◆ Understand how to promote additional services or products to customers

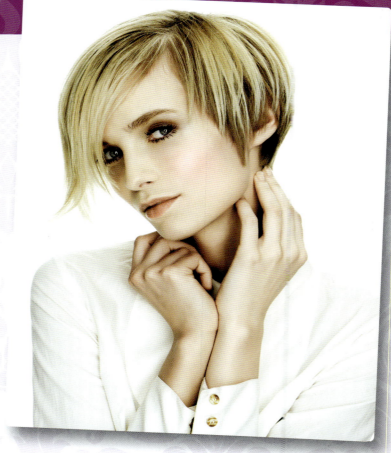

KEY TERMS

Benefits	merchandising	promotion
Features	multi-buys	shelftalkers
introductory discounts	point-of-sale material	special offers

Unit title

G18 Promote additional services or products to clients

Information covered in this chapter

- ◆ How to promote products and services
- ◆ How to make clients aware of the promotions
- ◆ How to gain client commitment as a result of salon promotion

INTRODUCTION

The services and products that salons provide to their clients are constantly being changed or updated. This happens so that they continue to meet customer expectations and keep abreast of the latest fashions and technology.

So, by offering new or improved services and products, your salon is able to:

- ◆ increase client satisfaction
- ◆ retain client loyalty for the future.

For salons, these two factors are directly linked and are therefore essential for a business to succeed. It is possible to make a really good job of satisfying our clients, but unless they continue to return (and within a reasonable timescale) the financial and on going success of the salon is drastically affected. So we need to stimulate the clients' loyalty by encouraging them to:

- ◆ buy our other services, products and treatments
- ◆ return on a regular basis
- ◆ share their experiences with other people.

Identify additional services or products that are available

Good customer service is being customer-focused. It is centred upon the needs of the client and is reflected within all of the aspects that are involved in routine salon operations: the telephone response times, salon refreshments and magazines, visually pleasing interiors and the polite and friendly staff. It is your duty to be upbeat, outgoing and positive when you communicate with the clients.

Salon services and products

Most salons have tariffs and **point-of-sale material** that provide information about the services and products they provide. This is a good way of providing information to clients as they can easily be seen and provide a talking point in the salon. But printed material is not always at hand or available, particularly when services and product ranges are being continually updated.

You need to be aware of changes and additions, so that you can provide advice on available services or products that would benefit your clients. You also need to keep up to date on all the features and benefits of newly introduced services and products. If you find that there are recent additions in the salon that you haven't seen before, you will need to ask your manager or supervisor for more information.

The products available in your salon can come from a lot of different sources and suppliers and this can often make it harder to keep abreast of new lines or product developments. But this is often the way that salons have to operate in order to cover a constantly changing, comprehensive range of options at a competitive price.

Products are not wallpaper!

Products should never be treated as wallpaper. They are not decorative items used to cheer up a 'dingy' corner, they have far more important purposes. Retail displays are an expensive investment for the salon and stock resting on shelves is an expensive cost. Products provide a useful, additional input to the salon's income and many salons look for a significant proportion of their turnover to be derived from these sales.

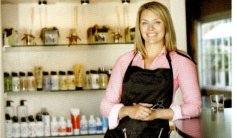

There are hidden benefits to the purposes of retailing which you may not have thought about. The promotional displays have an integral part in supporting the salon's image. If you think about it another way, the salon *only* purchases products for use and resale that are befitting the quality of services that your salon wants to be *identified* with. It therefore enables the clients to gain an extension of the salon experience, in the products that they take home.

Features and benefits – the things that clients are interested in

In order for you to promote and ultimately sell your salon's services, treatments and products, you need to recognize how they are viewed by clients. To do this you need to consider each service or product in terms of its features and its benefits and how these aspects would meet the needs of your clients:

◆ '**Features**' are the functions, i.e. what the service, treatment or product does.

◆ '**Benefits**' are the results of the functions, i.e. advantages, what the service or product achieves.

For example, suppose you recommend a client to spend £11.50 on a conditioning treatment. Why should they do this? What are the benefits of the service?

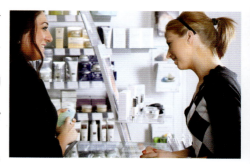

◆ The feature is: it re-conditions dry, damaged hair.

◆ The benefits for them are: it improves the dryness and helps to smooth damaged lengths; therefore it will improve handling, make the hair easy to manage and comb and enhance the hair further with shine and lustre. So these benefits justify the investment on their hair.

Knowledge of service and product features enables you to sell your clients the benefits. You thereby create a need, and once the client has accepted the need, you are in a good position to make the sale.

The first step is therefore for you to gain a thorough knowledge of each service and product available in the salon, and to translate this knowledge into an understanding of the features and benefits for each one.

Inform clients about services or products

New clients that come in to our salons are part of a very special group. They have probably found us through the network of already satisfied customers. Those satisfied customers feel confident enough in our expertise to promote our skills and services by recommending us to their friends and colleagues.

If recommendation is such a powerful channel of communication, why don't we use it more?

Well we can. The perfect time to talk about the variety of services and treatments available to clients is when they are in the chair in front of us. Recommendation is the simplest way of extending the range of services to our clients and enhancing the professional relationship.

The most effective way of introducing clients to products that will benefit them is to use them on their hair in the salon. This style of introduction creates a close relationship between:

◆ something that the client needs (with the added benefit of)

◆ seeing how it is applied (through to)

◆ the results that it achieves.

This style of **promotion** is improved further by not only showing the product to the client but by passing it to them so that they can experience the product by:

◆ holding it and

◆ smelling the fragrance.

ACTIVITY

Promoting business

The services and products that the salon provides to its clients generate the income that the business exists on. If the clients do not return on a regular basis, the business will fail. Therefore, client loyalty is vital to the success of the business and this can only happen if the client is satisfied with the services they receive.

Give three ways in which you think client loyalty may be maintained.

Now give suggestions for how to promote the business to its clients.

How do we inform clients of what we have to sell?

In-salon promotions are the most popular way of conveying *messages* to the clients which, in turn, become a topic of conversation whilst they are having their hair done. However, any form of salon activity costs money and that outlay has to be budgeted for.

So the first part of the process is to find out what the promotion is about? If it is linked to a new product introduction, then there will be some form of supporting resources to help inform the clients. Whenever a new product or range of products is introduced, the manufacturer will produce a variety of point-of-sale material that provides people with professionally produced information, posters, etc. to help with its launch. The amount of supporting material tends to be distributed in line with the levels of purchases made by the salon.

So, a small independent salon that has bought an entry-level introductory deal from the supplier may only have a small amount of supporting material or resources to use within the salon, whereas another, larger, chain-type salon will be bulk-buying a larger amount and will get more resources to help promote the product.

Implementation stages of product or service promotion

The following information provides you with a checklist for the stages of putting an in-salon promotion into practice.

- ✓   Find out the budget

- ✓   Make individuals aware of the product's features and benefits

- ✓   Let staff know what their roles and targets are

- ✓   Implement the promotion

- ✓   Evaluate the effectiveness of the promotion

The budget is set by management and may include the initial outlay figure for purchasing the products as well as the additional cost of setting up the promotional activities. Everyone involved should be informed well in advance of the promotion about the nature and purpose of the event. This provides staff with a clear idea of what the newly introduced products do, their application and how they benefit the clients, and the product selling costs.

Usually on a product launch there would be an introductory period that may tempt customers with special offers or deals.

The most popular promotions are usually in the form of:

- ◆   **introductory discounts** – where products are available for a set period at a lower price

- ◆   **multi-buys** – typically two-for-ones or get three for the price of two

- ◆   **special offers** – buy all three and get a free beach towel or scarf.

Staff need to be made aware of the promotional plan, any incentives linked with the promotion and their personal targets for the introductory period. Each member of staff might have an individual role to play in the overall team plan. For example, the junior may ask the client if they want to try the new conditioner on their hair at the basin. From this a client gets the chance to gain their first experiences of the product.

The promotion continues at the styling position where display materials – e.g. show cards or leaflets – inform the client of the benefits from using the product. This is further backed up by the stylist's recommendation and advice. The client would be asked if they noticed and liked the *smell* of the conditioner when it was applied, or if they can *see* and *feel* the difference that it has made to their hair.

Then finally, before the client leaves, they *connect* again with the promotion when they see a well-put-together display in reception. The receptionist could now ask if the client would like to add the product to their bill so they can use it at home.

You can see from this example that it can be a whole-team approach. This is particularly important for larger salons where clients are handled by a number of different individual members of staff: this increases the likelihood of continuity being lost. In these situations, passed-on communications are paramount as useful sales can be lost.

Common senses When a promotion is implemented, a plan of action is put into effect and all successful promotions have to be *sensory events*. Effective selling is experiential; it provides the purchaser with a variety of experiences that they can:

- see
- touch
- smell
- hear or
- taste.

Our five senses provide the only ways in which people can be influenced in making a purchasing decision. The more sensory *channels* that are involved in the promotional environment, the more chances are that the customer will buy.

At the end of the promotional period the success and impact of the event can be evaluated by team discussion, reviewing sales reports and listening to feedback from the clients on how the promotion was received.

ACTIVITY

Using the senses

You can see how the senses are used when you go shopping. For example, what do you notice when you go into a shopping centre? The shops that sell toiletries open their doors so that the fragrance of the goods can fill the air.

Again, why do you think that supermarkets put their fresh produce or coffee shop next to the front door? It's so they can stimulate the clients' senses with the things that they can touch and smell.

How do you think the senses are used in your salon to help in the promotion of products? Write down the types of experience that the client would get from the introduction of a new styling product.

Promotional materials A typical product promotion will consist of:

◆ point-of-sale **merchandising** – central 'island', open cabinet, shelf displays

◆ **shelftalkers** – printed promotional slips/cards fixed to/dangling from shelves; 'mobile' ones that bob or bounce deliver best results

◆ eye-catching displays – these are instantly informative – locate them where they'll be seen at reception or centrally in treatment areas

◆ arrangement of popular lines at eye level with price details – use 'price watch' stickers

◆ linking displays with money off and other special offers – first visit, loyalty, recommend-a-friend discounts and promotional tie-ins with major local stores.

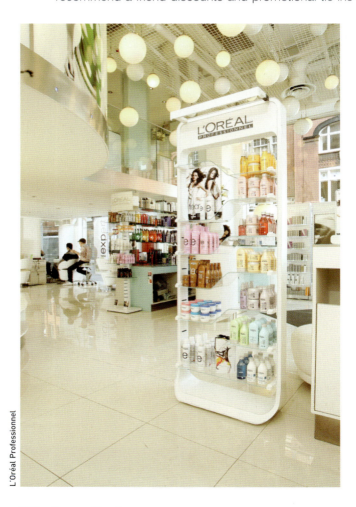

L'Oréal Professionnel

Window displays Window displays are an essential way of advertising services, their costs and displaying products. They are relatively inexpensive to dress, if they are maintained by salon staff. But care needs to be given to the quality of dressing, as public expectations of retail window space are generally high. Part of the secret to creating eye-catching displays is constant change. Therefore the display windows need to be changed frequently, if they are to have any impact on the passing trade.

New salon customers find us through a variety of different ways and the image of the salon created by the front window is part of that formula; although we shouldn't forget that reputation, location, advertising campaigns and, the most important, personal recommendation, all have a major impact too.

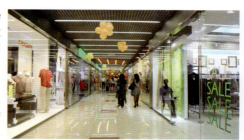

Website The most popular and interesting way to find out about what a business has to offer from a remote location is through its website. All salons have some form of Internet presence, even if it is only a Facebook page or Twitter account. And as managing the information upon a website gets easier, many salons can upload their own photographs, edit textual content and can provide engaging, interactive and fun ways to sell their services and products.

The website can be a very powerful marketing tool for any business and this will continue to be the fastest and most effective way of reaching customers for many years to come.

ACTIVITY

The selling process

Look at the list of things below then think about what you need to do or say to the client to complete the selling process.

The selling process	What can you do or say?
Giving advice	
Find out the client's needs	
Recognize client interest	
Recognize client disinterest	
Gain agreement	

Gain client commitment to using additional services or products

Recognizing interest – buying signals

You need to be able to differentiate between genuine interest and a polite and friendly, but negative response. Just because someone responds in a polite or friendly way it is not an indication of 'I want to buy that'.

Genuine interest is expressed in at least two ways:

1 The client will *ask* how that will benefit them, e.g. 'Would that be suitable for my type of hair?' or, 'How does that work?'

2 The client will *show* their interest by taking the product and holding it for closer examination, or through their positive body language.

Therefore when you introduce or recommend the client to a new service or product, you will need to look for the signs of interest mentioned above.

TOP TIP

A client cannot only show their interest through body language, they can show their lack of interest too!

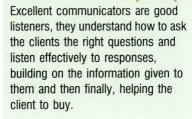

TOP TIP

Genuine interest is expressed by the client wanting to know more and/or showing it by what they do.

For more information on question styles, open questions, closed questions and body language, see **Chapter 3**, pages 42–59.

BEST PRACTICE

Excellent communicators are good listeners, they understand how to ask the clients the right questions and listen effectively to responses, building on the information given to them and then finally, helping the client to buy.

Anything other than these signs could indicate a lack of interest and you should be careful how you proceed. There is little point pursuing the issue if you are receiving little or no response; even if you think it's the best product or service that they could have. The last thing that you want to be seen as is 'pushy' or a 'commission seeker'. It won't help your professional standing and it may tarnish your professional relationship too!

Communication

So from the information already covered in this section you can see that there are many ways in which we communicate with our clients. Establishing an effective communication between you and the client is the most important aspect that determines your success in your role. The relationship between stylist and client is built on quality of service, professional advice, trust, support and a listening ear. Good communication ensures productive and effective action. On the other hand, poor communication can lead to misunderstandings, misinterpretation and mistakes.

Verbal and non-verbal communication

ACTIVITY

Features and benefits
Put yourself in the clients' position; think about how they view and experience the salon's services, treatments and products.

1. What is meant by the term 'features'?
2. Now explain what is meant by the term 'benefits'.

Now in terms of features and benefits, give the features and benefits to the client for the following services:

1. A new haircut.
2. A semi-permanent colour.
3. A conditioning treatment.
4. Temporary 'clip-on' hair extensions.

Good and bad selling techniques

Key factors indicating GOOD selling techniques

◆ Listening, asking questions, showing interest

◆ Using the client's name

◆ Empathy (putting yourself in the client's place), establishing a bond

◆ Recognizing non-verbal cues (dilated pupils = 'I approve'; ear-rubbing = 'I've heard enough')

◆ Identifying needs; helping clients reach buying decisions

◆ Knowing your products/services

◆ Highlighting the results or user benefits; demonstrating these where possible

◆ Thinking positively, talking persuasively, projecting confidence and enthusiasm.

Key factors indicating BAD selling techniques

◆ Doing all the talking

◆ Not listening, not 'hearing' unspoken thoughts, arguing

◆ Interrupting – but never letting the clients interrupt you – thus losing an open opportunity for giving extra information

◆ Hard selling, 'spieling' (working to a script)

◆ Threatening – 'You won't get it cheaper anywhere else', knocking the opposition

◆ Manipulating – 'Oh dear, I'll miss my sales target'

◆ Knowing nothing about the product

◆ Treating 'no thanks' as personal rejection

◆ Blinding clients with science

◆ Staying mainly silent waiting for an order

◆ Insisting the client should buy the product.

For more information on consumer legislation see Appendix 3.

Consumer legislation

The rights of your customers should not be compromised; they are protected from fraudulent and sharp practice by a variety of consumer laws.

SUMMARY

Remember to:

✓ use positive communication techniques

✓ maintain client confidentiality

✓ listen to clients and understand their needs

✓ promote the range of services, products and treatments with the salon

✓ use positive body language and the reasons why it plays such an important part in good customer service

✓ Remember the clients' legal rights – know your legislation

Knowledge Check

For this project you will need to gather information from a variety of sources.

For the following legislation find out how:

◆ the Health and Safety at Work Act

◆ the Data Protection Act

affect the way that services can be provided to clients.

In your project pay particular attention to the aspects that would have impact on a business and the implications if this legislation were not considered.

ASSESSMENT OF KNOWLEDGE AND UNDERSTANDING

A selection of different types of questions to check your sales and promotion knowledge

Q1 Selling opportunities occur when the features and _____ of products are explained.

Fill in the blank

Q2 Business develops without promotion or advertising.

True or false

Q3 Which of the following are types of in-salon promotion?

Multi selection

Radio advertising	☐	1
Hairdressing competitions	☐	2
Hairdressing demonstrations	☐	3
Point of sale material	☐	4
Reception displays	☐	5
Merchandising	☐	6

Q4 PR is a term which refers to professional media handling.

True or false

Q5 What is the most cost-effective way of selling services to clients?

Multi choice

External demonstrations	O	a
Internal promotions	O	b
Client consultation and advice	O	c
Point of sale material	O	d

Q6 Merchandising is a retailing strategy.

True or false

Q7 Which of the following are laws protecting consumer purchases?

Multi selection

The Consumer Protection Act	☐	1
COSHH	☐	2
Trades Descriptions Act	☐	3
RIDDOR	☐	4
The Prices Act	☐	5
The Data Protection Act	☐	6

Q8   The vendor must ensure that goods they sell are of _____   Fill in the blank
quality.

Q9   When handling complaints avoid which of the following?   Multi choice

Maintaining eye contact with the client   O a

A discussion in a quieter area of the salon   O b

Telling the manager about the event   O c

Folding your arms and being defensive   O d

Q10   A prospective client forms their first impressions of salon staff in less   True or false
than ten seconds.

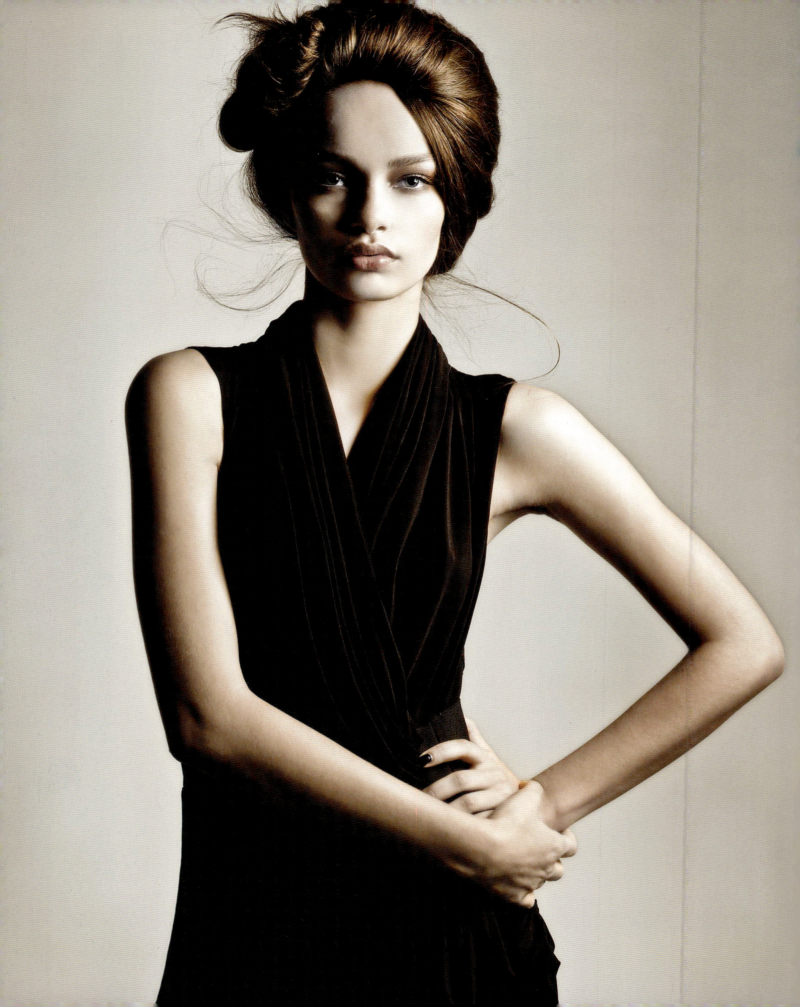

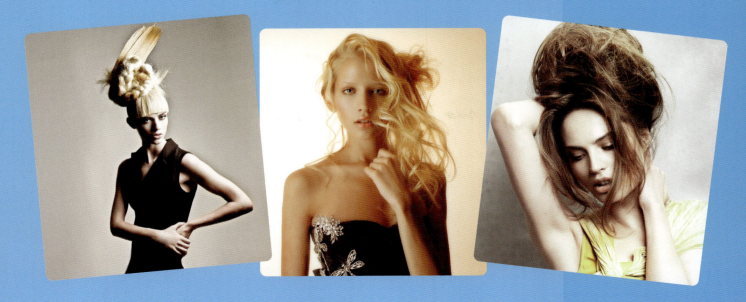

PART TWO
Technical services

This section of the book now covers the remaining technical services that salons provide to their clients.

6 Consultation and advice

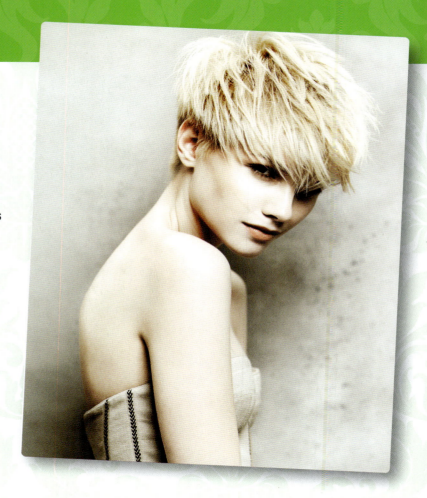

LEARNING OBJECTIVES

◆ Be able to identify what clients want

◆ Be able to analyze the hair, skin and scalp

◆ Be able to advise clients and agree services and products

◆ Understand the salon's services, products and their prices

◆ Know how to perform hair, skin and scalp analysis

◆ Know how to perform tests prior to services and treatments

◆ Be able to record information relating to the client's consultation

KEY TERMS

chemically treated

contra-indication

cortex

cowlick

cuticle

dermis

double crown

epidermis

follicle

graduations

hair colour

hair tendency

hair texture

hygroscopic

influencing factors

nape whorl

oblong

outlines

oval

paraphenylenediamine (PPD)

porous

porous hair

relaxing

round

square

strand test

tapered neckline

tones

trichologist

widow's peak

Unit title

G7 Advise and consult with clients

Information covered in this chapter

- Hair tests
- Hair and scalp disorders
- Client consultation processes and techniques
- Contra-indications to services and treatments
- Basic structure of hair and skin
- Hair growth stages and patterns

INTRODUCTION

Consultation is arguably the most important service provided in a hairdressing salon, although the professional advice it produces for its clients often seems undervalued in relation to other professional sectors. But make no mistake; the service of consultation is fundamental to all other services that take place within the salon and, without it, hairdressing and barbering cannot survive.

If consultation is rushed, you run the risk of unexpected outcomes or unpredictable disasters. On the other hand, when too much time is taken, it will eat into the planned service time, and this causes a 'knock-on' effect that will make the stylist (or client) run late or force the stylist to rush the job.

BEST PRACTICE

Effective communication relies upon listening to the client, hearing what they have to say, responding to them positively in what you say, and backing that up with the right body language.

BEST PRACTICE

You have to earn respect; your client is already paying for it.

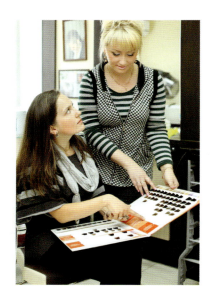

TOP TIP

Visualization is a rare skill; being able to see what something will be like before actually doing it is often very difficult for stylists, let alone clients.

TOP TIP

'Advising clients' means listening to what they have to say about their hair, asking appropriate questions and coming up with suitable suggestions for styles and treatments.

The consultation service

It is essential that you get the balance right and enough time must be given to:

◆ gain the client's trust and professional respect

◆ use visual aids either brought by the client or available from the salon

◆ conduct an analysis of the starting situation

◆ discuss the client's expectations in line with your analysis

◆ negotiate and then agree the best course of action

◆ provide home care maintenance and management advice.

Identify what clients want

Hairdressing is about relationships – and professional relationships are built over time and through good communication.

So in consultation, use your communication skills to find out what the client wants in a clear and mutually understood way. It's not that our clients want to mislead us; it's more to do with the fact that most people find that explaining an idea is very difficult.

Most people have no self-visualization. That means that they haven't an ability to imagine what a style would look like on them, and this can be a huge problem for those trying to give advice. Seeing what the clients are seeing is everything, so you have to find a way of *seeing through their eyes*.

Good, effective communication

A good communicator will use a mixture of techniques; this is a sort of 'toolbox,' a mixture of effective communication skills that covers the following.

1   *Listening and hearing*. This is the ability to hear and understand what the client is saying. This is essential when you need to review what has been said later, when you finally agree on the service and course of action to take.

ACTIVITY

Communication

1.   Can you think of the gestures, posture or expression that would portray at least three types of negative body language?

2.   List at least six different ways of communicating.

3.   Explain briefly what communication means to you.

2   *Speaking clearly*. It is important that you are clear with what you say and that you are not misunderstood by the client. During consultation you will be asking questions and trying to find enough information in the time available to make the right decisions for your client. You will be weighing up what the client wants against the

limitations that arise during the analysis. You will be getting the client to agree on the various possible options and planning the necessary course of action.

3   *Understanding body language.* The most difficult aspect of consultation is *reading between the lines*. Your ability to understand situations based upon what has been said or not said, is exceptionally useful. There are times when your client will look in a certain way, or say something that makes you stop and think. In these situations, your ability to read the situation, i.e. your perceptiveness in picking this up and responding appropriately, will have a huge impact on what happens next.

4   *Finding help*. There will be times during consultation when you will find that you aren't sure of what the client means, or possibly, not sure of what you see. If you make an inaccurate assessment of these factors it could lead to a disaster. It is vitally important that you clarify the situation at every point by confirming back to them what you *think* you have understood.

Further information can be found in other parts of this book: G17.3 Communicate information to clients, page 49 and G18.3 Gain client commitment to using additional services or products, page 93

Asking questions to find out what the client wants

1   You need to ask the right sorts of questions to get the information that you need.

2   You need to ask those questions in a way that your client understands.

The main types of question styles are covered below.

Open questions These are good to use if you want to gain more in-depth information from the client. They start with 'who', 'what', 'when', 'why', 'where' and 'how'. Examples:

◆   What products do you use on your hair?

◆   When did you last wash your hair?

◆   How often do you use the straightening irons on your hair?

Closed questions These are useful for a quick 'yes' or 'no' elimination response. Examples:

◆   Have you had permanent colour on your hair before?

◆   Would you like me to do it in your lunch hour today for you?

◆   Are you against moving the parting from the centre?

Feeling questions These types of questions focus upon the client and are good to use when you are trying to gauge a personal opinion or feeling. Examples:

◆   How do you feel about taking the length back up to the shoulders?

◆   Do you want me to talk you through the home care for this style now?

◆   What do you think about a complete colour change today?

TOP TIP

If you find that your line of questions isn't getting the information that you need, try asking again but in a different way. E.g. 'Well, how do you feel about changing the colour?' or, 'What other things do you find that also work well on your hair?'

'Choices' questions These can be considered to be leading as they request the client to make a response based on a set number of options. Examples:

◆ Would you prefer the smaller intense leave-in treatment, or the normal after shampoo conditioner?

◆ Shall we see if there is time today to do it all, or would you rather make a separate appointment for the highlights after the cut?

◆ Where would you like to wear the parting, in the centre where it is now or move it across so that you can have a sweeping fringe?

Whatever style of question you choose to use, you must make sure that:

◆ you identify any limitations or influencing factors that affect your styling options

◆ the client understands what you are saying/doing

◆ you allow the client time to consider the options that you provide

◆ you urge the client to give you as much information as possible

◆ you listen, *hear* and understand the client's responses

◆ you confirm what you hear before moving on to the next aspect of the consultation.

Questioning styles

Open/closed questions

Open questions will result in explanations or descriptions. **Closed** questions will result in short answers such as 'yes' or 'no'.

Feeling questions

Feeling questions ask 'how do you **feel** about a fringe?' 'What do you **think** if I restyle it today?' 'Do you **want** more volume?'

Questioning styles

Choices questions

'Would you like to keep the parting in the centre, **or** would you like to try it on the side for a change?'

No misunderstandings

You may need to ask things in different ways. If a client seems puzzled or confused, stop, go back and ask again in a different way. Misunderstandings can happen at any time but the most common reasons are:

◆ not listening to the client

◆ client's levels of understanding

◆ stylists using jargon: technical terms that the client won't know

◆ clients using hairdressing terms incorrectly, e.g. 'I like my hair layered a lot'

Make sure that you seek clarification or confirm points as they are discussed; show that you understand by nodding in agreement. When you get to a point in the consultation where you are not sure about something, re-ask your questions in a different way to probe further.

Identify the limitations or influencing factors

Some of these will crop up in conversation, but the main **influencing factors** are going to arise during your visual examination of the hair and scalp. So whether you do your inspection first or later will depend on the service that you are going to do, or how comfortable the client is with the consultation process.

Allow time for the client to express their wishes and consider your advice. Give the client time to prepare what they want to say. Many people will bring pictures from magazines or from the Internet which will give an impression of what they have in mind. But often those people feel embarrassed to take it out of their handbag when they get to the salon, so why not ask. 'Is there is anything that you have seen or brought with you?'

Don't rush them into making swift decisions; you need to *take them with you every step along the journey*. If they do feel rushed or that you are 'pushy' you will be alienating them from the outset. That's a difficult position to be in as you will be creating a tension during the service that would be uncomfortable for anyone to be in.

> **TOP TIP**
> It's easy to confuse clients if you start using technical terms. Keep it simple.

Using visual aids in consultation

Pictures 'A picture paints a thousand words' – the term may be overused, but it's very true. Pictures convey aspects of hairstyles or effects that are very difficult to put into words. They cut straight through technical jargon and establish a basis for things that you and the client can see and confirm.

Pictures are an immensely important visual aid and another form of language that hairdressers understand very well. One reason for this is hairdressers' understanding of **shape, proportion and balance**. As a stylist, you are trained in looking into pictures to see more than just an overall image. You see things like how volume is distributed, where hair needs to be shaped in a certain way and how colour can impact an overall effect. However, you can't expect the client to see these technical aspects too, so beware when pictures are used to express a feeling or a mood. You need to make sure that you are seeing the same things.

> **ACTIVITY**
>
> *Consultation*
> We can define consultation as a way of providing advice during a meeting.
>
> In order to carry out a thorough consultation there are a number of steps that should take place. Write down in order the sequence of events that should take place during client consultation.
>
> A.
>
> B.
>
> C.

> **TOP TIP**
> A picture is the quickest way of portraying themes, ideas, **tones** or moods.

Colour charts Colour charts are extremely useful for hairdressers. We rely on them every day. However, they are not always a very helpful medium for the client. We tend to treat others as we would want to be treated ourselves. This is a good philosophy, but there are times when our expectation of others is a little over-optimistic. Generally speaking, clients have very little ability for self-visualization, but that's why they are asking you for your opinions and advice.

Remember, colour charts tend to have very small samples of coloured wefts. Unless you can help the client visualize the:

◆ amount and placement

◆ colour intensity, and

◆ density and saturation of colour

then the value of using a colour chart as an example is greatly reduced.

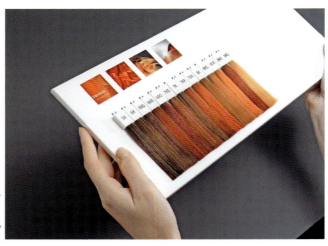

Image courtesy of Goldwell UK

Confirm and agree

Whatever methods you have used during your consultation, make sure that you confirm and summarize at all the points along the way. Only after you have both agreed a course of action can you take things to the next stage.

Lead the client through the consultation process

Take control of the situation; it is essential that you guide the client throughout the service. Your professionalism will be measured at the moment when the client realizes that it is you who is going to conduct the consultation. Everything is summed up (rightly or wrongly) by the client and you in a few moments and, contrary to customer service beliefs, you will not be able to satisfy the client fully unless you are in charge of this situation. You have to guide and steer the whole process in order to satisfy the client's expectations and those of your salon.

ACTIVITY

Body talk

What would be the visible signs of someone who:

1. Is being defensive?
2. Shows no interest?
3. Seems confused?
4. Wants to know more about your in-salon promotion?

Write down your answers in your portfolio.

Analyze the hair, skin and scalp

The analysis of the client's hair takes the form of a visual inspection. You need to brush and separate the hair in several directions in different areas over the head so that you can look for any signs that will either limit or modify the options available for your client.

You are looking for anything that could affect your decisions and this could relate to:

◆ **hair texture** – the thickness of individual hairs; is it coarse, medium or fine?

◆ hair length – is it layered, graduated or all one length?

◆ hair growth patterns – what directions does the hair grow in at the front, or the nape or over the crown?

◆ **hair tendency** – is the hair straight, wavy or curly?

◆ hair amount – how much hair do they have, how is it distributed over the scalp?

◆ hair condition – is the hair **chemically treated**, natural, dry or damaged?

◆ **hair colour** – is the colour natural or has it been highlighted or the colour changed in some way?

◆ hair problems – damaged **cuticle**, split ends, etc.

◆ face shape – is the shape **oval**, **round**, **oblong** or **square**?

◆ infections and infestations – are there any adverse signs or contra-indications?

◆ tests – elasticity, skin, colour, etc.

◆ lifestyle – manageability and the time available to maintain the look.

ACTIVITY

For discussion

Empathy and sympathy – is there any difference?

Discuss with your colleagues the differences between these emotions and why they are useful.

BEST PRACTICE

During consultation with your client, take enough time to find out what they want.

ACTIVITY

For discussion

Discuss with your fellow staff members how different client personalities will affect the style and method of consultation. Discuss also how you can vary the consultation delivery to ensure that a mutually beneficial outcome is derived.

BEST PRACTICE

Trust is hard earned. Gaining a customer's trust and loyalty takes time. Once you have earned this, the bond remains fragile, so handle with care.

The aspects to consider

Structure of hair and skin page 108	**Cortex**, cuticle, medulla, physical properties of hair and skin, hair **follicle**
Growth cycle of hair pages 113–116	Anagen, catagen, telogen
Hair texture page 114	Coarse, medium, fine
Hair tests pages 115–118	Skin/Patch test, strand test, colour test, test cutting, test curl, curl check, peroxide test, incompatibility test, elasticity test, porosity test
Infectious skin and scalp pages 119	Impetigo, scalp ringworm (tinea capitis), head lice (pediculosis capitis)
Non-infectious skin and scalp page 121	Folliculitis, dandruff (pityriasis capitis), alopecia, seborrhoea, psoriasis, eczema
Hair defects page 124	Split ends (fragilitis crinium), damaged cuticle, trichorrexis nodosa, monilethrix
Head and face shapes page 126	Oval, round, rectangular, square, heart-shaped
Other important physical features pages 127–128	Hair growth patterns, ears, nose, eyes, etc.

Structure of hair and skin

The hair shaft

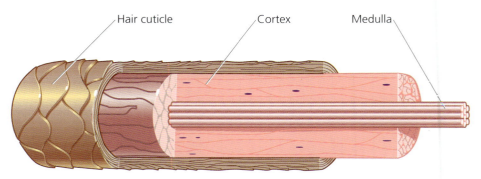

Hair cuticle   Cortex   Medulla

Hair The cross-section taken through the hair lengthways shown in the diagram provides us with a microscopic view of the three specific layers.

Cuticle The cuticle is the outer layer of colourless cells which forms a protective surface to the hair. It regulates the chemicals entering and damaging the hair and protects the hair from excessive heat and drying. The cells overlap like tiles on a roof with the free edges pointing towards the tips of the hair. The amount of layers is proportional to hair texture. Hair with fewer layers of cuticle is finer than coarser hair types which have several layers. Hair in good condition has a cuticle that is tightly closed, limiting the entry of moisture and chemicals. On the other hand, hair that is in a dry or porous condition has damaged or partially missing cuticle layers. One simple indicator of cuticle condition relates to the time taken to blow-dry hair. Hair in good condition will dry quickly in proportion to the amount of hair on the head (density). The closely packed cuticle allows the dryer to chase the water from the hairshaft. **Porous hair** absorbs moisture and therefore takes far longer to dry and is unfortunately subjected to more heat, which exacerbates the problem.

Cortex The cortex is the middle and largest layer. It is made up of a long fibrous material which has the appearance of rope. If looked at more closely, each of the fibres is made up of even smaller chains of fibres. The quality and condition of these bundles of fibres will determine the hair's strength. The way in which they are bonded together has a direct effect upon curl and ability to stretch (hair elasticity). It is within this part of the hair that the natural hair colour and permanent synthetic colour is distributed and perms make the permanent chemical changes.

Medulla The *medulla* is the central, most inner part of the hair. It only exists in medium to coarser hair types and is often intermittent throughout the length. The medulla does not play any useful part in hairdressing processes and treatments.

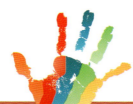

ANATOMY & PHYSIOLOGY
A closed smooth cuticle is the most important sign of healthy hair: hair imparts shine, dries more quickly, is resistant to chemical treatments and holds styles and colours better than hair with a raised/damaged cuticle.

Physical properties of hair

Hair in good condition naturally contains a certain amount of moisture that allows it to stretch and return, giving it elasticity. Hair that is dry and in poor condition is less elastic. Hair is **hygroscopic**: meaning it absorbs water from the surrounding air. How much water is taken up depends on the dryness of the hair and the moistness of the atmosphere. Hair is also **porous**. There are tiny tube-like spaces within the hair structure and the water flows into these by *capillary action*, rather like blotting paper absorbing ink. Drying hair in the ordinary way evaporates only the surface moisture, but drying over long periods or at too high a temperature removes water from within the hair, leaving it brittle and in poor condition. Damaged hair is more porous than healthy hair and easily loses any water, which makes it hard to stretch and mould.

Curled hair returns to its former shape as it takes up water (see alpha and beta keratin, Chapter 8, page 171), so the drier the atmosphere, the longer the curl or set lasts. Similarly, curling dry hair is most effective just after the hair has been washed because, although the surface is dry, the hair will have absorbed water internally. Blow-styling and curling with hot irons, heated rollers, hot combs and hot brushes all have similar temporary effects.

TOP TIP

Hair in good condition has moisture that helps to give it elasticity and shine.

Hair health and condition

So, the moisture levels within the hair are essential for maintaining good condition. We can see the evidence of this moisture from the shine that we associate with great-looking hair. 'Bad hair' denotes poor condition and the lack of shine is due to the unevenness of the hair's surface, i.e. the cuticle. A roughened cuticle surface is an indicator of either physical or chemical damage. Each of these states is difficult to correct. In mild cases of dryness, treatments can be applied to improve the hair's manageability and handling. In more serious situations of porous hair, the hair's ability to resist the ingress of chemicals and moisture is severely impaired. There are no long-lasting remedies for this so regular reconditioning treatments must be used.

So the health and the condition of the hair is your starting point. Whatever happens next should be a process of improving what went on before. A client will expect the service or treatment that you advise to be a step in the right direction. You will need to look for each of the following properties and aspects.

Features of hair in good condition

- Shine and lustre
- Smooth, tightly packed cuticle layers
- Strength and resistance to snapping
- Good ability to stretch and return to the same length (elasticity)
- Good natural moisture levels.

Features of hair in poor condition

- Raised or open cuticle
- Damaged torn hair shaft
- Split ends
- Low strength and resistance
- Over-elastic, too stretchy, snaps easily
- Dry, porous lengths or ends.

Physical hair damage is caused by

- Harsh or incorrect usage of brushes and/or combs
- Excessive heat from styling equipment.

Chemical hair damage is caused by

- Incorrect over-timing of all colouring and perming treatments
- Effects of hydrogen peroxide
- Over-lightening and highlighting services
- Excessive overuse of colouring/tinting products
- Perm products that are too strong or over-processing
- Chlorine from swimming pools.

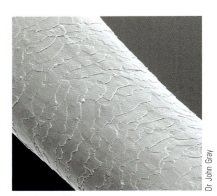

Good condition

Dr John Gray

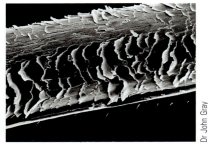

Poor condition

Dr John Gray

Weathering

◆ Hair is also damaged by excesses of ultraviolet radiation found in sunlight.

And generally speaking

◆ The normal and abnormal working of the body has a direct effect on the hair and scalp. Good health is reflected in good hair and skin. A balanced diet with plenty of fresh foods contributes to good health.

◆ Disease and drugs used in the treatment of disease take their toll on the hair and skin.

◆ Genetic factors affecting hair growth determine hair strength and texture.

◆ The hair of women is usually at its best during pregnancy.

◆ Deterioration of the hair and skin after giving birth is usually due to stress and tiredness.

The skin

The skin is the largest organ of the body and if laid flat would cover an area of about 21 square feet. It forms the barrier to a multitude of external forces and is made up of many layers.

The epidermis The **epidermis** is the front line of defence. This outer protective layer of the skin is called the *stratum corneum* and is a hard, cornified layer, consisting of 15 to 40 layers of flattened skin cells or corneocytes, which constantly migrate up from deeper regions and fully replace themselves about once a month. The corneocytes are filled with keratin and a fatty *lipid* that make a barrier to prevent loss of water through the skin.

TOP TIP

It is far easier to keep good-conditioned hair in good condition than it is to try to correct hair in bad condition.

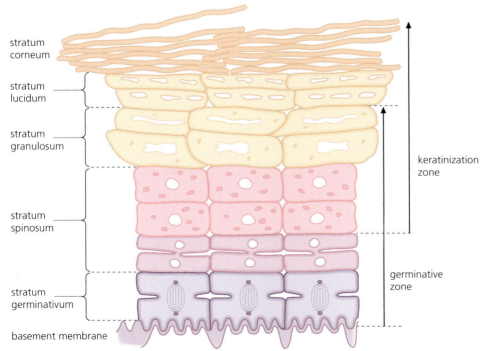

Layers of the epidermis

stratum corneum

stratum lucidum

stratum granulosum

keratinization zone

stratum spinosum

germinative zone

stratum germinativum

basement membrane

The dermis The **dermis** is the thickest layer of the skin. It is here that the hair follicle is formed. The dermis is made up of elastic and connective tissue and is well supplied with blood and lymph vessels. The skin receives its nutrient supply from this area. The upper part of the dermis, the *papillary layer*, contains the organs of touch, heat and cold, and pain. The lower part of the dermis, the *reticular layer*, forms a looser network of cells.

The subcutaneous fat The subcutaneous fat lies below the dermis. It is also known as the *subcutis*, or occasionally as the *hypodermis*. It is composed of loose cell tissue and contains stores of fat. The base of the hair follicle is situated just above this area, or sometimes in it. Subcutaneous tissue gives roundness to the body and fills the space between the dermis and muscle tissue that may lie below.

The hair follicle Hair grows from a thin, tube-like space in the skin called a hair follicle.

◆ At the bottom of the follicles are areas well supplied with nerves and blood vessels, which nourish the cellular activity. These are called *hair papillae*.

◆ Immediately surrounding each papilla is the *germinal matrix* which consists of actively forming hair cells.

◆ As the new hair cells develop, the lowest part of the hair is shaped into the *hair bulb*.

◆ The cells continue to take shape and form as they push along the follicle until they appear at the skin surface as *hair fibres*.

◆ The cells gradually harden and die. The hair is formed of dead tissue. It retains its elasticity due to its chemical structure and keratin content.

Sebaceous glands The oil gland, or *sebaceous gland*, is situated in the skin and opens out into the upper third of the follicle. Natural oil, i.e. *sebum*, is secreted into the follicle and onto the hair and skin surface.

The hair in the skin

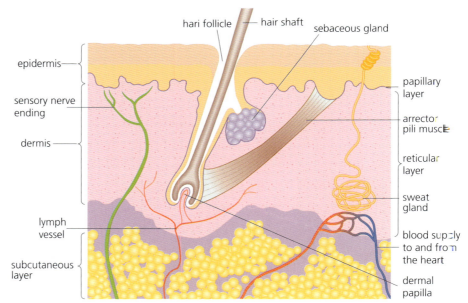

Sebum helps to prevent the skin and hair from drying. By retaining moisture it helps the hair and skin to stay pliable. Sebum is slightly acid – about pH 5.6 – and forms a protective antibacterial covering for the skin.

Sweat glands The sweat gland secretes sweat which passes out through the sweat ducts. The ends of these ducts can be seen at the surface of the skin as sweat *pores*. There are two types of sweat gland: the larger, associated closely with the hair follicles, are the *apocrine glands*; the smaller, found over most of the skin's surface, are the *eccrine glands*.

Sweat is mainly water with salt and other minerals. In abnormal conditions sweat contains larger amounts of waste material. Evaporation of sweat cools the skin. The function of sweat, and thus the sweat glands, is to protect the body by helping to maintain the normal temperature.

The hair muscle The hair muscle, or *arrector pili*, is attached at one end to the hair follicle and at the other to the underlying tissue of the epidermis. When it contracts it pulls the hair and follicle upright. Upright hairs trap a warm layer of air around the skin. The hairs also act as a sensor of touch: for example, you soon notice if an insect crawls over your skin.

Hair growth

Hair is constantly growing. Over a period of between one and six years an individual hair actively grows, then stops, rests, degenerates and finally falls out. Before the hair leaves the follicle, the new hair is normally ready to replace it. (If a hair is not replaced then a tiny, bald area occurs.) The lives of individual hairs vary and are subject to variations in the body. Some are actively growing while others are resting. Hairs on the head are at different stages of growth.

Stages of growth The life cycle of hair is as follows:

◆ *Anagen* is the active growing stage of the hair, a period of activity of the papilla and germinal matrix. This stage may last from a few months to several years. It is at this stage of formation at the base of the follicle that the hair's thickness is determined. Hair colour too is formed in the early part of anagen.

◆ *Catagen* is a period when the hair stops growing and cellular activity decreases at the papilla whilst the follicle shrinks.

◆ *Telogen* is the final stage, when there is no further growth or activity at the papilla. The follicle begins to shrink and completely separates from the papilla area. This resting stage does not last long. Towards the end of the telogen stage, cells begin to activate in preparation for the new anagen stage of regrowth.

The new anagen period involves the hair follicle beginning to grow down again. Vigorous papilla activity generates a new hair at the germinal matrix. At the same time the old hair is slowly making its way up and out of the follicle. Often the old and new hair can be seen at the same time in the follicle.

Stages of hair growth

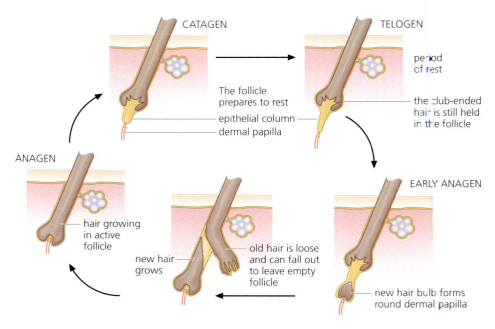

In some animals most of the hairs follow their life cycle in step, passing through anagen, catagen and telogen together. This results in moulting. Human hair, however, develops at an uneven rate and few follicles shed their hair at the same time. (If all hairs fell at the same time we would have bald periods.)

Hair texture

Individual hair thickness is referred to as hair texture and the main types are:

◆ very fine hair

◆ fine hair

◆ medium hair

◆ coarse hair.

The main differences between the hair textures relate to the number of layers of cuticle.

Hair types

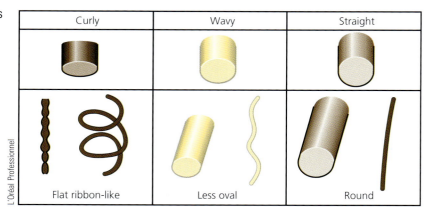

L'Oréal Professionnel

Hair and skin tests

There are a number of tests that you can carry out to help diagnose the condition and likely reaction of your client's skin and hair. These tests will help you to decide what action to take before, during and after the application of hairdressing processes.

You will need to carry out and record all these results in line with your own salon's policy for conducting tests.

Development/strand test A **strand test** or hair strand colour test is used to assess the resultant colour on a strand or section of hair after colour has been processed and developed. It is carried out as follows:

1 Most colouring products just require the time recommended by the manufacturer – check their instructions.

2 Rub a strand of hair lightly with the back of a comb to remove the surplus colour.

3 Check whether the colour remaining is evenly distributed throughout the hair's length. If it is even, remove the rest of the colour. If it is uneven, allow processing to continue, if necessary applying more colour. If any of the hair on the head is not being treated, you can compare the evenness of colour in the coloured hair with that in the uncoloured hair.

Colour test This test is used to assess the suitability of a chosen colour, the amount of processing time required and the final colour result. Apply the colour or lightening products you propose to use to a cutting of the client's hair and process as recommended.

Skin sensitivity test (patch test) The skin test (i.e. patch test) is used to assess the reaction of the skin to chemicals or chemical products. In the salon it is mainly used before colouring. Some people are allergic to external contact with chemicals such as PPD (found in permanent and quasi-permanent hair colour). This can cause dermatitis or, in more severe cases, permanent scarring of skin tissue and hair loss. Some are allergic to irritants reacting internally, causing asthma and hay fever. Others may be allergic to both internal and external irritants. To find out whether a client's skin reacts to chemicals in permanent colours, the following test should be carried out at least 24 hours prior to the chemical process.

1 Select a dark base shade in the colour range you are going to use (darker shades contain more PPD' and will show a skin sensitivity more readily).

2 Clean an area of skin about 8mm square behind the ear (or in the fold of the arm).

3 Apply a little of the colour (without hydrogen peroxide) to skin and do not cover.

4 Ask your client to report any discomfort or irritation that occurs over the next 24–48 hours. Arrange to see your client at the end of this time so that you can check for signs of reaction.

5 If there is a *positive response*, i.e. a skin reaction such as inflammation, soreness, swelling, irritation or discomfort, do not carry out the intended service. Never ignore the result of a skin test. If a skin test showed a reaction and you carried on anyway, there might be a more serious reaction which could affect the whole body.

BEST PRACTICE

Tests are a vital part of general hairdressing services. If they are missed or ignored you and the salon run the risk of a potential disaster.

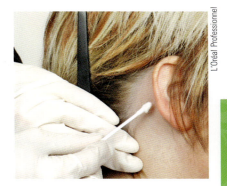

Sensitivity test

L'Oréal Professionnel

HEALTH & SAFETY

Skin testing is not just for new clients, it has now been found that clients can develop sensitivity to chemicals through prolonged use of the same or similar products. Therefore periodic testing for adverse reactions is essential and should be carried out routinely from time to time as recommended by the manufacturer.

6 If there is a *negative response*, i.e. no reaction to the chemicals, then carry out the treatment as proposed.

Warning: In recent years there have been a growing number of successful personal injury claims made against salons where the necessary precautions have not been taken.

TOP TIP

People who have had black henna tattoos are more likely to have a skin sensitivity or reaction to PPD. Ask your client if they have had one.

TOP TIP

Incompatibles (i.e. incompatible chemistry)

Henna is still widely used throughout the world as a hair- and skin-dyeing compound. In the UK people using natural henna will often add other ingredients such as coffee, wine, lemon juice, etc. to intensify the final colour. However, other countries also add compounds to henna; e.g. India and Turkey sometimes add iron ore deposits which are crushed into the powder to increase the 'reddening' effect. If this mixture were to come into contact with hydrogen peroxide (either through colouring or perming), a chemical reaction would take place and in that exchange permanent damage and breakage would occur.

Test cutting In this test a piece of hair is cut from a place on the head where it won't be noticed. The hair can then be processed to check its suitability, the amount of processing required and the timing, before the process is carried out. The test is used for colouring, straightening, **relaxing**, reducing synthetic colouring, i.e. decolouring, lightening and incompatibility.

TOP TIP

Sensitivity and PPD

This test is used to assess the client's tolerance of chemicals introduced to the skin – PPD. The abbreviation stands for **paraphenylenediamine**, the main ingredient within permanent colour that is a known irritant to skin and eyes and can cause an allergic reaction.

ACTIVITY

Incompatibility test

To do this you will need the following materials:

1. ammonium hydroxide (1 part) or ammonium thioglycolate
2. hydrogen peroxide 6%/20 vol (20 parts)
3. glass bowl
4. a small piece of hair treated with a product containing metallic salts
5. a small piece of untreated hair (cut from a friend or colleague).

Record your findings – what happened when the different hair samples were immersed in the solutions? What did you see?
For:

1. treated hair
2. untreated hair

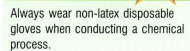

BEST PRACTICE

Always wear non-latex disposable gloves when conducting a chemical process.

Test curl This test is made on the hair to determine the lotion suitability, the strength, the curler size, the timing of processing and the development. It is used before perming.

Curl check or test This test is used to assess the development of curl in the perming process. The test is used periodically throughout a perm and for final assessment of the result.

Peroxide test This test is made on hair that has been decoloured or stripped of its synthetic colour. The test is used to assess the effectiveness of the process and to check that no synthetic pigment remains. Any synthetic colour remaining will oxidize later and darken again within two or three days. If the hair darkens after testing, remove all the chemicals from the test section, then reapply the decolourant. It may take several applications to strip all of the unwanted colour.

Incompatibility test Perm lotions and other chemicals applied to the hair may react with chemicals that have already been used, such as home-use products. The incompatibility test is therefore used to detect chemicals/elements which could react with hairdressing processes such as colouring and perming. The test is carried out as follows:

1 Protect your hands by wearing gloves.

2 Place a small cutting of hair in a small dish.

3 Pour into the dish a mixture of 20 parts of 6 per cent hydrogen peroxide and one part ammonium thioglycolate (general purpose perm solution). Make sure that you are not bending over the dish to avoid splashing the chemicals on to your face or inhaling any resultant released fumes.

4 Watch for signs of bubbling, heating or discolouration. These indicate that the hair already contains incompatible chemicals. The hair should not be permed, coloured or lightened if there are any signs of reaction. Perming treatment might discolour or break the hair and could burn the skin.

Pull test A pull test helps to evaluate excessive and/or abnormal scalp hair loss. It is particularly relevant to the attachment of hair pieces and hair extension services.

To conduct a pull test:

1 Gently pull small sections of hair whilst sliding the fingers from root to point on at least three areas of the scalp.

2 If more than 12 hairs per hand are shed, this could indicate an abnormal hair loss.

3 This is a **contra-indication** and the attachment service should not be provided.

Tensile strength test A test to determine the breaking point of hair. This test is carried out in a similar way to an elasticity test, although the strength of the internal structure of the hair is tested to breaking point.

TOP TIP

Hair that doesn't stretch has little or no level of natural moisture. The hair will not respond to chemical processing or styling in the same way that hair does with adequate levels of moisture.

TOP TIP

Natural moisture levels

The natural moisture levels in hair play a significant part in the way that hair responds to treatments and styling. If the natural levels can be retained following perming, colouring and lightening the client's hair will remain manageable, easier to detangle and able to hold thermal styling effects for far longer.

Deplete those natural levels and the hair becomes porous and will tangle easily, is less manageable and not able to hold a set for long. Pre-chemical treatments help to reduce the hair's moisture reduction.

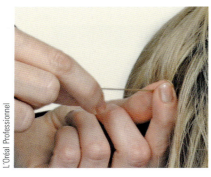

Tensile strength test

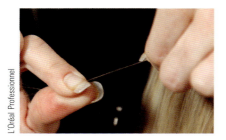

Elasticity test

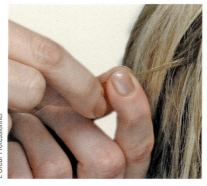

Porosity test

Elasticity test This test is carried out on a dry single hair and used to determine how much the hair will stretch and then return to its original position. It is an indicator of the internal condition of the hair's bonded structure and ability to retain moisture. By taking a hair between the fingers and stretching it you can assess the amount of spring it has. If the hair breaks easily, care needs to be taken before applying any hairdressing process and further tests are indicated – a test curl or a test cutting, for example. Natural healthy hair in good condition will be elastic and more likely to retain the effects of physical curling, setting or blow-shaping longer. It will also take chemical processes more readily. Hair with little elasticity will not hold physical shaping or chemical processes satisfactorily.

Porosity test The porosity test is used to assess the ability of the hair to absorb moisture or liquids – another indicator of condition. If the cuticle has lifted or is torn or broken, it will soon lose its moisture and become dry. It may be able to absorb liquids quicker, but its ability to retain them is reduced. If the cuticle is smooth, unbroken and tightly packed, it may resist the passage of moisture or liquids. By running the fingertips through the hair, from the **point ends back to the roots**, you can assess the degree of roughness. The rougher the hair, the more porous it will be and the faster it will absorb chemicals.

Hair and scalp diseases, conditions and defects (contra-indications)

Diseases of the hair and scalp may be caused by a variety of infectious organisms and particular tell-tale signs or symptoms enable us to identify them. An initial examination should be carried out before any hairdressing process occurs, so that any adverse conditions can be identified. If this is not done a variety of serious outcomes can occur. However, not all hair and scalp conditions are dangerous; some non-infectious conditions can easily be addressed within the salon.

ACTIVITY

Parts of the skin

The skin is the outer covering of the body. It is a complex organ, made up of different layers and contains many parts: oil (sebaceous) and sweat glands, hair muscles, blood and nerves. Complete the table below by explaining what these parts of the skin are and what they do.

Parts of the skin	Explain what this is and what it does
Epidermis	
Dermis	
Hair follicle	
Sebaceous gland	

Infectious (contagious) diseases

Bacterial diseases				
Condition	Symptoms	Cause	Treatment	Infectious
Folliculitis Inflammation of the hair follicles.	Inflamed follicles, a common symptom of certain skin diseases.	A contact bacterial infection, or due to chemical or physical action.	Medical referral to GP	Yes
Impetigo A bacterial infection of the upper skin layers.	At first a burning sensation, followed by spots becoming dry; honey-coloured, crusts form and spread.	A staphylococcal or streptococcal infection.	Medical referral to GP	Yes
Sycosis A bacterial infection of the hairy parts of the face.	Small, yellow spots around the follicle mouth, burning, irritation and general inflammation.	Bacteria attack the upper part of the hair follicle, spreading to the lower follicle.	Medical referral to GP	Yes
Furunculosis Boils or abscesses.	Raised, inflamed, pus-filled spots, irritation, swelling and pain.	An infection of the hair follicles by staphylococcal bacteria.	Medical referral to GP	Yes

Courtesy of Mediscan
Courtesy of Mediscan
Prof. Andrew Wright, Dermatologist Bradford
Prof. Andrew Wright, Dermatologist Bradford

Viral (contagious) diseases

	Condition	Symptoms	Cause	Treatment	Infectious
Courtesy of Mediscan	**Herpes simplex** (cold sore) A viral infection of the skin.	Burning, irritation, swelling and inflammation precede the appearance of fluid-filled blisters, usually on the lips and surrounding areas.	Possibly exposure to extreme heat or cold, or a reaction to food or drugs; the skin may carry the virus for years without exhibiting any symptoms.	Medical referral to pharmacist	Yes
Courtesy of Mediscan	**Warts** A viral infection of the skin.	Raised, roughened skin, often brown or discoloured. There may be irritation and soreness. Warts are common on the hands and face.	The lower epidermis is attacked by the virus, which causes the skin to harden and skin cells to multiply.	Medical referral to pharmacist	Yes

Animal parasite (contagious) infestations

	Condition	Symptoms	Cause	Treatment	Infectious
Courtesy of Mediscan	**Head lice (pediculosis capitis)** Infestation of the hair and scalp by head lice.	An itchy reaction to the biting head louse, 'peppering' on pillow-cases and minute egg cases (nits) attached to the hair shaft close to the scalp.	The head louse bites the scalp feeding on the victim's blood. Breeding produces eggs, which are laid and cemented in incubation until the immature louse emerges.	Referral to a pharmacist	Yes
Courtesy of Mediscan	**Scabies** An allergic reaction to the itch mite.	A rash in the skin folds around the midriff and on the inside of the thighs, extremely itchy at night.	The itch mite burrows under the skin where it lays eggs.	Medical referral to GP	Yes

Fungal (contagious) diseases

	Condition	Symptoms	Cause	Treatment	Infectious
 Dr John Gray	**Ringworm (Tinea Capitis)** of the head.	Circular bald patch of grey or whitish skin surrounded by red, active rings; hairs broken close to the skin, which looks dull and rough. The fungus lives off the keratin in the skin and hair. This disease is common in children.	Fungal infection of the skin or hair.	Medical referral	*Yes*

Non-infectious (non-contagious) diseases

Conditions of the hair and skin

	Condition	Symptoms	Cause	Treatment	Infectious
 Courtesy of Mediscan	**Acne** Disorder affecting the hair follicles and sebaceous glands.	Raised spots and bumps within the skin, commonly upon the face in adolescents.	Increased sebum and other secretions block the follicle and a skin reaction occurs.	Medical referral to GP	No
 Contains public sector information published by the Health and Safety Executive and licensed under the Open Government Licence v1.0	**Eczema and dermatitis** In its simplest form a reddening of the skin.	Ranging from slightly inflamed areas of the skin to severe splitting and weeping areas with irritation and soreness.	Many possible causes, eczema often associated with internal factors, i.e. allergies or stress. Dermatitis a reaction or allergy to external factors	Medical referral to GP	No
 iStock © Ken Roberts	**Psoriasis** An inflamed, abnormal thickening of the skin.	Areas of thickened skin, often raised and patchy. Often on the scalp and also at the joints (arms and legs).	Unknown	Medical referral to GP	No

Conditions of the hair and skin

	Condition	Symptoms	Cause	Treatment	Infectious
 Courtesy of Mediscan	**Dandruff (Pityriasis capitis)**	Dry, small, irritating flakes.	Fungal (yeast-like) infection, or physical or chemical irritants.	Anti-dandruff treatments	No
 Courtesy of Mediscan	**Seborrhea**	Very greasy, lank hair and greasy skin, making styling difficult.	Over-production of sebum.	Astringent shampoos	No

Alopecia (hair loss)

	Condition	Cause			Infectious
 Prof. Andrew Wright, Dermatologist, Bradford	**Alopecia areata**	The name given to balding patches over the scalp. Often starts around or above the ears, circular in pattern ranging from 1–2.5cm in diameter.			Trichological referral
 Courtesy of Mediscan	**Traction alopecia**	Hair loss as a result of excessive pulling at the roots from brushing, curling and straightening. Very often seen with younger girls tying, plaiting or braiding long hair.			None

Alopecia (hair loss)			
Courtesy of Mediscan	**Alopecia totalis**	Complete hair loss sometimes as a result of alopecia areata spreading and joining up across the scalp.	Trichological referral
Courtesy of Mediscan	**Cicatrical alopecia**	Baldness due to scarring of the skin arising from chemical or physical injury. The hair follicle is damaged and permanent baldness results.	
Courtesy of Mediscan	**Male pattern alopecia**	Premature male pattern baldness occurs in teens or early 20s. Senile pattern baldness occurs in late 30s–50s. Hair recedes at the hairline or loss at the crown area. Condition is hereditary (passed on in families).	Remedies currently being developed

Defects of the hair

Defects of the hair			
	Condition	**Symptom**	**Cause**	**Treatment**
Dr John Gray	**Split ends (Fragilitis crinium)** Fragile, poorly conditioned hair	Dry, splitting hair ends	Harsh physical or chemical treatments	Cutting off or special treatment conditioners

Defects of the hair

	Condition	Symptom	Cause	Treatment
 Redken	**Monilethrix Beaded hair**	Beadlike swellings along the hair shaft, hair often breaks at weaker points.	Irregular development of the hair forming during cellular production.	None
 Dr John Gray	**Trichorrexis nodosa** Nodules forming on the hair shaft	Areas of swelling at locations along the hair shaft, splitting and rupturing the cuticle layer.	Harsh physical or chemical processing.	None, although cutting and conditioning may help.
 Courtesy of Mediscan	**Sebaceous cyst** Swelling of the oil gland	Bumps, lumps and swellings on the scalp containing fluid, soft to the touch.	Sebaceous gland becomes blocked allowing a build-up of fluid to take place.	Medical referral
 Liz Hirst, Wellcome Images	**Damaged cuticle** Broken, split, torn hair	Rough, raised, missing areas of cuticle; hair loses its moisture and becomes dry and porous.	Harsh physical or chemical processes.	None, although cutting and conditioning may help.

ACTIVITY

Match the circles

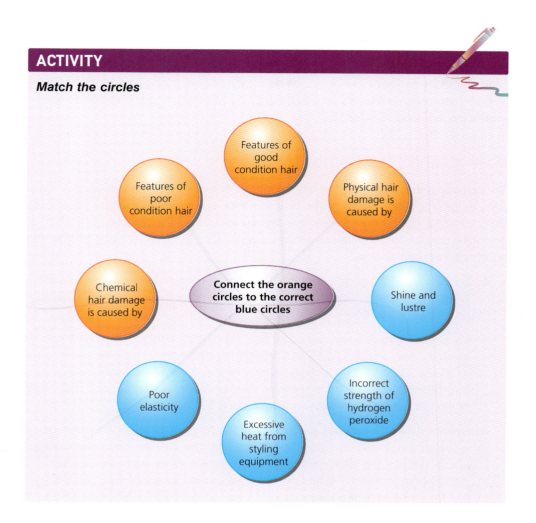

Factors and features that influence styling options

During consultation you will be considering all the aspects of the client's physical features. Is there anything that doesn't work? Is the client happy with the existing style? They may point to areas which you feel are wrong or unnecessary, so you need to be able to express your technical appraisal in a clear, simple way without confusion. Avoid using any technical jargon or trade terms.

Consultation is *customized* for the client. It is personal and individual on each and every occasion. We therefore have to consider technical and personal image aspects:

- ◆ cutting and final shape of the hair
- ◆ volume or colour which will enhance the style
- ◆ finishing options of blow-drying or dressing the hair
- ◆ hair type, hair growth, natural colour and face shape
- ◆ their personal image, lifestyle and personality
- ◆ amount of time they can give to their hair.

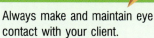

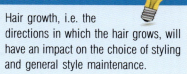
Look for responses to your suggestions The client's facial expression reflects their mood and how they are feeling. You need to pick up on these expressions and react to them appropriately. This will help to understand the client's wants and needs more easily. Expression is an important part of communication; remember, even if your client looks disgruntled or is scowling, you will need to use a friendly, pleasant expression to encourage them to relax.

Hair growth patterns

The hair's movement refers to the amount of curl or wave within the hair lengths. However, its growth pattern denotes the direction from which it protrudes from the scalp. Natural hair fall can be seen on wet and dry hair and strong directional growth will have a major impact on the lie of the hair when it is styled. So it is essential that it is taken into account during consultation.

◆ *Double crown* The client with a double crown will benefit from leaving sufficient length in the hair to over-fall the whole area. If it is cut too short, the hair will stick up and will not lie flat.

◆ *Nape whorl* A nape whorl can occur at either or both sides of the nape. It can make the hair difficult to cut into a straight neckline or tight 'head-hugging' **graduations**. Often the hair naturally forms a V-shape. **Tapered neckline** shapes may be more suitable, but sometimes the hair is best left long so that the weight of the hair over-falls the nape whorl directions.

◆ *Cowlick* A cowlick appears at the hairline at the front of the head. It makes cutting a straight fringe difficult, particularly on fine hair, because the hair often forms a natural parting. The strong movement can often be improved by moving the parting over so that the weight over-falls the growth pattern. Sometimes a fringe can be achieved by leaving the layers longer so that they weigh down the hair.

◆ *Widow's peak* The widow's peak growth pattern appears at the centre of the front hairline. The hair grows upward and forward, forming a strong peak. It is often better to cut the hair into styles that are dressed back from the face, as any 'light fringes' will be likely to separate and stick up.

Face and head shapes The shape and contours of the head are formed by the parietal and temporal bones. The back of the head and nape are formed by the occipital bones, which can be concave or convex: (curving inwards or outwards.) The frontal bone forms the shape of the forehead.

The face shape is made up of straight or curved lines, and sometimes a mixture of the two. Straight, fine shapes appear angular and chiselled or firm and solid. They can be triangular, rectangular, square or diamond-shaped. Curved line shapes appear soft and may be round, oval, pear-shaped or oblong. Shapes which have some straight and some curved lines are defined as heart shaped or soft square shaped.

To create a pleasant balance, the hairstyle and face shape need to be compatible. Generally speaking, an angular haircut will not suit a soft, rounded face. A soft hair shape will not complement a chiselled face. Hair shape **outlines** can be made to look quite different from the front by simply changing a parting from side to centre. Side partings tend to make the face appear wider, whilst centre partings close down the width of a wide forehead.

An oval face shape suits any hairstyle. Round faces need height to reduce the width of the face. A centre parting can also help to reduce width. Long facial proportions are improved with short, wider hairstyles. Square-shaped faces need round shapes with texture on to the face to soften them. Longer lengths beyond the jawline improve the balance and proportion.

Ears, nose and mouth Often ears are out of balance, which can affect the cut if you use them as a guide. Generally, large ears or even large lobes are accentuated by hair cut short or dressed away from the face. It is often better to leave hair longer over the ears unless it is an essential part of the style's impact.

Your client may wear a hearing aid and this may be a sensitive issue. Some clients wish to have all signs of an aid hidden, but others do not mind and even display it. You should discuss this with your client carefully and with sensitivity; they may feel too embarrassed to bring up the subject themself. The size of the aid will need careful consideration when completing the total image.

The position, shape, size and colour of the nose and mouth are very important in the facial expression. The angles that are created can be softening or harsh and must not be ignored when the image is being planned. Hair shape and make-up can contribute to create the required effect.

TOP TIP

The eyes are the focal point of the face. Use them within the style's construction.

What colour and shape are your client's eyes?

What are the eyebrows like?

Does your client normally wear spectacles?

TOP TIP

Checklist

◆ What are the shape, position and size of the client's ears?
◆ What is the shape and size of the client's nose and mouth?
◆ Are these features a major concern to your client?
◆ What is your client's facial and head shape?
◆ Are there any significant features that need to be accounted for?
◆ Small faces need 'opening up' while larger faces need narrower framing effects.

TOP TIP

The eyes are the focal point of the face. Good images in magazines use this aspect to sell everything from clothes to hairdressing. Your client will be drawn to strong images, but are they wearable in everyday life? The majority of 'hair shots' use hair in ways across the eye line to create artistic impact. These may be stimulating but not feasible. You must make a point of this during your consultation.

TOP TIP

Head shapes can have a major impact on the final profile of the style you are attempting to create. For example, a flatter crown or back of the head is made more noticeable when a contoured, layered cut is selected as the chosen hairstyle.

TOP TIP

Make-up

How much make-up is your client wearing?

What image are they trying to portray: natural, classic and businesslike, dramatic or romantic?

ACTIVITY

Hair growth patterns

Hair growth patterns do have an impact on the way that hair can be styled. For each of the listed growth patterns below, write down in what ways this will influence your styling options.

Widow's peak
Nape whorl
Double crown
Cowlick

TOP TIP

Have you taken the length and width of the client's neck into consideration?

Neck and shoulders The length, fullness and width of the neck will affect the fall of the back and nape hair. Longer necks allow better positioning of long hair. They are complemented by high, neat lines; for example, mandarin collars or polo-neck tops. Short necks need to be uncluttered, with short hair and low collars. Long and thin necks are more noticeable with short styles and will therefore be better suited to longer hair around them. Shorter necks can be counterbalanced with height or upswept hairstyles.

Body shape and proportions The body shape also needs to be considered. You need to carefully balance the amount, density and overall shape of the hair to your client's physical body shape. This is particularly important if your client considers their shape or size a particularly important factor. For example, a small, clinging hairstyle would look wrong on a large body shape.

Lifestyle, personality and age

Remember that people are restricted by what they do for a living or what they like to do in their spare time. Usually, people who work in environments where they have face to-face contact with clients have to be more particular about the image they portray. This is a very important factor in style selection.

From a leisure point of view, you should find out whether the client does a lot of sport or exercise. If so, the hairstyle will have to be versatile and able to withstand a lot of washing and possibly heat styling. Also, think about how the style could be handled to create a number of different effects when the client is going out. If you are styling for a special occasion, it is worth asking what dress will be worn. A beautiful gown needs to be accompanied by an elegant hairstyle. However, this style will need to be altered for normal wear.

- Many clients want practical and manageable styles for work.

- Nurses, doctors and caterers, among others, may require styles which keep the hair off the face, or they may have to wear face and head coverings at work.

- Dancers and sporty people need hairstyles which will not get in their eyes and obscure their vision.

- Fashion models may require elaborate styles for special photographic or modelling sessions or displays.

Character and personality can often override physical features when you are choosing a style for your client. A self-confident client will be able to wear looks that a self-conscious client cannot. Make sure you take this into account so that mistakes are not made. Is your client confident and outgoing, or shy, timid and retiring, not wishing to stand out in a crowd? Are they professional and businesslike?

And what age group does your client fall in to? There are basic rules that apply to people at certain ages:

- *Children* – simple, practical shapes (although parents often try to suggest fashions).

- *Teenager* – fashionable, trendy and willing to try new things.

- *Young married* – something suitable for work, attractive easier to maintain styles.

- *Parents* – practical and attractive styles, often shorter styles.

- *Middle-aged* – softening shapes to disguise wrinkles.

- *Older women* – softening shapes.

- *Business people* – fashionable cuts.

- *Older men* – simple, practical styles.

These are only general guides – there will always be exceptions to the rules.

Advising clients and agreeing services and products

Being able to recommend services and products to clients relies upon having a good working knowledge of what your salon provides. This range of services and products changes from time to time and you will need to keep abreast of those changes.

You will need to know:

- the ranges of services and products that are suitable for your clients' needs

- the prices and timings of those services and prices of the products available

- how to keep abreast of current fashions.

Making suitable suggestions and recommendations

Suitability relies upon matching the client's needs with the correct selection of services and products that your salon offers. We are all familiar with the salons that make a name for themselves by turning people out looking all the same. Similarly, there are other salons that have a seasonal collection of work and really push their clients into wearing the current look, just because they think it's good PR for the salon.

Both of these types of environments may be easy or fun to do from the stylist's point of view, but the client hasn't been considered at any point in the process. So sadly, in these sorts of salons, there is no consultation taking place. They just process people like a *mechanical production line*.

So, from your point of view as a junior stylist it would be unprofessional to recommend a shoulder-length bob to a client who had long hair down their back, just because you were really good at doing classic bobs!

The same goes for recommending products too; you may have a core of favourites that the salon uses and those are really good on your hair. Great, you have a product regimen that works for you. But that's as far as it goes. Your client has individual and particular needs and it is your job to match their needs with the features and benefits of products that your salon provides.

You may also think that the packaging of the new range really looks good and it smells great too. But do these features actually benefit your client?

Most people need products to do a job for them, like sorting out dry and damaged lengths or providing volume and lift. Remember, it's not what it looks like that makes it work; it's what's inside the bottle that really counts.

TOP TIP

Points of consideration to ask the client: How much time will they have available to style their hair?

How easy is it for them to replicate the same effect?

Are products essential for maintaining the look?

How often do they wash and condition their hair?

Always look at people as individuals; match their needs to those products that offer benefits that suit them.

When you do recommend a specific remedy as a course of treatments, don't forget to explain the benefits of prolonged, continual applications as opposed to a 'one-off' treatment. Although people generally want their problems sorted out immediately, this is seldom the case. You need to subtly express the values of continual usage even if the visible signs seem slow to work. A good way of doing this is to make a note on their client records that prompts you to review the results next time. This makes sure that you do a good job in remembering your client's specific needs and also helps to get them to return in the normal reappointed time frame.

Discussing costs and durations for services

You need to be aware of:

◆ the time it will take to provide the discussed service(s)

◆ the cost for the service(s) to the client

◆ any additional costs that could be involved to complete the service

◆ the costs of any products or treatments that could be purchased for home use

◆ any special offers in force at the time.

Most salons have a standard tariff that shows the costs of their services and in most cases the price shown is the price it will be, but that isn't the same in every case. It would be impractical for a salon to try and produce a tariff that covered service costs for every hair type, hair length and hair density! Just think, the price list would be several pages long and it would be so confusing for you to read, let alone the clients

So the standard price list covers the main services for the average range of people. This might extend to pensioners as well as children, but it will definitely cover the average range of men or women in between.

You need to be aware of the time it takes to complete a task for any service across the range and a good idea of what that will cost. Your clients have a right to know what they are spending before they commit to having the service or product.

Are there any hidden costs? Clients don't like unpleasant surprises. If your salon does have additional costs that aren't clearly displayed you would be better off stating them from the outset. For example, if you offer a client a coffee they might think that it is complimentary. Similarly, if you say that you are going to put a new treatment on their hair while they are at the basin, will there be an additional cost for that?

Retail products Most salons offer a comprehensive range of retail services that supplement the services that they offer. Keep up to date with the ranges that your salon offers. If your client shows an interest in the products on display or asks how they can benefit them, you need to be ready to provide those answers without: 'Err, umm, I don't know what that does'.

It will undermine your professionalism and it won't improve the likelihood of making a sale. If you aren't sure about the costs or benefits of a product, say to the client; 'I'll find out for you, let me see if Sally is free'.

Agreeing the course of action

When you have covered everything in your consultation, you need to summarize the points back to the client.

You could say:

> 'So, Mrs Jack, we've talked about the time and cost of your cut and blow-dry. Let me just run through what we are going to do. We will take 'X' off the length of the hair and introduce some layers to give it more texture and movement, then I'll finish it off with a smooth blow-dry look and apply some of that serum I was telling you about. Is that correct?'

Whatever your summary is, you must ask a question at the end of it. Unless you have the client's expressed wishes before you start then you haven't given them the opportunity to accept or decline your plans. In other words they haven't agreed the services or products and they have every right to dispute this at the end!

ACTIVITY

Home-care advice

Good home and aftercare advice is about giving the client the correct advice on looking after their hair.

This will include advice on:

◆ products

◆ tools and equipment

◆ future salon services.

1. What advice should you give regarding products?
2. What advice do you need to provide regarding tools and equipment?
3. What advice could you provide regarding future salon services/treatments?

Special services and situations

Some services also need additional preparation or special conditions before they can be carried out. For example; your salon may do hairpieces for hair-up work; some salons may do added clip-on hair extensions; others may offer the complete bonded extensions systems. In any of these cases it would be unlikely that all the necessary materials to do all of these services will be in stock. So you need to be able to tell your client exactly when those items will be available, the differences, benefits and pitfalls, how long it will take, how they will look after them and how much it will cost.

You will also need to check to see if a deposit is needed. Often in situations where there is a large investment of salon time or stylist's time, then other preparations need to be arranged in advance and it would be normal practice to take a deposit.

There are other special situations too. You may wish to offer a colouring service to a new client, but you know that you will have to conduct your skin test first. So you will need to tell the client what they can expect and also what you need to know should there be any adverse contra-indications. All this needs to be pointed out well in advance.

Keeping abreast of current fashions

Your knowledge should be up-to-date and there are numerous ways in which you can do this:

- ◆ trade shows and exhibitions
- ◆ courses and seminars
- ◆ trade magazines
- ◆ fashion magazines
- ◆ TV and the Internet.

You should keep in touch with what's happening in the celebrity world. These well-known icons create fashion; they are prepared and groomed by personal stylists who are employed by production and promotional companies so that they are always in the eye of the public. People are stimulated by the entertainment industries and the media are always following the lives of celebrities from film, TV and music. The success of magazines such as *OK* and *Hello* is due to the attention they pay to these peoples' lives and what they are up to.

Your customers will expect you to be aware of what is happening in these sectors and you will need to be ready to advise whether these new looks are going to suit them. In many cases they will not and you have to be ready to provide alternatives. You may have to consider many other alternatives, but try to incorporate something from the theme. If the main impact of the style that your client wants requires a fringe, but you feel that by taking the bob-line short to the chin is going to make their face appear too 'podgy', what about incorporating the fringe into a longer version of the look?

As you can see, there is always another way of tackling the problems. When you can't provide what the client wants, always offer suitable alternatives.

Referrals (see adverse hair and scalp conditions)

There will be situations where the client's anticipated service cannot be provided.

This could be due to:

- ◆ adverse hair and skin problems
- ◆ your salon doesn't do that particular service or treatment.

Specialist remedial referral
Some hair and scalp conditions can be treated in the salon, but many more will require specialist remedial attention. You need to know which ones are handled by the various specialists.

For example, a mother who brings a child in for a haircut who obviously has nits cannot be dealt with in the salon. You need to be sympathetic and not over-reactive. If you suspect an infestation has occurred, *go and find* a senior member of staff. They will help you to explain the benefits to the mother of looking out for infestations on a regular basis and the signs that she would probably see, i.e. small whiteish/grey nodules attached to the hair close to the scalp, generally around the back and nape, or evidence of the louse itself as a peppering of brown speckles over the child's pillow at night and itching.

BEST PRACTICE

If you are not sure what the problem is and it looks medical, the client will need a referral to a pharmacist or their GP.

For more information on adverse hair and skin conditions see page 118–124.

But that is as far as your comments should go. Your supervisor or senior stylist will need to refer them to a pharmacist so that the mother can purchase a remedy to apply herself at home.

A client with eczema may be aware of their condition, but you may be concerned that a planned service may aggravate the condition further. A referral to their doctor first is preferable, if only to eliminate the concern that your planned service won't make the condition worse.

If you find a condition that you are not sure about, get your senior stylist or supervisor to intervene. They will probably say to the client, 'I'm not sure what the problem is but I do think you should get it checked out before we continue our planned services'.

ACTIVITY

Contra-indications

What would you do and say if:

1. A client was found to be infected with head lice?

2. A client had cuts or abrasions on their scalp?

3. A client wanted a service that you felt because of their condition, should not be carried out?

4. During the consultation you suspected that metallic salts were present within the hair and the client wanted to have a chemical process?

TOP TIP

If you need to refer clients to a **trichologist**, you can find a listing through the trichological institute on the Internet at **www.trichologists.org.uk**.

Salon referrals

You need to keep abreast of the salons in your area that offer special services that your salon doesn't, services such as trichological analysis, hair extensions, hair transplants, wigs and hairpieces. But remember with referrals you must follow your salon's policy for external redirection. You may not be permitted to do this yourself; speak to a senior or supervisor before you say anything to the client.

ACTIVITY

With a work colleague pretend that you have a selection of clients waiting to pay their bill at reception. Taking turns now calculate a variety of bill totals for a range of your salon's services, treatments and products.

Keep notes on the services etc. that each of you have stated to one another, so that you can check each other's ability to add up the imaginary clients' bills.

For more information see *Data Protection Act (1998)* in Appendix 1.

For more information about client confidentiality see Chapter 4, unit G4 Reception Page 60

Client records

Keeping proper client records is essential for good salon management and to ensure clients receive a service appropriate for their individual needs. The records also give vital information should there be any subsequent client complaint, or worse, if there were any pursuance in a legal case against the salon.

Different salons use different systems for recording information. Some salons use hand-written cards whereas others use computerized systems. The information required will change from salon to salon.

Remember this is personal and private information, it must be handled confidentially and you have a duty to uphold the rights of your clients if you keep their personal information on file.

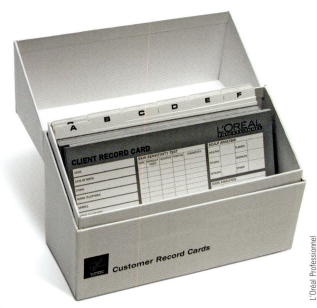

L'Oréal Professionnel

Client record cards

BEST PRACTICE

Make sure that records are found prior to consultation and used to check on previous client history. Update the records in line with your actions taken after consultation.

TOP TIP

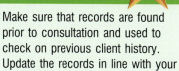

If you don't tell the client how to maintain their hair after the salon visit, how do you expect them to achieve a similar result at home?

BEST PRACTICE

Consultation checklist

✓ Listen carefully to what the client wants
✓ Use visual aids to assist the consultation process
✓ Tell the client possible effects or pitfalls
✓ Give good reasons for your suggestions
✓ Ensure that the client understands what is being said
✓ Agree on a final and suitable course of action
✓ Make it clear if follow-up appointments are necessary
✓ Carry out the agreed service or treatment
✓ Encourage the client to re-book the next visit before they leave
✓ Record the details for future reference.

SUMMARY

Remember to:

✓ listen to the client's requirements and discuss suitable courses of action

✓ follow the safety factors when working on clients' hair

✓ use positive body language and the reasons why it plays such an important part in good customer service

✓ identify the factors that affect the variety of choices available to the client

✓ promote the range of services, products and treatments with the salon

✓ recognize the adverse conditions that prevent salon services

✓ conduct the tests that are needed and avoid the risks of not taking appropriate action

✓ record the outcomes of the tests for future purposes.

Knowledge Check

For this project you will need to gather information from a variety of sources. List the services, treatments and products that are available in your salon. Then for each one listed explain:

1 what the features and benefits are to the client

2 how you would go about explaining these to clients

3 the costs of each of these.

ASSESSMENT OF KNOWLEDGE AND UNDERSTANDING

A selection of different types of questions to check your consultation and advice knowledge.

Q1	The three stages of hair growth are anagen, _____ and telogen.	Fill in the blank
Q2	The cortex is the outermost layer of the hair.	True or false
Q3	Which of the following are infectious diseases? (select all that apply)	Multi selection

Impetigo	☐ 1
Scalp ringworm	☐ 2
Alopecia	☐ 3
Head lice	☐ 4
Psoriasis	☐ 5
Eczema	☐ 6

Q4	The natural colour of hair depends on the amount of melanin within it.	True or false

Q5   Which of the following is commonly known as split ends?   Multi choice

Trichorrhexis nodosa   O a

Monilethrix   O b

Tinea capitis   O c

Fragilitas crinium   O d

Q6   Dandruff is a condition of the scalp usually caused by fungal infection.   True or false

Q7   Which of the following tests are carried out *during* technical services?   Multi selection

Skin test   ☐ 1

Strand test   ☐ 2

Development test curl   ☐ 3

Incompatibility test   ☐ 4

Porosity test   ☐ 5

Test cutting   ☐ 6

Q8   The layer of the skin below the epidermis is called the _____.   Fill in the blank

Q9   Which face shape suits most hairstyles and lengths?   Multi choice

Square   O a

Oblong   O b

Oval   O c

Triangular   O d

Q10   During consultation and hair analysis, a contra-indication will not allow the planned service to be carried out.   True or false

7 Shampooing and conditioning hair

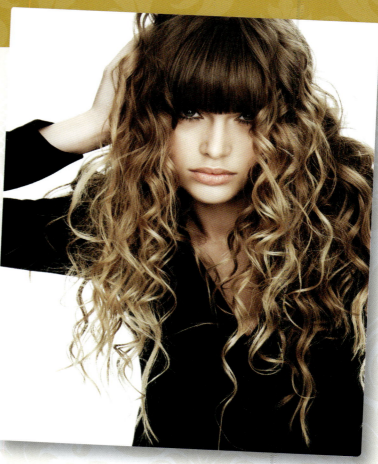

LEARNING OBJECTIVES

◆ Be able to maintain effective and safe methods of working when providing the services

◆ Be able to shampoo the hair and scalp

◆ Be able to condition and treat the hair and scalp

◆ Know how to work safely, effectively and hygienically when providing the services

◆ Understand the basic science for shampooing and conditioning

◆ Know the products and equipment that the salon uses

◆ Know how and when to use a variety of massage techniques for shampooing and conditioning

KEY TERMS

anti-oxidant
dermatitis
detergent
dry hair
effleurage
friction
hydrophilic
hydrophobic
manufacturer's instructions

oily scalp
penetrating conditioners
perm solutions
personal protective equipment
pH balance
plastic apron
polyvinyl or nitrile disposable
   gloves
pre-perm treatments

restructurants
rotary massage
salon services
steamer
surface conditioners
surface tension

Unit title

GH8 Shampoo, condition and treat the hair and scalp

Information covered in this chapter

- Different types of products and how they work
- A range of hair types and conditions
- How to work safely, effectively and efficiently
- How shampoos work and how pH values affect hair
- How shampooing, conditioning and treatments are carried out
- The massage techniques involved in shampooing and conditioning

INTRODUCTION

The shampooing and conditioning service forms part of most hairdressing processes and when they are done properly the service provides an invigorating and stimulating experience for the client.

The action of shampooing cleans the hair by removing dirt, grease, skin scale, sweat and product build-up, leaving the hair ready for blow-drying, setting or perming. Conditioning treatments are applied to smooth the cuticle layer, provide protection for the hair, improve handling and combing, make the hair look healthier and help the hair to resist external elements.

Maintain effective and safe methods of working when shampooing, conditioning and treating the hair and scalp

This part of the chapter covers the following aspects of the service:

◆ cleaning and maintaining the shampoo/conditioning area

◆ preparation and protection of both you and the client

◆ working efficiently, safely and effectively

◆ recognizing different hair and scalp requirements

◆ maintaining records.

Cleaning and maintaining the shampoo and conditioning area

Your health and safety and that of the client are vitally important. Because of this you should make sure that you always follow the manufacturer's instructions when handling any chemicals or equipment. Shampoos and conditioners are chemicals and therefore you must wear adequate protection to reduce risks from skin conditions such as **dermatitis**. Always wear the **personal protective equipment** (PPE) provided by the salon such as, **polyvinyl or nitrile disposable gloves** and a **plastic apron**.

Because of the risks to health and safety, the wash-point area must be kept clean and tidy at all times and all items of waste should be removed and disposed of in a covered bin. Always use the cleaning materials provided by the salon to clean the wash-point areas, this will ensure that only hygienic sprays etc. are used in areas where there is a risk to public health and prevents infection from spreading.

The basins are in continual use and the clients may be coming and going back to these during different services. For example, a client who is having a cut and blow-dry will have their hair washed at the beginning of the service, whereas a client having a colour will arrive at the basin much later in the process. So, with all these different types of services going on, lots of different situations occur. A client who has had a perm may have all their cotton neck wool removed at the basin; this may be saturated with alkaline chemicals and must be removed safely and properly.

Always keep a check on the levels of wash-point products and materials during use; towels, shampoos and conditioners will eventually run out and these will need replenishing at different times throughout the day.

Preparation and protection for you and the client

The client's clothes must be protected from spills and splashes at all times whilst they are in the salon with a clean, freshly laundered gown. Similarly, a fresh clean towel is placed around the shoulders and can be fixed with a sectioning clip so that it doesn't slip or fall away during the shampoo/conditioning process. You should also keep a look out through shampooing and conditioning processes for the position of the towel in relation to the basin and the client's neck. If there isn't enough towel between the basin and neck then water can seep down the client's neck and wet their clothes. On the other hand, too much fabric may initially feel comforting to the client, but will soon get saturated and again the client will feel uncomfortable and their clothes will get wet. In certain situations, you will need to apply a plastic cape on top of the towel as this provides extra protection, particularly for chemical services or special conditioning treatments.

It is very important that after sitting the client at the basin, you make sure that they are comfortable and that their back and neck are fully supported by the position that they are in at the basin. When the client is correctly seated, the basin forms a supportive barrier at the nape of the neck that neither pinches causing discomfort, nor does it allow water to leak over the rim.

Your standing position is equally important from your safety point of view too. You should be standing close enough to the basin to be upright when either in a *side or front wash position* (your arms and shoulders are positioned above the torso and hips without having to twist or lean forwards) or from in a *back wash position* (your arms and shoulders are directly above your hips and feet and slightly behind the position of the client's head when they are laying back). You need to maintain this posture throughout the shampoo or conditioning process otherwise you will be exposing yourself to the risk of injury and longer term back condition or fatigue.

Working efficiently, safely and effectively

During the shampoo process you will be controlling the water pressure to make sure that it is fast enough to rinse the hair properly, but slow enough so that it doesn't spray the client's face at the same time. You will also be keeping a regular check on the water temperature too. Many water systems are affected by other staff drawing water at the same time, as well as other appliances elsewhere in the building, such as washing machines, toilets and sink, all drawing from the same water supply. This can make the water temperature fluctuate at the wash-point very quickly and you need to be sensitive to those changes in temperature so that the client doesn't get burned!

Keep an eye on the clock; you must remember that all wash-point activities are part of a wider hairdressing service, the stylist will need the client back in the styling chair as soon as possible so that they don't overrun and that they don't make the client or stylist late.

Water is essential to all the salon's services and shampooing alone can take five to ten litres for each wash. So it is vitally important that this valuable and expensive resource is not unnecessarily wasted. Always use water sparingly and never leave the taps running between shampoos, even if it is just the cold water!

> **TOP TIP**
>
> Shampooing and conditioning should be a relaxing, enjoyable experience when it is done well; conversely, if it is done badly, it will imply something negative about the other **salon services** that follow.

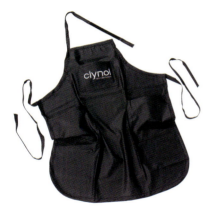
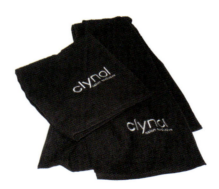

Many hairdressing procedures create potential blockages and for this reason salons are very careful about the materials put down the drain. Beneath each basin is a waste trap. This fitting serves two purposes:

1   it forms a seal that stops vapours and smells coming back from the sewerage system

2   it provides a safeguard for stopping hair and debris from entering into the sewerage system.

In addition, if a client loses an earring during shampooing it can be retrieved by undoing the waste trap. But since this procedure could be difficult and is certainly disruptive during opening hours, some salons now also use plastic hair traps which are inserted from above. These are ideal for stopping any small items from penetrating further below. Make sure that they are regularly cleaned and free of tangled hair. This will keep the drainage clear and stop water backing up in the basin!

Recognizing different hair and scalp requirements

Choosing a shampoo Shampoos come in a variety of forms, including creams, semi-liquids and gels, and a range of different sizes too.

There are many different types of shampoo bases (the substances that form the bulk of the shampoo) and some are kinder and gentler on the skin than others. The balance of these various shampoo ingredients is important; for example, the **detergent** content in shampoos for an **oily scalp** is higher than those for normal and **dry hair**. So too is their ability to deal with different hair types and conditions.

Shampoos are named after the ingredients or essences within them: henna, camomile, rosemary, jojoba, aloe vera and mint are just a few typical varieties available in the supermarkets today. Choosing the right shampoo for the hair condition or following service is important. If the wrong choice is made the hair may become difficult to manage afterwards: it may become brittle, flyaway, static, oily or even dry.

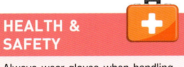

HEALTH & SAFETY

Always wear gloves when handling chemicals. This will reduce the risk of contact dermatitis.

ACTIVITY

See if you can match the shampoos on the right with their appropriate applications on the left. We have done the first one for you.

Moisturizing shampoo	Dandruff
Medicated shampoo	Fine, lank hair
Volumizing shampoo	Dry or porous hair
Colour-protecting shampoo	Coloured or highlighted hair

If the shampoo doesn't remove all of the styling products that have been previously applied, they could block products used as part of the next service that you want to carry out. For example, hair wax that is applied on a daily basis adheres to the hair and creates a product build-up. This must be removed in order to achieve a final satisfactory result.

'Classic' popular shampoo types

Type	Effects on the hair
Aloe vera	A popular, mild natural base ideal for healthy hair and scalps that can be used on a frequent basis
Camomile	Better on oily scalps; has a natural lightening effect
Clarifying	Strong, deep-acting, often used prior to chemical services to remove build-up of styling products and dirt
Coconut	Contains an emollient which helps dry hair to regain its smoothness and elasticity
Jojoba	A natural base better on normal to drier hair types
Lemon	Contains citric acid; ideal for oily scalp types or for removing product build-up
Medicated	Helps to maintain the normal state of the hair and scalp; contains antiseptics such as juniper or tea tree oil
Mint	A natural base suited to normal to slightly oily scalps, often used as a frequent use shampoo
Oil	Can contain a range of natural bases such as pine, palm and almond; these are used to smooth and soften drier hair and scalps
Soya	Helps to lock in moisture for the hair and scalp
Tea tree oil	A natural essential oil, which is like an antiseptic which will fight infections on the scalp

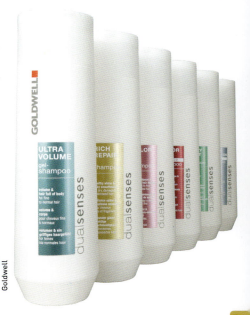

Goldwell

Preparing to shampoo – checklist

✓ Prepare the client with a clean fresh gown and towel.

✓ Look at the client's hair and scalp to find out the condition.

✓ Ask questions such as: 'What products do you use at home?' 'How often do you shampoo your hair?' 'How often do you style your hair?'

✓ Look for any signs of infection, infestation or injury that would stop you from carrying out any other hairdressing processes.

✓ If you recommend any treatments, confirm them with the client before you apply them and advise the client of any additional time and costs involved.

Making the right choices about shampooing

The right choice of shampoo depends on the following factors:

◆ *Type, texture and condition of hair*:

   ◆ *fine hair* (without product build-up) requires a single wash shampoo that will not make it too dry or fluffy. Choose a shampoo that will add body and volume;

◆ *coarse hair* usually requires two washes with a shampoo that will tend to soften it and make it more flexible;

◆ *thicker hair* usually requires two washes with shampoo that will penetrate and make good contact with all the hair and scalp;

◆ *frequency of shampooing* – If hair is washed once or more daily, choose a shampoo specially designed for frequent use;

◆ *water quality* – If the water in the salon is in a hard water area, more shampoo is needed to form a good lather. In soft water areas shampoos foam more easily, so less shampoo is required to do the job.

◆ *shampoo purpose* – Is the shampoo intended just for cleaning or is it to treat the scalp, condition the hair or colour the hair?

◆ *planned services* – What are you going to do with the hair later? Some shampoo ingredients (Pro V or dimethicone) produce a flexible coating on the hair shaft. This could be beneficial in adding protection and locking in moisture or, conversely, in the case of conditioning-type shampoos and most conditioners, it could prevent or prolong the processing of some treatments such as perms.

BEST PRACTICE

Make sure that you match the correct products to the identified hair and scalp conditions. If you use the wrong products you will probably make the condition worse than it is. If in doubt ask a senior or your supervisor.

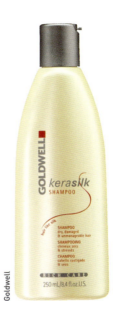

Goldwell

TOP TIP

If oily deposits remain on hair they may cause a barrier to other chemical processes. If you believe that the client's hair has build-up, you can use a clarifying shampoo as a deep cleanser first.

ACTIVITY

Shampooing is a process that can differ between salons: what is the preferred process for shampooing in your salon and how long should it take? Write down your response in the space provided.

1.

2.

3.

4.

If you see something you aren't sure about – seek assistance!

There will be times when you don't recognize a certain hair or scalp condition. In these situations always seek help from a senior stylist or your supervisor. If you suspect a contra-indication that could put the salon at risk from cross-infection or infestation, you need to report it immediately and quietly, and without over reacting, to a senior member of staff.

How do conditioners work?

Conditioners use a combination of chemical and electrical (ionic) properties to achieve their effects. They can balance and counteract the effects that the chemical services and physical processes have upon the hair. There are two ways in which they bond with the hair:

◆ *Absorption* – This relies upon the natural state of the hair. Dry and porous hair has many tiny spaces within the hair's internal structure. These areas suck in the conditioning agents by capillary action, just as water is drawn into a sponge.

◆ *Attraction* – This occurs after the hair has been shampooed. The action of the detergent on the hair during shampooing ensures that all product, dirt and dust are removed. When these particles are removed it leaves the surface of the hair in a 'charged' state. This prepares the hair for the conditioner which is now attracted to the sites upon the hair that have been electrically charged. (This ionic attraction principle can be explained another way. Do you remember how you stick balloons to the wall or ceiling at a birthday party? After blowing the balloons up, you rub them vigorously on the sleeve of your jumper. This removes electrical particles and now makes the balloon stick to anything it comes into contact with, just like a magnet!)

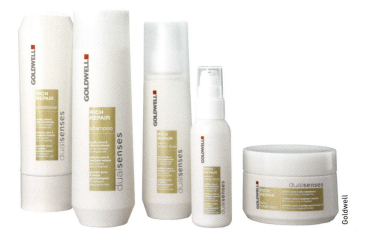

Goldwell

Different types of conditioner

There are three different types of hair conditioners:

◆ surface conditioners

◆ penetrating conditioners

◆ scalp treatments.

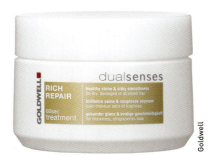

Goldwell

Surface conditioners These conditioners do not enter the hair but remain on the cuticle surface. Their main purpose is to coat the hair and improve the look and feel by adding shine and moisture. Some of these conditioning rinses are used after perms and chemical straighteners to return the hair back to its natural **pH balance**. This group of conditioners would normally contain:

◆ vegetable and mineral oils

◆ lanolin

◆ fats and waxes

◆ mild acid formulations which close the cuticle, could be citric or acetic-based.

Penetrating conditioners Penetrating conditioners have deeper-acting benefits. They enter the hair shaft through the cuticle layer and are deposited into the cortex by capillary action. This suction of the product is like a natural magnetism, drawing the product in to the cellular spaces within the hair. These penetrating conditioners, often called **restructurants**, are designed to temporarily repair the physical structure of the fibres within the cortex and damaged areas within the cuticle layers. Apart from smoothing the hair and adding shine, they tend to make the whole hair structure much stronger. (Examples are hair strengtheners such as L'Oréal's Kerastase Ciment Anti-Usure or Wella's Liquid Hair.)

BEST PRACTICE

A protective conditioner is used before chemical processes to prepare the hair and even out the porosity of the hair before the process is carried out.

BEST PRACTICE

A corrective porosity balancing conditioner is used after chemical processes to replenish moisture and shine or to return the hair back to its natural pH-balanced state.

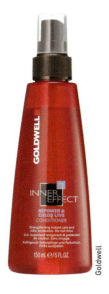

Goldwell

Their composition is more chemically complex. They are based on:

◆ *proteins*, natural vegetable ingredients and amino acids

◆ *humectants*, which lock in moisture to the hair

◆ *emollients*, add flexibility by softening, smoothing and moisturizing the hair

Scalp treatments

Other than improving the look, feel and condition of hair, the final group of conditioners are designed to remedy a variety of skin problems. These scalp-active treatments are chemical preparations that are developed to target specific disorders. Therefore, your correct analysis of the client's scalp condition is essential. You will need to be able to identify and distinguish between:

◆ dry scalp conditions

◆ dandruff problems

◆ excessively oily scalp conditions.

Dry scalps A dry scalp can have some of the symptoms of dandruff, such as flaking on the surface of the epidermis, but if wrongly diagnosed, the corrective treatment may make the problem worse. A dry scalp can occur for a number of reasons.

It may be due to:

◆ a natural moisture imbalance within the client's skin

◆ shampoos or styling products

◆ other chemical services.

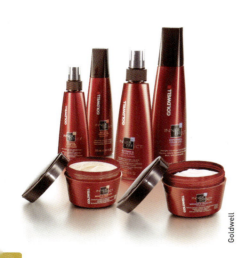

Goldwell

A dry skin condition is often a chronic or long-term problem; you should recommend a scalp-active treatment that will nourish and moisturize the scalp, whilst getting an agreement with the client that this is followed up at home as well. The type of treatment will depend upon the condition of the hair too. If the client has a dry scalp it doesn't necessarily follow that the hair will be dry too. This will have a bearing on how the treatment is to be applied. If the hair is normal and healthy you would not want to overload it with heavy moisturizers and emollients, so a more 'topical', carefully applied solution is required. Your client will also need to learn that not all products are the same. An application that is generally applied and combed through will have little effect! The product must target the problem and therefore the hair will need to be divided and the application should be made directly to the scalp.

Dry scalps can occur from intolerances or sensitivity to hairdressing products. A client can get a reaction when they use something different on their hair. Ask them whether they have tried something new. A typical cause would be newly introduced styling and finishing products such as 'root lift' mousse or heavy definition waxes. However, even a simple change of shampoo can cause dryness.

A dry scalp can also occur after chemical treatments. Many of the solutions we use in hairdressing have a quenching effect upon the skin. Alkaline solutions create this continual drying 'thirst' upon the scalp, so this is particularly relevant to perming and chemical straighteners. However, a reaction can be caused by any exposure to chemicals and you can prevent this by taking particular care when you apply any chemical service to the client.

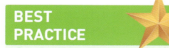

BEST PRACTICE

Always use balancing conditioners after any chemical processes.

Dandruff Dandruff can sometimes in its simplest form be mistaken for a dry scalp. Unfortunately, if you wrongly diagnose this condition, you will either make the problem worse or have no effect at all.

Normally, the skin cells produced in the lower dermis take up to 30–45 days to work up through to the surface of the epidermis. Once there, the cells are shed daily in the form of a fine visible dust. In the case of dandruff, though, this process becomes erratic.

In the diagram you can see that, as the layers of dermal cells work up towards the surface of the epidermis, they eventually 'lift' and come away as 'shedding'. This is commonly noticeable as 'scurf', white skin cells, when you brush or comb the client's hair. More often, it is deposited onto their clothes.

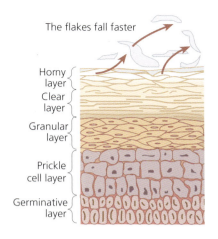

The flakes fall faster

Horny layer
Clear layer
Granular layer
Prickle cell layer
Germinative layer

Dandruff or *Pityriasis capitis* is caused by the overproduction of skin cells. It initially appears as small white flakes that loosen and continually shed from the scalp, rather as is the case with dry skin. A secondary condition occurs if the problem isn't rectified: the scalp becomes infected and larger, yellower, waxy flakes now appear that usually stick to the scalp. When dandruff has progressed this far you often smell it too! This condition is often more prevalent in people with oilier scalps.

In tackling this problem in its earliest stages, you should ask the client if they have or have had a dry skin condition. If they say no, then the scurf is probably due to this skin production imbalance. This can be rectified over a period of time by regular home use of the correct shampoos and conditioners.

If the dandruff has progressed to the second stage, it must be treated initially in the salon, and then with a follow-up at home over a longer period of time. The first objective would be to combat the infection, then to clear the scalp of the scaly build-up. This degree of infection cannot be rectified by one scalp-active application. It will usually involve a course of treatments often in liquid forms applied onto pre-sectioned hair, directly onto the infected areas.

Oily scalps An oily scalp, or 'seborrhoea', is caused by overproduction of natural oil (*sebum*) from the skin. The sebaceous gland in a normal state produces moderate amounts of oil, which is generally sufficient to lubricate the hair shaft and create natural moisture for the skin. This moisture, in turn, keeps the skin supple and helps to 'lock in' flexibility and elasticity. When the glands work overtime, then the imbalance of moisture becomes a nuisance. This is seen as excessively greasy hair and scalps that require frequent washing to give lank hair volume and body.

The normal approach to combating oily scalps is to shampoo it every day. When a client is asked how often they wash their hair and they give the answer 'at least once a day', there is a strong likelihood that there's a reason behind it. Sometimes people wash their hair every day because they fall into the routine of doing it when they take a shower. This is particularly obvious if they have easy-to-manage hairstyles, their lifestyle dictates it or they just have short hair.

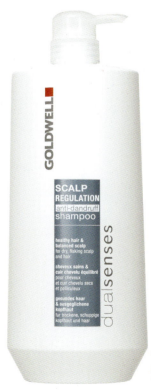

Goldwell

However, when you do notice that the frequency of washing is more than just a habit and a problem exists, then there are a number of medicated preparations that are designed to sort it out.

These astringent-type lotions will cause the skin to contract slightly and this will temporarily constrict the glands and reduce the production of oil. A treatment like this could initially be undertaken in the salon but, to have any long-lasting effect, it will have to be followed up at home.

Before and after chemical services

Where the cuticle has been damaged, the hair cortex becomes more porous, like a sponge soaking up any chemicals applied to the hair. Older hair is more likely to be damaged than newer growth. The porosity must be reduced before hair can be successfully permed or coloured. Pre-straighteners or **pre-perm treatments** will balance the porosity evenly through the hair. This enables the chemical service to be carried out in the confidence that no parts of the hair will be unduly damaged through the action of additional chemical application.

The pre-colouring treatments have a similar effect. These products will 'fill' the damaged sites along the hair shaft, repairing the cuticle layer and maintaining an even absorption, i.e. 'take-up', of colouring products into the cortex.

After chemical services the hair may need re-balancing. The normal state of hair is slightly acidic (pH 5.5) and many of the processes use caustic (ammonium-based) or corrosive (acid-based) compounds. In these situations it is always advisable to use an *acid-balancing conditioner*. Acid-balancing conditioners will act either as an **anti-oxidant** (to remove unwanted 'free oxygen', which may be left in the hair after using hydrogen peroxide in operations such as neutralizing, colouring and lightening) or to reduce the alkaline state of hair with mild acidic compounds following perming and straightening.

ACTIVITY

Answer the following questions in the space provided:

Q1 What types of products are available in your salon?

Q2 What shampoo would you use for dry or porous hair in the salon?

Q3 What shampoo would you use for fine or lank hair in the salon?

Q4 What shampoo would you use for an oily scalp in the salon?

TOP TIP

When treating conditions of very oily scalps or dandruff, it is best to try one product at a time, giving it the full opportunity to do its job. It is all too easy to give up on a new introduction before it has had time to make a significant difference.

Maintaining records

At the end of the process you need to update all treatment records, including what shampoos and conditioners were used, for future purposes. It is hard to remember what has been used on a client from one salon visit to another and someone else may be conducting the wash-point operations next time. Apart from this, even if you do attend to the client next time, it is unlikely that you will remember everything that you used previously and this may be particularly embarrassing if the client specifically asks for the same regimen again.

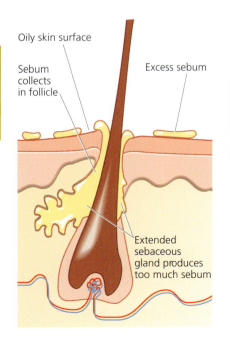

Oily skin surface

Sebum collects in follicle

Excess sebum

Extended sebaceous gland produces too much sebum

Shampoo the hair and scalp

Because shampooing (and conditioning) are chemical services, you should wear disposable nitrile or polyvinyl gloves. The risk of dermatitis is increased significantly during these processes, particularly when hands are constantly wet. Take protective measures to look after your hands and make sure that you don't get dermatitis. (See dermatitis page 151.)

Special note: shampoo equipment

Most references in this book refer to the backwards-style wash-point; these make up 90 per cent of all typical salon shampooing equipment. In salons where there is insufficient space or room to move clients around, or for the type of service being offered, such as shaving in barber's shops, the front or forwards wash is still used. Although this may not be the most pleasurable way to provide services to the client it still addresses specific needs; particularly if the client has a neck complaint and cannot lie backwards.

HEALTH & SAFETY

Some specific injuries or neck complaints prevent the client from lying back at the basin. In some cases this has led to clients passing out when pressure is applied to the back of the neck. Ask your client if they know of any reason why they cannot lay their head back into the basin.

STEP-BY-STEP: SHAMPOOING TECHNIQUE

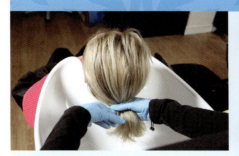

1 Prepare the client with a clean fresh gown and towel

Sit the client at the basin and detangle their hair

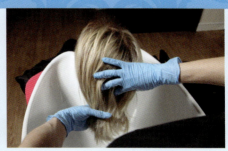

2 Loosen the lengths and make sure that all the hair is in the basin and none is caught around the nape area

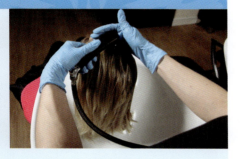

3 Check and adjust the water pressure and temperature. Ask the client if it is OK

Create a shield with one hand and dampen the hair working from the front to the back

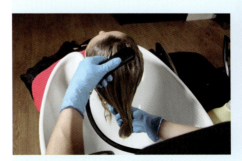

4 Ensure that all the hair is wet

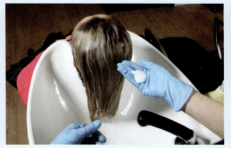

5 Select the correct shampoo for the client's hair, then apply a small amount from the dispenser to the palm of your hand

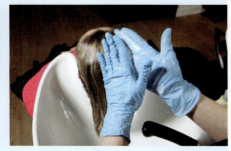

6 Spread evenly over your hands

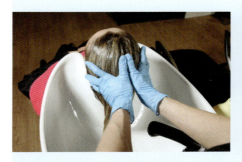

7 Apply the shampoo evenly to the hair with effleurage

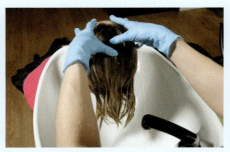

8 Start the rotary massage technique at the front with your hands in a 'claw-like' position

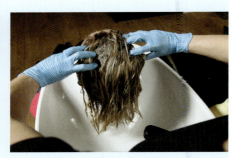

9 Gently move your fingers in circulatory movement around the head

Ask the client how firm a pressure they would like

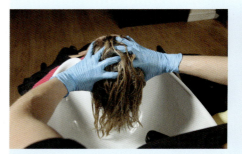

10 Work from the front, over the top, over the crown

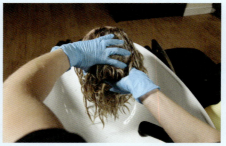

11 Continue to work down to the back of the head and then around to the sides

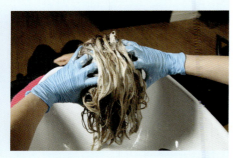

12 Work the massage until a lather increases. This will show that the hair is being cleansed

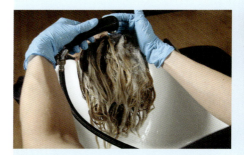

13 After shampooing, recheck the water temperature and pressure then rinse the lather away

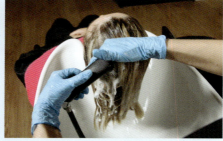

14 Repeat the whole process if a second shampoo is required

Normally on short hair one shampoo will do and take around five minutes

Longer hair will need a second shampoo and will take proportionally longer

Massage techniques used in shampooing

There are three types of shampooing massage techniques:

1 Begin shampooing with **effleurage**, gentle stroking movements with the flat of the hand that help to spread the products evenly.

2 Continue with firm but gentle **rotary massage** (circular movements). Let the fingertips glide over the scalp, whilst moving your hands towards each other in the centre (up from the sides, over the top and down into the nape). Move your hands in decreasing circles around the head to make sure you cover the scalp fully.

3 Occasionally change the rotary massage to **friction**, a quicker rubbing movement with the fingertips used to deep clean any difficult areas.

4 Finally, use soothing effleurage movements again to complete the shampoo process.

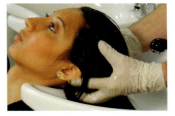

Shampooing: Rotary finger positions

What is dermatitis?

Dermatitis is a painful, itchy skin condition that affects the skin. Generally speaking, when hairdressers have this condition, it appears as a sore, sometimes moist reddening of the skin between and along the fingers and hands. The skin takes on this condition due to frequent contact with chemicals: shampoos, hair colourants, **perm solutions** and neutralizer. You must take adequate precautions to prevent this from happening. Always wear nitrile or polyvinyl disposable gloves for technical processes at the washpoint.

See Unit G20, page 13 for more information on dermatitis.

BEST PRACTICE

While shampooing:

◆ make sure the client is comfortable at all times

◆ be careful, especially with your hand positioning and massage technique, water flow and temperature, and the client's head and neck positioning throughout the process

◆ work in a clean, methodical and hygienic way.

After shampooing:

◆ make sure the water is turned off and replace the shower head in its place

◆ apply suitable conditioning treatment

◆ lift the hair away from the face and basin and carefully wrap in a towel. Place either side of the towel up and around the hairline, overlapping, and the remainder at the back, up and balanced evenly on the top

◆ lead the client from the basin area back to the work point

◆ remove the towel and comb the client's hair through.

See conditioning process page 156 for more information.

TOP TIP

Hard, linear and circulatory massage movements are uncomfortable for the client. Practise the right pressure with your colleagues at the salon.

TOP TIP

Always record the products that you have used on the client's record card so that they can be charged for and used again in the future.

TOP TIP

If your client is in the habit of washing their hair every day advise them to use a mild frequent use shampoo. Anything else may be too strong or may create a build-up in regular use.

TOP TIP

Regular brushing helps to remove products, dirt and dust from the hair.

BEST PRACTICE

Shampooing dos and don'ts

◆ Always use clean, fresh towels and gowns.
◆ Make sure that your hands and nails are hygienic and clean.
◆ Wear non-latex disposable gloves.
◆ Avoid splashing water or shampoo lather onto the client's face or near their eyes as the chemicals will cause discomfort if not injury.
◆ Always keep your hand in contact with the water whilst rinsing so that you can detect any sudden change in its temperature.
◆ Always direct the water spray away from the hairlines and into the basin.
◆ Carefully comb the hair after shampooing to remove any tangles.
◆ After using the basin, always clear and clean the area before it is used again.
◆ Turn off the water in between shampoos and conditioning to avoid wastage.
◆ Rinse and dry your hands afterwards to remove any shampoo or conditioning chemicals and reapply a barrier cream.

BEST PRACTICE

Wet hair can tangle very easily, which makes it very painful to comb through. So when you comb through your client's wet hair, you should always disentangle the ends first, then work back up through the lengths getting closer to the scalp. This makes the process simpler, it takes less time and it doesn't hurt either!

If you look at the ingredients on the packaging of shampoos you will find somewhere the term *SLS* or *TLS*. These are the common chemical terms for the detergents *Sodium Lauryl Sulphate* or *Triethanolamine Lauryl Sulphate*. Detergent in shampoo will, with prolonged use, cause contact dermatitis. You must take adequate precautions to avoid this happening. Barrier creams are an effective way to do this. They should always be applied to clean dry hands before any backwash activity takes place. They will need regular reapplication throughout the day to get maximum protection.

HEALTH & SAFETY

◆ Raising the client too quickly from the basin can be dangerous; for some, it may make them feel dizzy when they try to stand up and, for others, if they have had any neck problems, it could cause injury.
◆ Make sure that you do not apply too much pressure on the back of the neck or 'joggle' the client's head around by wrongly applying uneven pressure on either side.
◆ Always test the water temperature on the back of your hands before transferring the flow to the client's head. Look out for changes and fluctuations in water temperatures and pressures.

How does shampoo clean the hair?

Water by itself will not spread easily over the hair and scalp. This is because water molecules are attracted together by small electrical forces. These have their greatest effect at the water's surface, creating the effect called 'surface tension'. On hair, water by itself would form droplets. The detergent in shampoo reduces surface tension, allowing the water to spread easily over the hair and scalp, wetting them. *Detergents* are therefore *'wetting agents'* and shampoos contain detergents.

Each detergent molecule has two ends similar to a magnet. The 'hydrophilic' end is attracted to water molecules; the other 'hydrophobic' end repels water and is attracted to dirt and grease instead.

Detergent molecules lift the grease off the hair and suspend it in the water. This suspension is called an 'emulsion'. The grease holds the dirt so, as the grease is removed, the dirt loosens too. The emulsion containing the dirt is rinsed away with water leaving the hair clean.

> **TOP TIP**
>
> Good shampooing is physically soothing, psychologically calming and, overall, an enjoyable experience. A poor shampoo has the opposite effect!

ACTIVITY

You can always find out if your own shampooing practices are acceptable if you shampoo your colleagues' hair at work. Ask each other in what ways you need to modify or change your techniques.

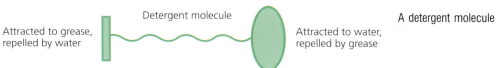

Detergent molecule

Attracted to grease, repelled by water

Attracted to water, repelled by grease

A detergent molecule

Detergent molecules surrounding grease

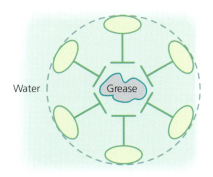

Water

Grease

pH values and effects

> **TOP TIP**
>
> **Acidity and alkalinity**
>
> Like many other chemicals, shampooing can affect the surface of the skin. This changes its natural pH balance and removes essential moisture. The pH scale measures acidity or alkalinity. It ranges from pH1 to pH14. Acid compounds have pH values 1 to 6 and alkalis have pH values of 8 to 14.
>
> A compound with a value of 7 is neither acidic nor alkaline and is therefore neutral.

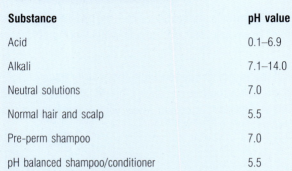

Approximate value of substances

Substance	pH value
Acid	0.1–6.9
Alkali	7.1–14.0
Neutral solutions	7.0
Normal hair and scalp	5.5
Pre-perm shampoo	7.0
pH balanced shampoo/conditioner	5.5

The normal pH of the hair and the skin's surface is 5.5. This is referred to as the skin's 'acid mantle'. The acidity is due in part to the sebum, the natural oil produced by the skin. Sebum production is an important skin function. Skin protects the underlying tissue, acting as a barrier; it prevents liquid loss from inside and keeps excess liquid outside the body. It also protects the body from infection. An acid skin surface inhibits, i.e. slows down, the growth of bacteria and makes them less likely to enter the skin. If the acidity of the skin is reduced and rises above pH 5.5, infection is more likely to occur.

Hairdressing procedures can affect this natural equilibrium, so pH-balancing products are used after perming and straightening, to return the skin to the natural acid mantle.

The pH of solutions can be measured by using a universal indicator, and a simpler indicator of acidity or alkalinity solutions can be made apparent by using pink or blue litmus papers.

Pink litmus paper used in alkali substances will turn mauve/blue. Conversely, blue litmus paper used in acid solutions will turn red.

If hairs are placed in an alkaline solution above pH 8.5 they swell and the cuticle lifts. In slightly acid solutions the cuticle is smooth and the hair is soft; in strong solutions of either acid or alkali the hair will break down and is destroyed.

Acids and alkalis are used in this way for high-lift colours. High-lift colours have added ammonia and this alkaline compound helps to swell the hair, enabling the colour to penetrate deep into the cortex of the hair.

Stronger alkaline compounds are available as hair-removing creams; these are applied to areas where the skin contains unwanted hair. The application is left for the prescribed time and is then wiped away, removing the hair with it. The skin is then rinsed and an acid-balancing skin conditioner is applied.

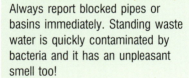

pH scale

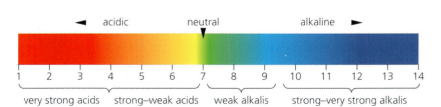

ACTIVITY

Example questions and model answers

Q1 How long should it take to complete the shampoo and conditioning service at work?

A1 We are allowed to take up to 'X' minutes for the whole process.

Q2 What is dermatitis and how do you avoid contracting it?

A2 Dermatitis is a skin condition that arises from direct contact with chemical substances. It has patchy red areas, often between the fingers or over the hands. In advanced stages, the areas are itchy and the surface of the skin can break. It can be avoided by wearing non-latex disposable gloves.

Q3 What types of protective wear are available for clients while they are in the salon?

A3. The salon provides gowns, towels and protective capes, which are worn whilst the services and treatments are carried out.

Q4 How would you advise your clients about choosing a shampoo?

A4 I would look at the hair and scalp to see the natural condition before I took the client to the basin.

ACTIVITY

Answer the following questions in the spaces provided:

Q1 Why is your posture important when you are shampooing and conditioning?

Q2 What safety considerations do you have to think about whilst the client is at the basin?

Q3 Why do you have to rinse the hair well after shampooing or conditioning?

Q4 Why do you need to keep the wash area clean and tidy?

Condition and treat the hair and scalp

Why do we condition the client's hair?

One of our primary roles as hairdressers is to improve and maintain the condition of our client's hair. If the cuticle surface of the hair is roughened or damaged the appearance will be dull. Clients want their hair to shine, therefore we have to improve the cuticle surface to make it as smooth as possible. We do this with help from conditioners and that way their hair will be easier to manage, easier to comb and easier to brush.

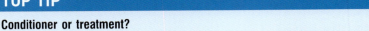

TOP TIP

Conditioner or treatment?

If your client does not routinely condition their hair, then the problem of dull hair is made worse. In a case like this, deeper-acting and longer-lasting treatments will be needed.

The principle of seeing shine can be thought of like this.

If you walk down the street, stop outside a shop window and look in, you will see your own reflection in the glass. The image of yourself is bounced back to your eyes from the smooth, flat surface of the glass. If the surface was roughened and uneven the image would be distorted and you would not be able to see a clear reflected image.

Now think of this in hair terms. The smoother the surface of the hair the better the shine. The duller the hair, the more roughened the surface is.

Conditioning: what should you be doing?

Question	First of all ask the client what has been previously done and what has been used upon the hair. If this is a regular client in the salon, check out the treatment history on their records.
Look and feel	Examine the hair and scalp closely. What condition is the hair in now? Look at the tell-tale signs – porous lengths and ends; loss of natural moisture and elasticity; dry, split or damaged ends or cuticle. Test for elasticity as good conditioned hair should be able to stretch and return to its previous length.
Advise	From what you see and feel, what would be the best course of action? A simple surface conditioning treatment? A salon-based deep-acting treatment? A prescribed course of treatment at home? Or a combination?
Agree	From the course of action you advise, get your client to see the benefits too. Explain how long the process will take, and also the costs involved.
Reassurance	Tell the client when to expect to see any marked changes and improvements. Explain that maintenance at home is just as important.
Maintenance	Prescribe any follow-ups. Explain how the hair should be managed at home or if products are needed to support the whole process.

ACTIVITY

What is your salon's procedure in respect of the following and what products would you use on each occasion?

1. Shampooing and conditioning hair prior to a cut and blow-dry?
2. Shampooing and conditioning hair prior to a perm?
3. Shampooing and conditioning hair after a highlighting service?

What are the benefits of using conditioners?

Professional products are formulated to protect and improve a range of different hair types and disorders. The main benefits of a good conditioner are that it:

◆ smoothes the cuticle edges

◆ improves the handling and combing when the hair is both wet and dry

◆ temporarily repairs and fills damaged sites along the hairshaft or missing areas of the cuticle or cortex

◆ provides shine, lustre and sheen

◆ creates flexibility and movement by locking in moisture

◆ balances the pH value of the hair back to a slightly acid 5.5.

Applying conditioner

Each conditioning treatment is specific to the task in hand. It is therefore extremely important to follow the manufacturer's instructions so that the product can do its job. Some (like a dandruff treatment) require the hair to be divided and lotions to be applied directly to the scalp. Others require heat assistance from hot towels or a steamer for deeper penetration into more damaged types of hair.

The following sequence provides guidelines for applying more deeper-acting penetrating-type conditioners.

STEP-BY-STEP: CONDITIONING

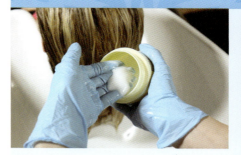

1 After shampooing, remove the excess moisture from the hair – now take a small amount of the product

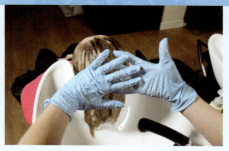

2 Spread the hair treatment evenly between your hands

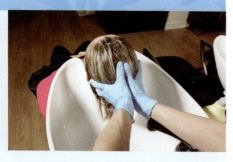

3 Apply the treatment to the hair evenly using effleurage

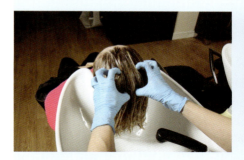

4 Now using deeper stroking movements – draw the treatment through the underlying sections of hair to ensure a comprehensive coverage

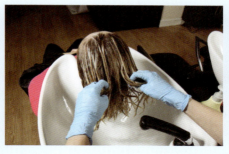

5 Use effleurage to massage the treatment into the hair

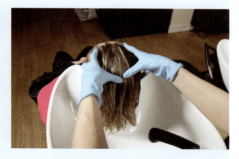

6 Remember that the treatment is a therapeutic service – with the product evenly applied, now work with petrissage movements from the frontal area

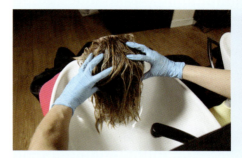

7 Over the top towards the crown

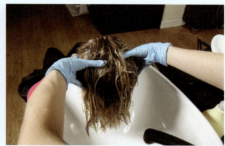

8 Then, back around the ears – through to the nape of the neck.

Repeat this sequence (6, 7 and 8) several times

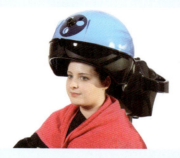

9 If the treatment needs to be developed with the aid of a steamer, move the client to a styling section to allow for full processing

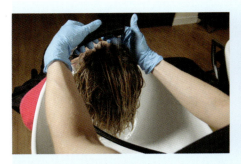

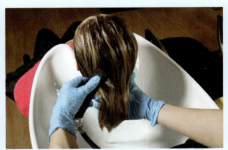

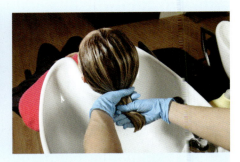

10 When the processing is complete – rinse away the excess at the basin. Remember to shield the client's hairline to avoid splashing their face

11 Rinse until the hair feels clean

12 After thorough rinsing – carefully squeeze out the excess

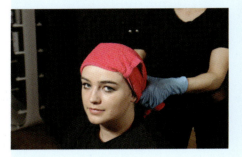

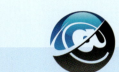

CourseMate video: Shampoo and Condition

13 Carefully envelop the hair in a clean towel and move the client to the styling section for further services

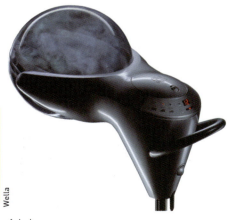

Wella

A hair spa

HEALTH & SAFETY

Steamers

Steam will only be produced when water is boiled at 100° centigrade. Therefore the moist heat can be very hot if the steamer is left unattended. Always check with the client to make sure that the equipment is not too hot.

Using heat during conditioning treatments

Using a steamer A steamer looks like a portable hood dryer with a water tank reservoir on the top. The water tank is removable and can be filled with tap water; the tank is replaced into the machine and a heating element boils the water when it is switched on. As the water boils within the machine the steam is transferred to the twin-walled, transparent hood part of the steamer. A series of small holes within the inner wall of the steamer allows steam to emerge and provide a hot, moist heat which is delivered to the person seated beneath.

The application of moist heat develops the treatment more quickly than if it were left at room temperature; it enables the product to penetrate more deeply into the hair, where, if it were left without heat, it might not work as well.

Precautions A steamer is an electrical piece of salon equipment, always check the condition of the plug and lead before turning it on.

When it is in use, keep an eye on the levels of water within the reservoir and always check with the client to make sure that the temperature is comfortable and not too hot.

Note The machine can be used for conditioning treatments and some lightening services, such as highlights and root-application oil lightener. When a steamer is used within a lightening service the moist heat principle develops the hair colour without extracting moisture from the hair and stops the product from drying out during the process.

Hot towels We can see that heat is used within treatments to help the product to penetrate further into the hair. Hot towels can be used as another alternative for applying heat during the processing of a treatment.

A towel is folded in half length-ways and folded again to make a long, thick band shape. The towel is then immersed into a sink of hot water and left to soak for a few moments. As the towel is removed, it is wrung out by twisting so that all excess water is removed and it is then placed around the client's head and secured so that the hair is totally enveloped within the towel. It can be left to develop for a period of time (according to the product manufacturer's instructions) and the towel and residual product can be removed and rinsed from the hair.

Scalp massage

Massage is a therapeutic method of manipulating the skin and muscles by either hand or machine. The effects of this may be:

◆ improved blood flow and the removal of fatty or bodily waste

◆ stimulation, re-energizing and invigoration

◆ soothing relaxation

◆ improved muscle tone.

Scalp massage has been a normal part of hairdressing services throughout history. It is common throughout Asia and has now become a beneficial supplement to the Western range of hairdressing services. There are several different types but the most popular used in Britain are Indian head massage and Oriental Shiatsu massage. Many salons view this as a major area for improvements to their service tariffs and offerings and there are several courses and texts available on the subject.

Contra-indications to scalp massage Scalp massage can be a therapeutic and/or stimulating service to clients, but not every client will benefit from it, or like the sensation that massage provides. Look for signs to see if the service can be provided and ask the client if they have any reasons that they know of that would not permit the service to be conducted.

Do not provide massage when:

◆ there are signs of cuts or abrasions on the scalp

◆ there are signs of reddening from conditions like eczema or skin sensitivity or skin allergies

◆ the client feels unwell or has a headache

◆ the client's scalp is naturally oily, as massage will stimulate the sebaceous glands further and make the hair even greasier

◆ there are any other adverse symptoms such as infections or infestations.

If you have any doubts about symptoms and contra-indications, always ask a senior member of staff for their assistance. You may be putting the salon at risk from legal action or pursuance if you don't follow this process properly. If you do offer scalp massage services and have covered the above contra-indications, make sure that you keep

BEST PRACTICE

Hot towels

If you do use the hot towel method for developing a treatment, always check that the temperature of the damp towel is not too hot, or that excess moisture is not dripping from it. The towel must be damp, but not wet.

TOP TIP

Effleurage is a smooth, soothing stroking action, performed with firm but gentle movements of the hands. You should use it before and after the more vigorous movements. It improves skin functions, soothes and stimulates nerves and relaxes tensed muscles.

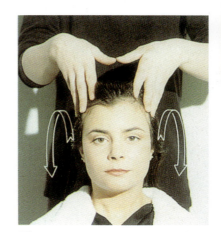

Effleurage

a record of your consultation and the responses made by the client after the service, for future reference.

Pre-shampooing scalp massage Scalp massage stimulates grease production and loosens dead skin cells and dirt from the pores. Given before shampooing, it provides a wonderful prelude to the other salon services. The time taken to do this depends really on you and the client. Some people can stand more stimulation than others. Older clients, for example, may have more sensitive scalps and will not benefit from ten minutes of manipulation. Conversely, other clients may find it more beneficial than the other services offered. It's a very personal thing.

Providing hand massage

1 Seat your client comfortably, with a clean fresh towel and gown.

2 Using effleurage first, draw your fingertips firmly but not too hard over the head. Your hands should move from the front hairline in an even pressure down to the nape several times.

3 Next use petrissage. Apply this lightly but firmly. With the fingertips, feel through the hair to the scalp and gently rotate on the scalp all over the head. Maintain an even pressure and balance throughout the process, covering all areas, slowly but with the same rhythmic momentum without exerting too much pressure.

4 Finally, use effleurage again to release the pressure of blood stimulated around the scalp during the previous movements.

5 Allow the client to sit quietly for a while to enjoy the benefits of the massage process.

Providing aftercare advice to clients

After completing the shampooing and conditioning treatments you should provide the client with some recommendations on how they can manage their hair themselves. This will ensure that:

◆ the client is able to gain similar benefits at home from those gained by attending the salon

◆ the client continues the care regimen of that provided by the salon.

Specifically, you need to tell them about:

◆ the ways and reasons for combing and brushing their hair

◆ different sorts of products that would be beneficial to them

◆ how often they should use these products at home.

The ways in which the client should comb and brush their hair

You need to tell the client how they can make their hair easier to manage and maintain a good condition for a longer period of time. Many contemporary effects involve some sort of styling or finishing product and we have already explained that shampooing aims to remove this type of product build-up. But combing and brushing should occur at other times too. Many clients aren't aware that they should be brushing or combing their hair on a daily basis, and that's regardless of whether they are washing it or not. The action of styling and most finishing products on the hair will lock the cuticle together in some

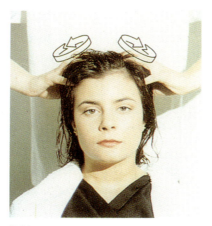

Petrissage

TOP TIP

Petrissage is a deeper, circular, kneading movement. It assists the removal of waste build-up and promotes the flow of nutrients to the skin and is normally used in conditioning and hand scalp massage.

TOP TIP

When disentangling long hair, always work from the points of the hair first, working backwards up the hair, towards the roots. This:

◆ makes combing far easier and quicker

◆ eliminates harsh, painful pulling

◆ reduces tearing and further damage to the hair

◆ minimizes any discomfort to the client.

way and it is this principle which enables the hair to stay in style/place. But unless this is detangled in the morning after lying on it, it will start to damage those areas that are locked together by tearing layers of cuticle away from the hair.

So it is essential that the hair is detangled. Initially this is done by separating the main tangles with the fingers and then when roughly loosened, the hair can be brushed or combed.

If the client has longer hair, tell them to start brushing near the ends of the hair first. If the hair is brushed from the root area first, all the locking points down the hair will be squeezed to the same point causing a large knotted area that will be really difficult to remove without damaging the hair. As the ends become free, the client can slowly work backwards, up the hair shaft to the mid-length and ends and then finally the roots.

Hair should always be combed or brushed downwards. If you have ever attempted to backcomb dry hair, you may have noticed some resistance. This is because the cuticles' free edges all point towards the ends of the hair. So when you push against them they will tangle together. But that makes combing hair out much simpler. When we comb through conditioners we always detangle the ends first, working back up the lengths. This helps the cuticle edges to slip over one another, making the whole process far less painful.

The different sorts of products that would be beneficial to the client

Your recommendations for products are based upon what you decided to use during the shampooing and conditioning process. Salons want their clients to make the most of the services that they offer and that includes the retail ranges that they may offer too. Most forward thinking salons use the same products at the wash-point as those available within their retail items; this backs up the salon's services by giving the client the opportunity to have similar experiences at home as they do in the salon.

You should always make a point of telling the client what products you are using on their hair and, more importantly, why you are using them. This is a professional protocol that stimulates interest and can lead to important additional sales too.

For more information on specific types of products see page 143.

How often the client should use these products at home

Finally, after providing the client with information about what products they should be using, you should also be giving them some idea of how frequently their product regimen should be used. Many people are locked into washing their hair on a daily basis and in most cases this is unnecessary. Very few people need to wash their hair every day but it becomes part of a habit, particularly if in having a shower every day they find it's just as quick to wash their hair too. If their own particular needs point towards not washing every day, then you should tell them. For example if the client has dry, porous and damaged hair, they certainly will not benefit from excessive washing, although the conditioning aspect will be particularly beneficial. Similarly, a client who has an excessively oily scalp may have to shampoo every day, but then may not benefit from using a regular surface conditioner. As you can see, each client must be considered on their own merits; they are individuals with individual needs. Your advice will go a long way to helping them counter their own particular problems.

SUMMARY

Remember to:

- ✓ prepare clients correctly for the services you are going to carry out

- ✓ shampoo and condition hair correctly, prior to all salon services

- ✓ 'brush up' on the science of how shampoos work on the hair to make it clean

- ✓ adhere to the safety factors when working on a client's hair

- ✓ wear *personal protective equipment* (PPE) to avoid contact dermatitis

- ✓ keep the work areas clean, hygienic and free from hazards

- ✓ work carefully and methodically through the processes of shampooing and conditioning the hair

- ✓ use positive body language as it plays such an important part in good customer service

- ✓ use only the correct shampooing and conditioning products appropriate to the task

- ✓ use good posture and avoid the consequences of poor posture.

Knowledge Check

This project relates to the techniques of shampooing and conditioning and the differences between types of conditioner.

Describe in your own words when you would use the following techniques:

- ◆ rotary

- ◆ effleurage

- ◆ petrissage.

How would you adapt the techniques for clients with very long hair?

What is the purpose of the following types of conditioner:

- ◆ Surface-acting?

- ◆ Penetrating?

Write your answers in your portfolio.

ASSESSMENT OF KNOWLEDGE AND UNDERSTANDING

A selection of different types of questions to check your knowledge.

Q1   Coarser, _____ hair takes longer to dampen than finer, oilier hair during shampooing.   Fill in the blank

Q2   Petrissage is commonly used during shampooing.   True or false

Q3   What factors should you consider during shampooing and conditioning? (select all that apply)   Multi selection

Water hardness	☐ 1
Water pressure	☐ 2
Water softness	☐ 3
Water temperature	☐ 4
Water wastage	☐ 5
Water wetness	☐ 6

Q4	Effleurage is a massage movement of circulatory movements.	True or false
Q5	The pH value of pH-balanced shampoos and conditioners is:	Multi choice

3.5–4.5	O a
4.5–6.0	O b
5.5–6.5	O c
7.0–7.5	O d

Q6	Dandruff is a condition of the scalp usually treated by shampoo.	True or false
Q7	Which of the following would take place after chemical processing? (select all that apply)	Multi selection

Pre-perm shampoo	□ 1
Anti-oxidant conditioning	□ 2
Medicated treatment	□ 3
Conditioning rinse	□ 4
Anti-dandruff shampoo	□ 5
Pre-perm treatment	□ 6

Q8	When conditioning long hair it is important to apply to the mid-lengths and _____.	Fill in the blank
Q9	A shampoo for dry hair would typically contain?	Multi choice

Critical acids	O a
Oils	O b
Medicating agents	O c
Anti-dandruff agents	O d

Q10	During conditioning it is always necessary to leave the treatment on.	True or false

8 Style and finish hair

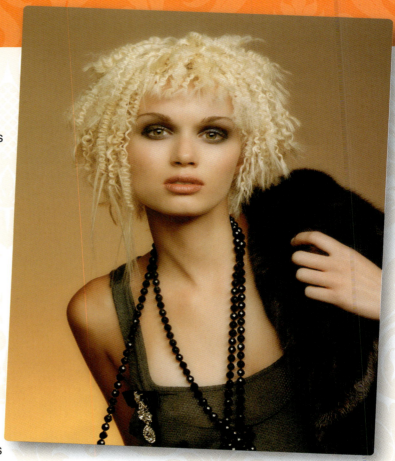

LEARNING OBJECTIVES

- ◆ Be able to maintain effective and safe methods of working

- ◆ Be able to blow-dry hair into shape

- ◆ Be able to finger-dry hair into shape

- ◆ Be able to finish hair with heated styling equipment

- ◆ Know how to work safely, effectively and hygienically

- ◆ Understand the effects of styling and finishing techniques on the hair

- ◆ Know how to use styling products and equipment

- ◆ Know how to provide aftercare advice to clients

KEY TERMS

alpha keratin	finger-drying	radial brush
beta keratin	paddle brush	scrunch-dry
contra-indications	polypeptide chains	vented brush
Denman brush	portable appliance testing (PAT)	
diffuser	product build-up	

GH10 Style and finish hair

Information covered in this chapter

◆ The different types of products and equipment used for styling, finishing and protecting the client's hair

◆ A range of styling techniques and methods that will create a variety of effects

◆ The basic science of alpha and beta keratin, i.e. the physical changes that take place during styling

◆ The home care advice that you should give

INTRODUCTION

This chapter looks at the aspects of blow-drying and finger-drying hair. Blow-drying has been the most popular styling technique for several decades, its popularity has grown in the belief that effects can quickly be achieved and that hair maintenance is low. In the hands of professionals, it seems so simple but like many other things in life, it is, when you know how.

So this section gives you the information to spread a little magic with your clients too!

Maintain effective and safe methods of working when styling and finishing hair

Client preparation – positioning

Client positioning has a lot to do with their safety as well as your safety too. If a client is slouched in the chair, they are a danger not only to themselves but to you too. Client comfort should extend to the point where it makes the salon visit a welcome and pleasurable experience. However, that is where it ends. The salon is not an extension of the client's own front room! They should not clutter the floor around the styling chair with bags, magazines and shopping. Anything that can safely be stored away should be: it is not only a distraction; it's a safety hazard too!

Salon chairs are designed with comfort and safety in mind; your client should be seated with their back flat against the back of the chair and the chair at a height at which it is comfortable for you to work. You need to be able to get to all parts of the head, so the chair's height should be adjusted to suit the particular height of the client. Don't be afraid of asking the client to sit up: it is in their best interest too!

Client protection

Make sure that the gown is still on and properly fastened around the neck. It should cover and protect the client's clothes and come up high enough to cover collars and necklines. Don't make the fastening too tight, but it should be close enough at least to stop things going down the back of the neck.

If you can style and dry hair with a towel around the client's shoulders, do so. But in some situations this is not possible as the length of the hair can get in the way of the styling or drying technique. Remember, other than plastic capes, the towel and gown are the main items of personal protective equipment for the client and therefore, the only things protecting them from the things that you do.

TOP TIP

Always dry the client's hair well to remove the excess water before combing, blow-drying or finger-drying

TOP TIP

Work with semi-dry hair
During styling this enables the natural tendencies of the hair to be seen.

See Unit GH8, pages 140–141, for more information on client preparation.

TOP TIP

Look out for ways and things that can make your client's visit more comfortable and pleasurable. This is the first step in providing a better customer service.

TOP TIP

Tell the client that you are adjusting the chair height, they might be a little shocked in the belief that it's going to give way!

ACTIVITY

Different salons have different ways of doing things. Find out what your salon's policy is in respect to:

1. Preparing the client prior to styling
2. Preparing tools and equipment ready for use
3. The use of styling products within the salon
4. Retail products and how they are communicated to the client

Write your answers to these points in your portfolio.

Your posture and work positioning

Hairdressing involves a lot of standing and because of this you need to be comfortable in your work. You should always adopt a comfortable but safe work position and sometimes comfortable and safe are not necessarily the same thing.

A naturally comfortable position for work should allow you to stand close enough to the styling chair without touching it. This should allow you to position your shoulders and body directly above your hips and feet and to distribute your weight evenly over them. You shouldn't have to twist at any point as you can easily work around the chair or get your client to turn their head slightly towards you. You should wear flat shoes, so that your body weight is comfortably supported on the widest parts of the feet. This will allow you to work for longer periods of time without risk of injury.

Always make a point of lifting your arms to check the work height for your client. If you have to raise your arms anywhere near horizontal during your work, you will find that your arms will start to ache very quickly. Make height adjustments to the styling chair, either up or down, but don't forget to tell the client what you are doing, as it might be a little shocking for them to find themselves being dropped suddenly!

Your personal hygiene

You may have already covered this in Unit G20, but here is a quick check reminder.

Make sure that you always:

- ✓ wash and dry your hands thoroughly before attending to any clients

- ✓ avoid wearing jewellery that can dangle or tangle in the client's hair

- ✓ wear comfortable (flatter and not open-toed) footwear

- ✓ be aware of bad breath – use breath fresheners if you do have a problem

- ✓ shower daily before going to work

- ✓ make sure your clothes are clean and fresh every day

- ✓ think about appearances, make sure that your hair reflects your job role

- ✓ avoid cross-infecting others through poor hygiene.

Working efficiently, safely and effectively

Working efficiently and maximizing your time is essential, so making the most of the resources available should occur naturally. But how can you do that? One way of making the most of the salon's resources is being careful in the way that you handle the equipment and the products that you use. Always try to minimize waste, be careful of how much product you use; it's pointless using an amount of mousse the size of a football, when a small orange is ample! It only needs a bit of care and control when you dispense the products. Only use as much as you need, remember: *the towels don't need excess styling products; it's just throwing money away!*

Think about tidiness, you must work in an organized way. You should have the things that you need at hand, and the equipment that you want to use in position and ready for action. You should be thinking about all of the things that you need before you need them. This is a good exercise in self-organization and shows others that you are thinking about your work.

Finally, keep an eye on the clock; you need to work to time, and that means providing the complete service in commercial timings.

HEALTH & SAFETY

Always wear non-latex disposable gloves when handling chemicals. This will reduce the risk of developing dermatitis.

HEALTH & SAFETY

Safe use of electrical equipment – the Dos and Don'ts

Do	Don't
Do check the plugs and leads to make sure they are not loose or damaged before they are used.	Don't use electrical equipment with wet hands.
Do replace equipment after every time it is used.	Don't use any piece of equipment for any purpose other than that for which it was intended.
Do unravel and straighten the leads properly before use.	Don't ravel up leads tightly around the equipment; it could work the connection loose.
Do switch off electrical items when they are not in use.	
Do check heated styling equipment such as straighteners and tongs before applying them to the client's hair.	

ACTIVITY

Product knowledge

Complete the table below to show how the list of products is (a) applied and (b) suitable for different hairstyling methods.

Product	How is it applied/used?	For what sort of styling methods is it suitable?
Mousse		
Setting lotion		
Styling glaze		
Serum		
Defining wax		
Heat protection		
Moulding créme		

Blow-dry hair into shape

This section covers the following topics:

- ◆ Consulting the client
- ◆ Influencing factors affecting styling

- ◆ Styling equipment
- ◆ Styling and finishing products
- ◆ Styling techniques.

Consultation

G7 Advise and consult with clients, in Chapter 6, covers all the things that you need to consider before carrying out any service. If you haven't covered the consultation yet, read that chapter first. Otherwise see the checklist below to review the main points for blow-drying and finishing hair.

Consultation checklist

Look out for	Things you could ask the client	Why ask this?
Hair shape	How would you like your hair styled?	You can see if the style is achievable from the length and layering patterns as you brush through the hair and what sorts of products you will need to help style it.
Contra-indications	Have you had any problems with your hair or scalp recently?	If the client has had problems it gives you a lead to investigate further.
Hair type and tendency	Is your hair naturally wavy (or curly)?	If there is movement in the hair you need to find out if it is natural to get an idea of which brushes you need to use and whether you will need to use other heated styling equipment too.
Amount and texture of the hair	Does your hair take long to dry and style?	Thicker hair and some hair textures take longer to dry. You need to find out if there are any condition issues first.
Head and facial shape	Do you find that some styles suit you better than others?	Find out whether the client naturally chooses and wears styles that are aesthetically correct for them.
Natural growth patterns and partings	Is this the way that your hair usually falls?	If the natural parting is not where the client wants it, you need to point out the pitfalls of working against the natural fall of the hair.
Hair condition and the way that it lies	Do you normally use a finishing or defining product on your hair?	Will the final look be improved by definition, serums or other finishing products?
Likes and dislikes, visual aids/ pictures	Would you like something along these lines or do you prefer a simpler style?	You must get the client to confirm the desired effect before you start.

Influencing factors affecting styling

The client's physical features and their lifestyle have an impact on the choice of styling. Their face and head shape may not be suitable for what they have in mind. Similarly, if their job or leisure activities affect their options, then you do need to point these factors out.

See Unit G7 Advise and consult clients pages 100–136

Face shapes

Oval face shape

An oval-shaped face suits any hairstyle, so these facial types present the fewest problems and style selection limitations.

Round face shape

Generally speaking, round face shapes need height to compensate for the width of the face. Hairstyles that are cut to a level just below the ears tend to draw a focus to that point and therefore longer lengths at the side are a better option.

Long facial shape

Shorter profile lengths improve longer facial shapes with added width as opposed to added height.

Square face shape

Squarer face shapes need rounder styled edges with texture on to the face to soften the corners or heavier jawlines. Longer lengths also are favourable; these tend to create a frame focus elsewhere.

Triangular or 'Heart' shaped face

The width of the face can be compensated for with height. However, the triangular face tends to be accompanied by a pointed chin. Avoid short perimeters with solid angles, as this will exacerbate the problem. Compensate with longer lengths at the sides with fullness and movement.

Styling equipment

Blow-dryers The blow-dryer is one of the most commonly used items of equipment in the salon. There is a huge range of models available, with a variety of power outputs, speeds and heat settings. Ionic hairdryers can even reduce the 'flyaway' effect that is produced by static electricity when hair is heated in a colder environment.

A good professional hair blow-dryer should:

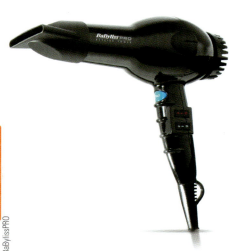

BaBylissPRO

Blow-dryer

- ◆ have at least two speeds and two heat settings
- ◆ have different shaped nozzles to channel the heat onto the brush or comb
- ◆ have a lead long enough for it not to tangle around the chair or client
- ◆ be powerful enough to dry damp hair quickly (1300w–1500w)
- ◆ have a cool shot button – to enable hot hair to be fixed (set) into shape around a brush
- ◆ not be too long so that it is balanced in the hand and can be held away from the client's hair during drying

◆ be light enough so that it can be manipulated easily and used for long periods without tiredness

◆ be quiet enough so that it allows natural conversation with the client.

Why work with damp partially dried hair?

In blow-drying or setting, the hairstyle is fixed as the **alpha keratin** changes to **beta keratin**. This takes place at the point where hair changes state from moist to dry. So when blow-drying, **finger-drying** and setting it is better to work with hair that is damp. It cuts down the time of drying and maximizes the work efficiency and amount of time spent on each client. Hair that is saturated still has to be dried, and using the blow-dryer and scorching the hair dry is damaging and unprofessional.

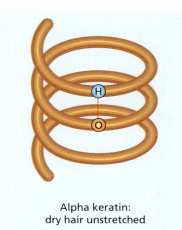

Alpha keratin:
dry hair unstretched

Before shampooing hair, the hydrogen bonds hold the **polypeptide chains** close together.

Hair in this natural **unstretched** state is called alpha keratin.

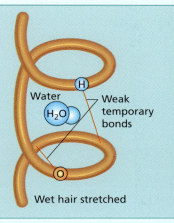

Wet hair stretched

When hair has been shampooed, many of the hydrogen bonds are broken.

This allows the hair to be stretched around a roller or brush.

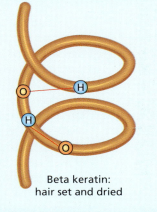

Beta keratin:
hair set and dried

When the hair has been **stretched** and dried into position (and allowed to cool) the hair is said to be in a beta keratin state.

In a beta keratin state, the hydrogen bonds are reformed to new locations on the polypeptides.

This is the principle of the temporary set.

HEALTH & SAFETY

Portable appliance testing (PAT)

All items of electrical equipment have to be tested and certified fit for use by a competent person. The items are tested, labelled and recorded and a compiled list is made available for inspection.

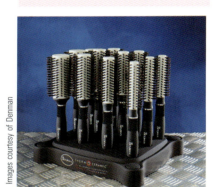

Images courtesy of Denman

More information on the effects of humidity on hair and the physical changes that take place within the hair can be found in Unit GH11 Set and dress hair, pages 184 & 215.

ACTIVITY

Give your answers to the following questions:

1. Why is hair always dried from roots to points?
2. When blow-drying why should the nozzle be parallel with the head?
3. Why is it important to keep the dryer moving during blow-drying?
4. What size mesh of hair should you work with when drying?
5. What effect does cold-shot have when blow-drying?
6. Why should you rough-dry the hair before you start?

TOP TIP

The cool-shot switch on a dryer is really useful for fixing in stronger volume or end movement into hair. After the hair has been heated, with the brush still in position, the cool shot immediately cools the hair, fixing the 'set' hair into position (just as allowing set hair to cool down after the rollers have been carefully removed makes the set last longer).

When a dryer is not in use there should be a safe position to store it. In daily salon use this could be a metal (ring) dryer holder attached to the side of the workstation; and after use, put away tidily.

Brushes Choosing the right tools to get the desired effect is essential. Different brushes do different jobs; if you use the wrong type of brush it will have a negative effect on the finished look.

The length of the hair and the desired effect dictates the type of brush you need to use. The table below gives a quick overview of what types are available and how they are used.

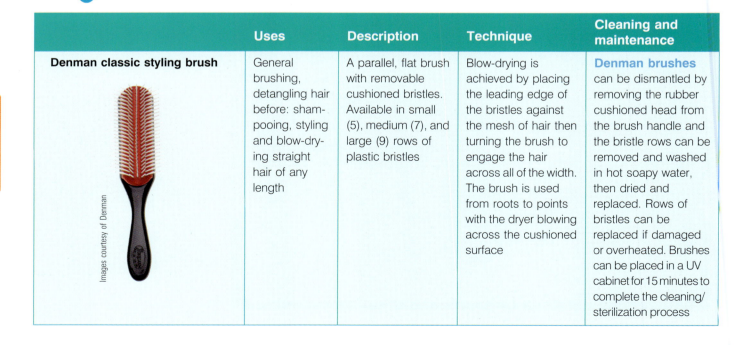

	Uses	Description	Technique	Cleaning and maintenance
Denman classic styling brush	General brushing, detangling hair before: shampooing, styling and blow-drying straight hair of any length	A parallel, flat brush with removable cushioned bristles. Available in small (5), medium (7), and large (9) rows of plastic bristles	Blow-drying is achieved by placing the leading edge of the bristles against the mesh of hair then turning the brush to engage the hair across all of the width. The brush is used from roots to points with the dryer blowing across the cushioned surface	**Denman brushes** can be dismantled by removing the rubber cushioned head from the brush handle and the bristle rows can be removed and washed in hot soapy water, then dried and replaced. Rows of bristles can be replaced if damaged or overheated. Brushes can be placed in a UV cabinet for 15 minutes to complete the cleaning/sterilization process

Images courtesy of Denman

		Uses	Description	Technique	Cleaning and maintenance
Vented brush	 E A Ellison & Co Ltd	General brushing, blow-drying straight short and mid-length hair	A parallel, flat brush with a double row of rigid plastic bristles (short and long) affixed to a brush head that is not solid, allowing air to pass between the bristles	Blow-drying is achieved by placing the leading edge of the bristles against the mesh of hair then turning the brush to engage the hair across all of the width. The brush is used from roots to points with the dryer blowing across the surface	**Vented brushes** can be cleaned by raking out any loose or tangled hair from the bristles, then washing in hot soapy water. The brush is then dried before use. Brushes can be placed in a UV cabinet for 15 minutes to complete the cleaning/sterilization process
Paddle (flat) brush	 Images courtesy of Denman	General brushing, detangling hair and pre-dressing hair	A flat brush with a wide head, usually with a cushioned head, and with wider teeth than a Denman. Sometimes the bristles are natural in composition, but generally they are plastic	Paddle brushes are generally too wide to use for blow-drying although sections can be dried by placing sections of hair upon the brush and drying by drawing down from the roots to the points of the hair.	**Paddle brushes** can be cleaned by raking out any loose or tangled hair from the bristles, then washing in hot soapy water. The brush is then dried before use. Brushes can be placed in a UV cabinet for 15 minutes to complete the cleaning/sterilization process
Radial brushes	 E A Ellison & Co Ltd	Blow-drying with volume, lift, wave and curl on shorter or longer length hair	Radial brushes are round in cross-section and come in a wide variety of sizes. The bristles are usually made of plastic although pure bristle brushes are still available. The inner body of radial brushes are often made of metal, allowing the brush to heat up and improving the drying speeds of the underneath hair within a section.	Blow-drying volume and movement is achieved by placing meshes of damp hair around the brush and drying the hair in position from both sides. When dry, the curl or movement can be affixed or set into position by applying a cool shot to increase the durability of the set	**Radial brushes** can be cleaned by raking out any loose or tangled hair from the bristles, then washing in hot soapy water. The brush is then dried before use. Brushes can be placed in a UV cabinet for 15 minutes to complete the cleaning/sterilization process

	Uses	Description	Technique	Cleaning and maintenance
Diffuser (although not a brush it is a piece of equipment used to style the hair)	**Scrunch-drying** and finger-drying hair to optimize the natural or permed movement within the hair	A diffuser is an attachment for a blow-dryer that suppresses the blast of hot air and turns it into a multi-directional diffused heat	The hair is styled with the fingers by either pressing into the cupped diffuser to dry or by working through the hair with the fingers until the hair is dried with the required amount of texture or definition	**Diffusers** are cleaned by spraying with an antibacterial spray then wiped with paper towels

Styling and finishing products

Choosing suitable products: you need to be aware of all the products that your salon uses and when and what effects they will achieve on different hair types and lengths.

ACTIVITY

Brushes

What are the differences between using the following brushes during blow-drying?

Brush	What sort of style is it used for?	What effect does it give?
Denman		
Small diameter Radial		
Large diameter Radial		
Paddle		
Vented		

ACTIVITY

In your portfolio explain each of the following:

1. alpha keratin
2. beta keratin
3. why hair should be allowed to cool before brushing through or finishing
4. the effects of humidity on hair
5. the effects of excessive heat upon hair
6. what advice on hair maintenance you could give to the client.

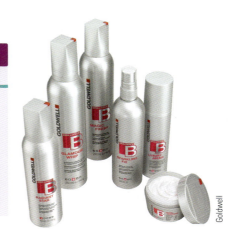

Goldwell

The table below shows the main ranges of styling products and what they do:

Styling Products

Product	What is it for?	How is it applied?	When do you use it?
Styling mousse Goldwell	A general styling aid for adding volume and providing hold	Apply a blob the size of a small orange evenly to the lengths	Use on dampened hair before sectioning and drying
Root lift mousse L'Oréal Professionnel	A special mousse that has a directional nozzle allowing you to apply foam at or near to the roots	Lift and separate sections of dampened hair so that the root area is exposed. Hold the can so that the nozzle aims the foam near the root	On hair that needs body but doesn't require setting hold at the mid-lengths and points

Product	What is it for?	How is it applied?	When do you use it?
Styling gel/glaze	A wet look firm hold finish on shorter hairstyles	Apply a small 'pea-size' amount from the fingertips all over evenly (You can always add more if necessary)	Not easy to blow-dry with but can be used in finger-drying and scrunch-dry techniques
Moulding clay	A dual purpose product for styling or finishing that bonds the hair with firm hold	(On damp hair) apply a small 'pea-size' amount from the fingertips all over evenly. (On dry hair) apply with fingertips to the points of the hair for texture and definition (You can always add more if necessary)	Used to give a firm textural bond on most lengths of hair
Definition crème	A finishing product that provides control on unruly hair	(On dry hair) Apply small 'droplet' amounts a little at a time with fingertips (You can always add more if necessary)	Used throughout the lengths of the hair for smooth control and conditioning

Product	What is it for?	How is it applied?	When do you use it?
Definition wax	A slightly greasy finishing product that provides textural effects to short to longer hair	(On dry hair) apply small 'pea-size' amounts a little at a time with fingertips (You can always add more if necessary)	Used throughout the ends of the hair for style definition and/or textural effects
Serum	A slightly oily finishing product that provides improved handling and shine	(On dry hair) apply small droplet amounts a little at a time with fingertips (You can always add more if necessary)	Used throughout the lengths of the hair for smooth control and better conditioning
Hairspray	A finishing product that is available in a variety of holds/strengths from either a pump or aerosol spray	Apply mist to hair from about 30–40 cm away from the hair for a 'fixed' hold on dry hair	Used as a final fixative, as an overall sealer or applied as a scrunching, textural finish

Product	What is it for?	How is it applied?	When do you use it?
Dry wax	A non-greasy finishing product that provides textural effects on short to longer hair	(On dry hair) apply small 'pea-size' amounts a little at a time with fingertips (You can always add more if necessary)	Used throughout the ends of the hair for style definition and/or textural effects

Note: always follow the manufacturer's instructions when handling styling and finishing products.

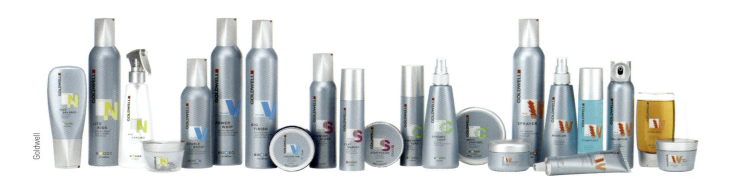

Goldwell

Styling techniques

Blow-drying hair Blow-drying is the most popular way of styling hair; it involves the tensioning, drying and positioning of hair into place with just a hand dryer and a brush. The technique requires a reasonable amount of dexterity and is quite difficult to pick up at first.

Prior to blow-drying the hand dryer is fitted with a heat- and air-focusing nozzle; this stops the dryer from randomly blasting the hair (and anything else) in a haphazard way. As the style is progressed, the nozzle can be moved around so that the client's scalp can be shielded from the potentially damaging, very hot blast and other sections of hair (awaiting styling) are not disturbed by the jet stream.

The idea is to start at the bottom or nape area and work upwards; fastening any hair not being styled out of the way neatly. Then as you work upwards to the next section the newly styled, dried hair is only placed upon previously dried sections. This organized way of drying prevents dry hair being re-moistened by damp hair and makes the finished style last.

When the client's hair is ready for styling the excess water must be removed so that:

◆ only damp and not saturated sections are worked upon

◆ the benefits of any styling products are not lost and diluted by excess water

◆ the client's hair is not unduly or excessively overheated

◆ the client remains comfortable and dry throughout the process rather than getting wet and cold.

> **TOP TIP**
>
> Hairdryers only blow out what they suck in from the other end.
> Always make sure that the filter is attached to the back of the dryer, as this will prevent your client's hair from getting sucked in. This is not only embarrassing for you, it is dangerous and unpleasant for the client too.

> **TOP TIP**
>
> Clean the gauze filters out on the back of the hand dryer regularly. This will prolong the dryer's life and enable it to work more efficiently too.

See the styling product table on pages 175–178.

Applying the styling product

After consultation and preparation you should towel-dry the client's hair and then, with a wide-tooth comb, carefully find the parting and detangle the hair lengths. Remember, if the hair is long you will need to work from the points through the lengths towards the roots.

You need to work upon hair that is damp rather than wet, so pre-dry any areas that need it first.

Then, select your product (depending upon your styling needs) and apply to the hair.

Distribute the product evenly throughout the hair, trying not to overload any particular areas and work through the lengths so that the product is evenly distributed upon the hair.

Drying the hair – roots to points (the way that the cuticle lies)

You should only work on relatively small areas at any one time; ideally these sections should not be any larger than the 'footprint' area of any type of brush that you will be using. If the sections are too large you will not be able to dry each mesh of hair properly and this will affect the durability of the finished look.

Be careful not to overheat any sections of the hair while you are drying, the effects would be long term and very detrimental to the condition of the hair.

Start the blow-dry at the lower back by sectioning out of the way any surplus hair and securing it with a clip. Then, taking your dryer in one hand, offer the dryer across to the section so that you can see whether the angle of the nozzle will create a parallel jet stream of air to the angle of the hair. Then, after any adjustments, take your brush in the other hand and introduce the bristles to the hair somewhere near to the root area. Pick and turn the brush so that the hair is caught across the bristles, turn on the dryer and now aiming across the brush, follow the brush downwards with the dryer, holding it about 10–15cm away.

Focusing the jet stream

The hair can only dry if the blast from the dryer is working over the surface of it. So bearing this in mind carefully aim the flat, jet stream of heated air across the surface of the brush, shielding the heat from the back (scalp side) of the brush. As you move the brush down, move the dryer down so that it mirrors the position of the brush at always the same distance away. Blow-drying from root to point ensures that the water is *chased* away from the hair and that the cuticle lays flat. This reduces 'fluffy' frizziness and will smooth the hair cuticle to improve shine.

If you are using a radial type brush you will find that you need to take a section (like that of rollering) and wind the hair around the brush. Again, focus the jet stream over the curved surfaces of the brush, but this time from both sides. This will enable the hair to dry around the brush forming part of the wave. Then after drying and while still warm, use a cool shot from the dryer (or use blast only without heat settings) to 'freeze' the wave into place. (This fixes the style with more durability like in setting; when rollers are allowed to cool down before removal and final brushing and dressing out.) If you do not allow the meshes of hair to cool it will result in a less firm result and will not last as long.

Finally, with the section dry you can take down another mesh, ready for drying into position.

Working with tensioned hair You have to maintain an even tension to the meshes of hair throughout the blow-drying service. This ensures that the hair will dry with a smooth, sleeker effect without frizzes or crimped areas. If you do create a kinked, uneven result, you can lightly spray down the hair with water and start again. Look out for the hair in the sectioning clips waiting to be dried too: If the hair has a natural tendency to wave or curl it might disfigure it before you can style it. Again, lightly mist it down with water and start over.

Blow-dry styling dos and don'ts

Dos	Don'ts
Do dry off the hair well so that it's moist but not wet before starting the blow-dry.	Don't leave damp towels around the client's shoulders.
Do take small enough sections that you can control and dry evenly throughout.	Don't leave the dryer running whilst you resection the hair.
Do try to direct the flow of air away from the client.	Don't use the top heat setting unless it's really necessary.
Do adjust the chair height so you can reach the top of the client's head without overstretching.	Don't pass the brushes to the client for them to hold in between sectioning.
Do ask the client to adjust their head position if you need to.	Don't try to use the same hand for brush work on both sides of the head.
Do clip out of the way any sections that are not yet being worked on.	Don't over-dry the hair as this will cause permanent damage.

TOP TIP

Blow-drying with radial brushes is very similar to setting with rollers. If you dry the mesh of hair on base it will give you lift at the root area; whereas a section dried off base (dragging the roots) will keep the root area flatter.

STEP-BY-STEP: BLOW-DRYING WITH A RADIAL BRUSH

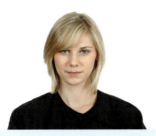

1 Gown and prepare your client, then shampoo and condition their hair

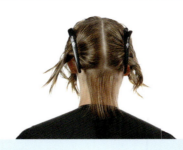

2 Rough-dry the excess moisture and detangle the hair

Start at the nape area and section off the lower perimeter length

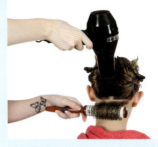

3 Wrap the client's hair around the brush and dry the hair from above and below to ensure that each section of hair is thoroughly dry before moving on

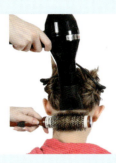

4 Be careful with the direction of the air from the dryer nozzle as it is easy to burn the client

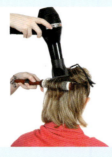

5 Carry on taking sections down and dry each one in a similar way.

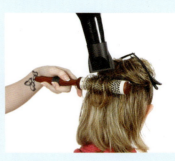

6 As the hair gets longer you will need to dry the root area first before attempting to dry the ends

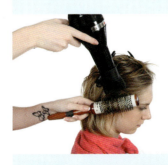

7 With the back done, move around to the sides.

Start with the lower sections first, building the shape and volume in the same way with the brush

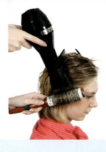

8 Work up through to the parting area and dry the fringe across, but with less volume

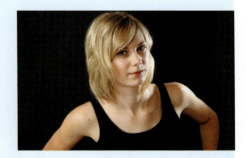

9 Final effect

STEP-BY-STEP: BLOW-DRYING LONG HAIR WITH A FLAT BRUSH

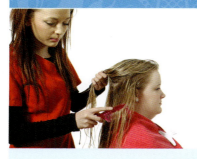

1 Move your client to the workstation and carefully disentangle their hair

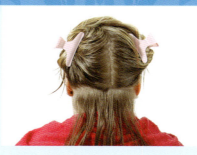

2 Starting at the bottom – take a horizontal section about 3cm above the nape hairline. Secure the remainder out of the way neatly

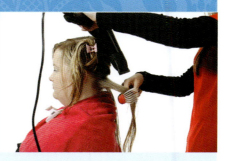

3 With nozzle attached and parallel with the section held in the brush, start drying from roots through to the ends

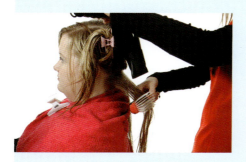

4 Remember to maintain an even tension upon the hair as you work through each section, taking care not to overheat or burn the hair

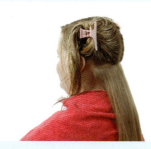

5 The dried section should look smooth and be evenly dried before you take down further sections to work on.

Repeat the process as you work up through the hair

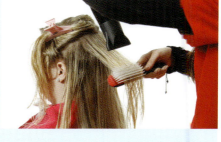

6 You should dry all of the back in the same way before starting the sides

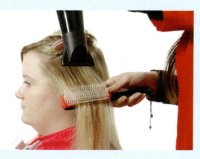

7 Moving around to the sides – start again at the lower sections, drying each one fully before moving on

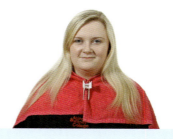

8 With all the hair dry – you are now ready to finish off with the straighteners

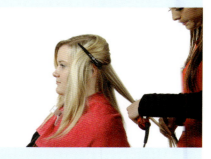

9 Start again at the back of the head at the lowest sections.

Make sure that the straighteners are not too hot (adjust the temperature according to the hair. E.g. finer hair needs less heat – 170–180° Coarser, curlier hair needs more heat 200°–210°).

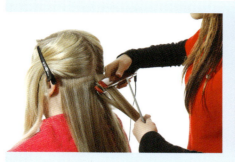

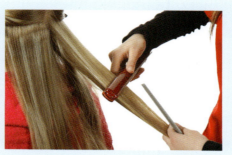

CourseMate video: Long Hair Blow Dry and Straighten

10 With the correct temperature, continue to work up through the sections – laying warm, recently straightened sections down on to previously straightened sections

11 Note: Be careful to use the straighteners correctly by passing the heated plates over the hair and downwards in one smooth, controlled pass over the hair at the same speed. Do not allow the straighteners to overheat any particular areas. You will damage the hair permanently!

STEP-BY-STEP: FINGER-DRY HAIR INTO SHAPE

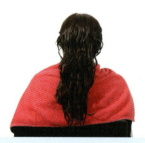

1 Towel-dry and remove excess moisture before you start

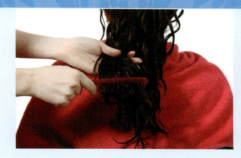

2 Detangle any knots with a wide-tooth comb

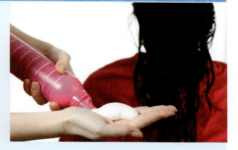

3 Apply some mousse to help hold the style

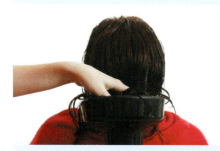

4 After rough-drying the hair, fit a diffuser on to the end of the blow-dryer and hold the lengths of the hair onto the diffuser prongs

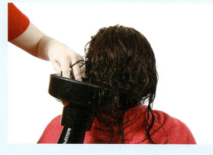

5 As the hair dries further, bulk the lengths together to finish drying the lengths
(This prevents the hair from separating too much and becoming fuzzy or fluffy)

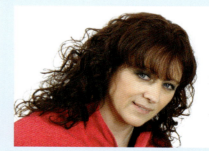

6 Final effect

ACTIVITY

Dos and Don'ts
Fill the table by indicating what the main dos and don'ts are for blow-drying.

Dos	Don'ts

Finish hair

After blow-drying the client's hair, you will need to do something to finish the look, even if it is only to brush the final effect through. More often than not, there is a lot more to do. This could be to:

◆ apply finishing products to the hair

◆ use other heated equipment to finish the effect.

Applying finishing products to the hair

Choosing the correct finish really depends on the look you are trying to achieve. It would be easy to get it all wrong at this stage and choose something that works against you. Sometimes it's the right product but wrongly applied, but more often than not, it's the wrong product correctly applied. Confused?

Most styling products like mousse or setting lotion do not create an immediate build-up upon the hair. They might be a little tackier than you had expected, or they might give a firmer hold than you had wanted. But in either case, when the hair is dry, a little too much won't have a critical effect on the desired outcome. However, if you apply too much serum or wax on the hair you will find yourself having to wash and start all over again!

This is easily avoided if you add product to your final effect in small steps. In other words, you build up the desired effect slowly by adding a little more until the result is achieved.

How do styling products make hair last longer?

Hair and, more importantly, hairstyles are affected by moisture, and moisture is in the air around us at different levels of what we call humidity. We know that if we get our hair damp that the style won't last and this effect is something in salons that we try to avoid.

Styling products laminate the hair with a moisture-resistant, invisible barrier. This stays on the hair and lasts until the next shampoo. In cases where heavier, denser finishing products have been repeatedly applied to the hair, then **product build-up** will occur. When this happens it will overload the hair and becomes difficult to remove, unless a clarifying shampoo is used.

Note * If your client is unaware of the effects that product build-up has on the hair you should advise them on how to manage their hair with other alternatives.

How do heat protecting products work?

In the preceding paragraph you can see how products work to protect the hair from moisture in the atmosphere; well that's not the only thing they can do. Blow-dryers can get very hot, but heated styling equipment is another thing altogether. Straightening irons and tongs have been very popular and many clients have been in the habit of using them, not just when the hair is shampooed and conditioned.

Heat-protecting sprays will put a heat-resistant layer upon the hair by doing two things:

◆ They improve the surface of the hair by smoothing it and enabling the heated equipment to slip over the surface without grabbing in any areas

◆ They resist higher temperatures from styling surfaces long enough for the hair bonds to be re-arranged in the new (temporary) shape.

See alpha and beta keratin, section on page 171 for more information.

Keeping the heated styling equipment clean

With prolonged use, the surfaces on tongs and straighteners can get product build-up themselves. This should always be looked out for as any residue of styling products such as wax, hair sprays, gels, serums, etc. will impair the slippy, smooth surfaces and create roughened areas that will grab and stick to the hair when they are hot. This is damaging as it could also burn the client's hair.

Using heated equipment

Using heated tongs, hot brushes and straightening and crimping irons
Electric curling tongs, heated brushes and straightening irons are a popular way of applying finish to a hairstyle. They are particularly useful in situations where:

◆ setting or blow-drying will not achieve the desired look

◆ the hair is not in a suitable condition to be dried into shape.

Sometimes you will not achieve the result that the client is expecting. When extra volume, movement or curl is needed on hair that lacks natural body, or is very fine, additional help is needed to create a lasting effect. Heated tongs and/or brushes provide a quick solution to do this. They can be bought in a variety of different sizes (i.e. diameters), which give different levels of movement.

Professional heated tongs (and many hair straighteners) usually have a thermostatic temperature control. This is particularly useful as you can *dial up* the heat setting required to achieve the desired effect for a particular hair type. This eliminates the chance of damage to the hair caused by excess heat.

TOP TIP

Some hair conditions are more suited to setting techniques. If the client's hair is too porous or lightened, dry setting or heated rollers would be a good alternative.

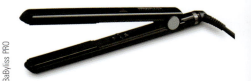

BaByliss PRO

STEP-BY-STEP: CURLING USING CERAMIC TONGS

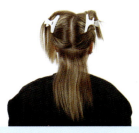

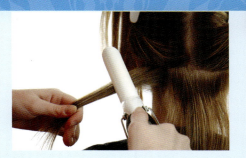

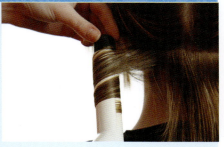

1 The majority of hairdressing services are started at the back

Section off and secure the hair at the nape

2 Dial up the correct temperature for the hair type then place the barrel of the tongs near the root end and start to turn

3 As you turn slightly open and close the tongs so that hair is drawn in to the barrel of the tongs

Note: This produces a far more effective spiral curl than trying to wind points to roots

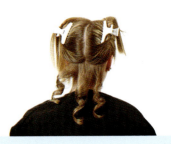

4 With the lower section done, carry on working up through the hair until all of the back is complete

By starting at the bottom you lay new warm curls down onto cooler, previously curled hair

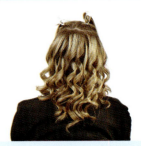

5 The back should start to look like this – continue the same patterning into the sides

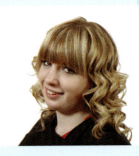

6 Final effect

CourseMate video: Spiral Tongs

TOP TIP

Hot styling tools can make hair static and flyaway. Heat protection sprays control this and protect the hair from being excessively overheated.

Straightening irons and particularly ceramic straightening tongs have been a very popular way of calming unruly hair. They work by electrically heating two parallel plates so that the hair can be run between them in one movement from roots to ends, smoothing out the unwanted wave or frizz in the process.

Ceramic straighteners have been particularly successful as they heat up in just a few moments and have a higher operating temperature than metal irons (180–210°C). This alarmingly high temperature would initially be considered as damaging to hair but, because they have the ability to transfer heat quickly and smoothly to the hair without *grabbing*, they are very effective in creating smoother effects. But because of their temperature you must check them before you introduce them to the hair so that you don't permanently damage the client's hair.

TOP TIP

Very hot styling tools without a non-slip coating or ceramic surface, can often tend to stick when they are introduced to hair that has styling products on it.

This grabbing effect can cause damage as the hair will bond to the edges of the equipment until it is removed. Always check the temperature settings before you use heated equipment and where possible, start at a lower temperature. Remember, you can always turn the temperature up.

When straightening is needed to complement the look on longer hair, it is often better to straighten each section as the blow-dry proceeds. If you start underneath, each section is completely finished before you move on up the head. The hair will stay flatter from the outset and each section is totally dry, stopping the hair from reverting to its previous state (i.e. reverting to alpha keratin).

The use of crimping irons tends to go through phases of popularity at least once every decade or so. They too have parallel fixed plates but these are wavy and produce flat 'S' waves on longer hair. They are a great styling accessory for competition and stage work as crimped effects are visually striking and very unusual. In staged hairdressing shows models with crimped hair will often accompany the look with strong fashion colours.

Unlike tongs and straightening irons, crimpers are not turned, twisted or drawn through the hair:

1 Each mesh of hair is started near the head and works down to the points of the hair.

2 The meshes should be no wider than the crimping irons and are crimped across the width of the plates.

3 After a few moments of heating each section of the mesh the crimpers are moved to the last wave crest created and pressed again.

4 This is repeated down the lengths of the hair until all of the hair is crimped.

5 The final look is not combed out or brushed, but allowed to fall in waved sections.

Crimping is not advisable on shorter, layered hair unless a frizzy, fluffy look is wanted. The most successful results are on longer, one-length hair.

Electrical equipment health and safety checklist

- ✓ Never get too close to the client's head with hot styling equipment
- ✓ Never leave the styling equipment on one area of hair for more than a few moments
- ✓ Always replace the styling tools into their holder at the workstation when not in use
- ✓ Always check the filters on the back of hand dryers to make sure that they are not blocked (this will cause the dryer to overheat and possibly ignite)
- ✓ Look out for trailing flexes across the floor or around the back of styling chairs
- ✓ Let tools cool down before putting them back into storage
- ✓ Always check for deterioration in flexes or equipment damage
- ✓ Never use damaged equipment under any circumstances

BEST PRACTICE

Heated equipment – advice for the client

Heated styling equipment such as straightening irons and tongs work at very high temperatures. When you are ready to use them, tell your client to keep their head still as any sudden movement or twisting could draw the hot surfaces closer to the scalp or even burn them.

TOP TIP

Care for tongs, straighteners and crimpers

When hairspray or styling products have been used on hair they can cause a build-up on the surface of electric tongs and straighteners. Over time, this will cause tacky or sticky points to develop upon the surface of the equipment when it is hot. Hair will stick to these areas and will cause damage. Sticky points on tongs and straighteners stop the equipment from gliding smoothly over the hair.

ACTIVITY

Revision of Facial shapes

For consultation purposes, as hairdressers, we tend to group clients into categories that follow a range of basic facial shapes. Look at the list below. What styling options or limitations does each facial shape provide?

Facial shape	Styling options/limitations
Round	
Oval	
Square	
Oblong	
Heart	
Triangular	

Styling and finishing products

Product		On short hair	Uses on medium-length hair	On longer hair
Mousse	A useful setting aid available in different strengths. Needs to be applied evenly through the hair lengths. Can be applied with a brush on longer hair	Apply a blob the size of a golf ball evenly to the roots and ends on damp hair to give volume and texture	Apply a blob the size of a small orange evenly to the roots and ends on damp hair to give volume and texture	Apply a blob the size of an orange evenly to the ends for styling hold
Setting lotion	Classic setting agent in liquid or semi-gel form. Needs to be applied evenly along the hair lengths	Apply half the contents of the bottle all over evenly for volume and styling hold	Apply the contents of a bottle all over evenly for volume and styling hold	
Styling/glaze	A firm setting agent that will produce a wet-look finish after drying	Apply a small amount all over evenly for firmer styling hold	Apply a moderate amount all over evenly for firmer styling hold	
Dressing cream	A non-greasy control cream for eliminating static from hair. Needs careful application as it is easy to overload finer hair types	Apply a small amount to your fingertips. Work through before combing out to give control, reduce static and calm down strays	Apply a small amount to your fingertips. Work through before combing out to give control, reduce static and calm down strays	

Product		On short hair	Uses on medium-length hair	On longer hair
Serum	An oil-based control agent for eliminating static and improving texture. Needs careful application as it is easy to overload finer hair types	Apply a small amount to your fingertips. Work through to flatten and add shine	Apply a small amount to your fingertips. Work through to flatten and add shine	Apply a small amount to different areas with your fingertips. Work through to flatten and add shine
Wax	A grease-based paste for defining texture	Apply a small amount to your fingertips. Work through to define and hold	Apply a small amount to your fingertips. Work through to define and hold	
Hairspray	A finishing product for fixing hair into place	Apply mist to hair from about 30–40cm away from the hair for a 'fixed' hold	Apply mist to hair from about 30–40cm away from the hair for a 'fixed' hold	Apply mist to hair from about 30–40cm away from the hair for a 'fixed' hold
Heat protection spray	Use in conjunction with electrically-heated styling tools. The product laminates the outer layer of the hair so that it is protected from damaging effects of heat		Apply to lengths after drying to provide protection from intense heat when using straightening irons	Apply to lengths after drying to provide protection from intense heat when using straightening irons

Provide aftercare advice

You are expected to know about blow-drying, the heated tools that you use and a range of styling and finishing products. This is so that you can advise your clients on their own hair maintenance. Look back through this chapter, and in particular the reference tables covering products and equipment.

For more information on providing advice, see Chapter 6 Consultation pages 100–136.

SUMMARY

Remember to:

- ✓ prepare clients correctly for the services you are going to carry out
- ✓ put on the protective wear available for styling and dressing hair
- ✓ listen to the client's requirements and discuss suitable courses of action
- ✓ adhere to the safety factors when working on clients' hair
- ✓ keep the work areas clean, hygienic and free from hazards
- ✓ promote the range of services, products and treatments with the salon
- ✓ clean and sterilize the styling tools and equipment before they are used
- ✓ work carefully and methodically through the processes of blow-drying hair
- ✓ take care when using heated styling equipment
- ✓ communicate what you are doing to the client as well as your fellow staff members.

Knowledge Check

For this project you will need to gather information from a variety of sources.

Collect together photographs, digital images and magazine clippings about styling, blow-drying, setting and dressing techniques.

Include styles for long hair as well as short; for weddings, special occasions and casual wear.

In your portfolio describe:

◆ how the styles were achieved

◆ why each is suitable for its purpose

ASSESSMENT OF KNOWLEDGE AND UNDERSTANDING

A selection of different types of questions to check your styling and finishing hair knowledge.

Q1   A round brush is also known as a _____brush.   Fill in the blank

Q2   Humidity in the atmosphere will make a blow-dried finish drop.   True or false

Q3   Which of the following items are examples of heated styling equipment?   Multi selection

Tongs	☐	1
Vented brush	☐	2
Crimpers	☐	3
Thinners	☐	4
Grips	☐	5
Straighteners	☐	6

Q4   The keratin bonds of stretched hair are said to be in the beta state.   True or false

Q5   Which chemical bonds within the hair are affected during heat styling?   Multi choice

Hydrogen bonds	O	a
Disulphide bonds	O	b
Sulphur bonds	O	c
Premium bonds	O	d

Q6   Ceramic straighteners can be used to curl hair.   True or false

Q7   Heated tongs will produce which of the following results and effects?   Multi selection

Increased body at the roots	☐	1
No body at the roots	☐	2
Curl at the ends	☐	3
Straighter effects	☐	4
Wavy effects	☐	5
Same as straightening irons	☐	6

Q8   A paddle brush is a type of _____ brush.   Fill in the blank

Q9   Which item of equipment would smooth and flatten frizzy, unruly hair best?   Multi choice

                                                        Curling tongs   O a
                                                 Ceramic straighteners   O b
                                                        Crimping irons   O c
                                                           Blow-dryer   O d

Q10   In blow-drying, the hair should always be dried from root to points.   True or false

9 Men's styling and finishing

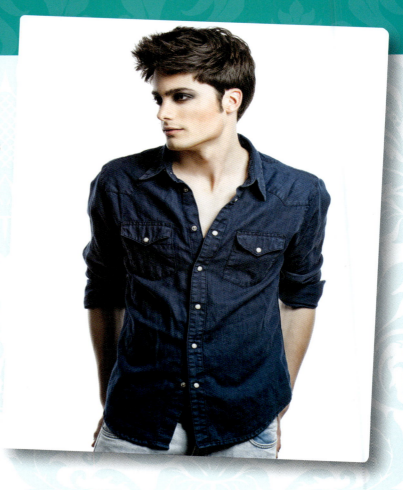

LEARNING OBJECTIVES

◆ Be able to maintain effective and safe methods of working

◆ Be able to dry and finish men's hair

◆ Know how to work safely, effectively and hygienically

◆ Understand the basic science that relates to drying and finishing hair

◆ Know how and when to use different drying and finishing techniques, products and equipment

◆ Know how to provide aftercare advice for clients

KEY TERMS

defining crème

dry wax

finger-drying

hair clay/putty

hair gel

hair varnish

humidity

styling glaze

Unit title

GB5 Dry and finish men's hair

Information covered in this chapter

◆ The types of products used for styling men's hair and how they work

◆ A variety of styling techniques that can create different effects

◆ The basic science of the physical changes that take place during styling

◆ The advice you should give to clients so they can maintain their own hair

INTRODUCTION

Men's hairstyling is becoming as demanding as women's hairdressing, gone are the days where every male sitting in the barber's chair has the same grade 2 clipper cut all over. Now men's grooming involves lots of different styling products and all the styling tools too, so you now have the opportunity to create exciting effects that will stretch your creative skills to the limits of your imagination.

Maintain effective and safe methods of working when drying hair

To avoid unnecessary duplication, many of the things that you need to know relating to preparation and health and safety are covered elsewhere in this book. For more information on these aspects, see the referenced pages below.

- ◆ *Preparing, protecting and positioning the client (pages 140–141, 166)*
- ◆ *Preparing and positioning the equipment ready for use (pages 18 & 268–269)*
- ◆ *Working safely and preventing infections (pages 16 & 270–271)*
- ◆ *Reducing risks – good salon safety and salon equipment (pages 6–16)*
- ◆ *Personal health and hygiene (pages 16–18)*
- ◆ *Reducing risks – contact dermatitis (pages 13–14)*
- ◆ *Reducing risks – handling chemicals (pages 13–14)*
- ◆ *Reducing risks – working with electricity (page 15)*

Main differences for drying and finishing men's hair

Most of the preparatory aspects for this outcome are similar to those of styling and finishing hair in unit GH10, although it is worth noting that some products and tools are developed with men specifically in mind, as their uses and applications are different to that on women's hair.

Taking 'on-board' these factors, the modern man creates his fashionable looks from a smaller, compact *toolkit* containing far fewer styling products than that which women use; he wants to create finished effects that are individual but achieved from products that do specific jobs.

Finishing products for men

Product	Application	Purpose	Suitability
Dry wax	Applied in small amounts by the fingertips into pre-dried hair	A moderately firm hold providing a non-wet look or greasy finish. Ideal for men who really don't like the look of product on the hair, but need the benefits of the control it provides	Suited to short and medium-length hair; the effects need to be created carefully and slowly by adding more as needed. It is very easy to add too much and overload the hair, particularly on finer hair types

Product	Application	Purpose	Suitability
Defining wax Wella	Work a small amount of product in your finger tips and sculpt into dry hair. Shape and rework as desired.	A strong defining clay that allows styles to be reshaped and recreated.	Ideal for textured looks and short hair, styles can be used to define key areas.
Hair varnish L'Oréal Professionnel	Applied in small amounts by the finger-tips into pre-dried hair. Care needs to be taken in applying the product evenly, throughout the hair.	A high-gloss look with a greasy texture. The styles created are moisture repelling. Ideal for men who do like product effects on their hair.	Suits short hair with long lasting, low maintenance looks, suitable for sports etc. Again the effect needs to be created slowly: it is easy to overload the hair and these types of product do produce a build-up on the hair.
Hair gel Wella	Distribute 1 or 2 pumps into your palms and work into the hair.	A styler that lifts, texturizes and tousles hair into many different styles with a pearl shine, finish and hold.	Can be used on dry hair. For extra lift in short hair, work into wet hair and blow dry.

Product	Application	Purpose	Suitability
Styling glaze *L'Oréal Professionnel*	Applied first to the hands and rubbed into wet or pre-dried hair all over. The hair is styled after and allowed to dry and fix into shape.	A wet look effect with firm to strong hold. Suitable for controlled or groomed looks with a mild, wet look effect.	Again like gel, you can't overload the hair as the look is based on 100 per cent coverage. The styles created are suited to short hair and are more resistant to moisture than gel but create less sculpted or highhair effects than gel.
Hair clay/putty *Wella*	Work a small amount of product in your finger tips into dry hair to design your desired shape.	A matt styling paste to create casually textured styles.	Suitable on dry hair to add definition.
Defining crème *Wella*	Work a small amount of product in your finger tips into dry hair.	A moulding cream to construct a rugged texture with a strong matt definition.	Ideal for short hair for an edgy, matt finish.

Product	Application	Purpose	Suitability
Hairspray	Applied to pre-dried hair by directional spraying from 30cm away.	Provides mild, moderate and firm hold, can be used as a final fixative or as a styling product when scrunched in.	Easy to apply, providing a long lasting effect on any hair length.

Note: Always follow the manufacturer's instructions and guidance for use when using any styling or finishing products

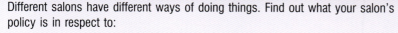

ACTIVITY

Different salons have different ways of doing things. Find out what your salon's policy is in respect to:

1. preparing the client prior to styling
2. preparing tools and equipment ready for use
3. the use of styling products within the salon
4. retail products and how they are communicated to the client.

Dry and finish hair

This section covers the following topics:

◆ consulting the client

◆ influencing factors that affect styling

◆ styling and finishing products

◆ styling techniques.

Consultation

G7 Advise and consult with clients (Chapter 6) covers all of the considerations that you should make before carrying out any hairdressing service. If you have not covered the consultation chapter yet read that section first, otherwise the following checklist will help you to review the main points.

Consultation checklist

Things to look for	Things you could ask the client	Why ask this?
Look at the hair shape	How would you like your hair styled?	You can see if the style is achievable from the lengths and layering patterns as you brush through the hair and what sorts of products you will need to help style it
Look for infections or infestations that will stop you from carrying on	Have you had any scalp problems recently?	If the client has had problems it gives you a lead to investigate further
Look at the type and tendency of the hair	Is your hair naturally wavy (or curly)?	If there is movement in the hair you need to find out if it is natural to get an idea of which brushes you need to use and whether you will need to use other heated styling equipment too
Look at the amount and texture of the hair	Does your hair take long to dry and style?	Thicker hair and some hair textures take longer to dry. You need to find out if there are any condition issues first
Look at the head and facial shape (see Unit GH10 pages 169–170)	Do you find that some styles suit you better than others?	Find out whether the client naturally chooses and wears styles that are aesthetically correct for them
Look at the natural partings	Is this the way that your hair usually falls?	If the natural parting is not where the client wants it, you need to point out the pitfalls of working against the natural fall of the hair
Look at the quality of the hair and the way that it lies	Do you normally use a finishing or defining product on your hair?	Will the final look be improved by definition, serums or other finishing products?
Likes and dislikes, visual aids/pictures	Would you like something along these lines or do you prefer a simpler style?	You must get the client to confirm the desired effect before you start

Choose the right equipment

Men's hairstyles tend to rely upon simpler effects. Admittedly, some men do dry their hair in a more formal, blow-dried way but the vast majority tend to create their desired effects from 'finger-drying' or 'scrunch-drying', with the added assistance of products to achieve the final effects they want.

Styling tools and applications

Denman classic styling brush

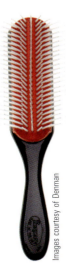

Images courtesy of Denman

Vented brush

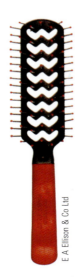

E A Ellison & Co Ltd

Paddle (flat) brush

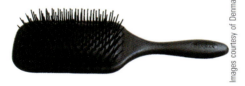

Images courtesy of Denman

Radial brushes

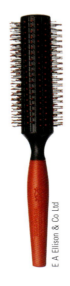

E A Ellison & Co Ltd

Diffuser

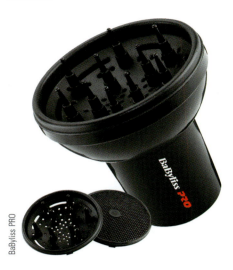

BaByliss PRO

To find out more about these brushes uses, techniques and tips for cleaning and maintenance see Chapter 8 pages 172–174

ACTIVITY

Product knowledge
For each of the products listed below, indicate for which styles and what hair lengths they are most appropriate.

Product:	Suitable styles and lengths
Soft wax	
Gel	
Moulding clay	
Pomade	
Mousse	
Hard wax	

Blow-drying

Believe it or not, the blow-drying technique of using a hand-held dryer and styling the hair with a brush started as a barbering service in men's hairstyling.

In a time where women's hairdressing salons were made up of private compartmentalized cubicles, the client would be consulted and attended to in total privacy by their stylist. On the other hand, men in barber's shops were seated in open, communal styling areas where communications between barber and client and client to other clients was commonplace.

In front of the seated male would be a front wash basin with a shelf and styling mirror above. On one side of the shelf, a leather strop would hang down for sharpening razors and on the other side there would be a heavy, retro-looking, chromed metal electric hand dryer.

Over the past 50 years most things have changed dramatically, but some have not. The history of the hand dryer is one, as in so many areas of life, in which an initial idea was taken from one particular environment, and then re-worked and re-invented to be supplanted in another.

Things you need to know about the basic science of drying and finishing hair:

1 The effects of **humidity** on hair, see chapter covering unit GH11

2 The physical effects of heated styling equipment on the hair structure, see chapter covering unit GH10

3 How the incorrect application of heat can affect the hair and scalp, see chapter covering unit GH10

4 Why hair should be allowed to cool prior to finishing, see chapter covering unit GH10

5 Why hair should be kept damp before drying, see chapter covering unit GH10

6 How heat protectors act to protect the hair, see chapter covering unit GH10

Finger-drying

Finger-drying is a less formal way of drying men's (or women's) hair into style. After removing excess moisture from the hair, some mousse can be applied to provide some body and texture to work with.

STEP-BY-STEP: FINGER-DRYING AND STRAIGHTENING

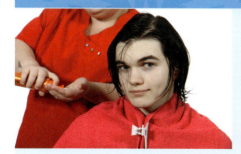

1 After shampooing and conditioning the hair, towel-dry any excess moisture before detangling.

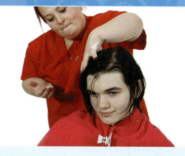

2 Then add your styling product evenly into the hair

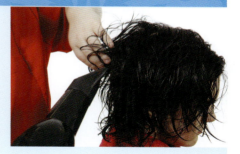

3 Rough-dry the excess moisture first to cut down drying time

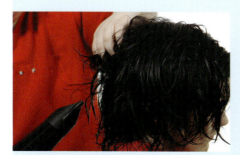

4 If you want to encourage movement into the hair, it will scrunch-dry better if it is drier rather than wetter

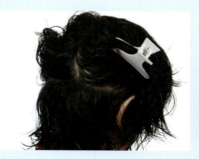

5 Now with the hair rough-dried, you can start at the back and section the hair off so that you work on smaller areas of hair

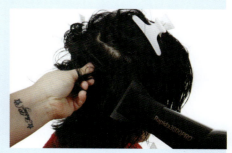

6 Rub the hair between the fingers and hold in a scrunch until dry.

As an alternative you could use a diffuser

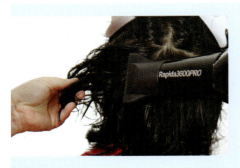

7 As the hair dries the movement will fix into place

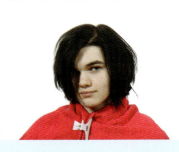

8 A very natural and casual finish. Alternatively, and for a straight finish you could use straightening irons

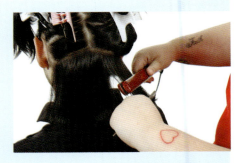

9 Re-section the hair and start at the bottom to pass the heated plates over each held mesh of hair

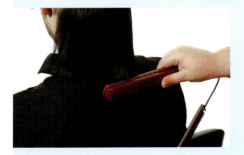

10 Take care to straighten the hair with one smooth motion without grabbing or jerking.

Be careful not to damage the hair. Heat protection is recommended

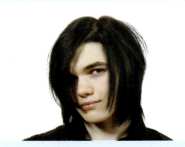

11 Same hairstyle but with a straightened effect. This provides more definition and can be textured further with wax or moulding paste.

The main idea of finger-drying is to use a blow-dryer with the fingers in a directional drying process, on generally shorter hair. Using the fingers provides three main benefits for this technique:

1 It allows a style to be shaped and moulded on hair that would normally be too short to dry with brushes.

2 It enables the stylist/barber to keep a check on the dryer heat as the fingers act as a temperature gauge for the client's head.

3 It provides stylists/barbers with a non-fussy styling option for the male client.

The checklist below covers the main considerations for finger-drying men's hair.

Finger-drying men's hair

◆ Always work with damp and not saturated hair – rough-dry if necessary

◆ Work on small areas/sections of hair

◆ Try to dry the hair in the direction of roots to points – it will dry more quickly and keep the cuticle layer smoother, making it look healthier and shinier

◆ Avoid burning the scalp – angle your dryer away from the head

◆ Move the position of your client's head in order to get around and cover all areas of the head

◆ Use both hands to dry the hair, so swap the dryer around; this allows you to work on both sides of the head effectively

ACTIVITY

Blow-drying vs. finger-drying
Complete this activity by answering this question:
In what circumstances is blow-drying more suitable than finger-drying as a way of finishing a client's hair?

STEP-BY-STEP: BLOW COMBING

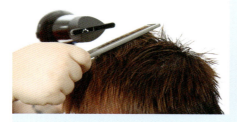

1 The blow comb is a drying technique that is really useful for adding lots of lift into men's short hair

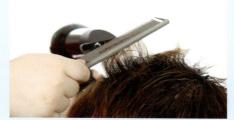

2 The hair is lifted with a cutting comb and the hot stream of air is introduced to the surface of the comb

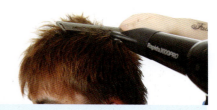

3 This is done all over the hair at any point where lift is needed

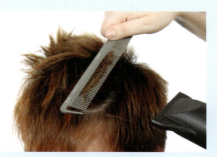

4 As the style progresses, you can see that a randomized form of lift and texture is created

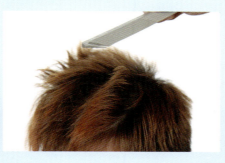

5 This close up shows you the amount of lift that can be achieved.
The final effect can be enhanced with wax or hair putty products

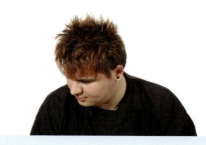

6 Final effect

Provide aftercare advice

You are expected to know about blow-drying, the heated tools that you use and a range of styling and finishing products. This is so that you can advise your clients on their own hair maintenance. Look back through this chapter and in particular the reference tables covering products and equipment.

For more information on providing advice, see Chapter 6 Consultation pages 100–136

SUMMARY

Remember to:

- ✓ prepare the client correctly before the service
- ✓ listen to the client's requirements and discuss their options
- ✓ always follow the manufacturer's instructions
- ✓ keep the work areas clean, tidy and hygienic
- ✓ promote the salon's product ranges
- ✓ always clean and sterilize the styling tools and equipment before use
- ✓ work in a careful and logical way when blow-drying or finger-drying hair
- ✓ take care when using heated styling equipment
- ✓ tell the client what you are doing, keep them informed of what is happening

Knowledge Check

For this project you will need to select two of your clients.

A. Client 1 should have short hair.

B. Client 2 should have longer hair.

For each of these clients:

1 Describe what your client's hair was like before you started.

2 Describe what techniques and tools were used to complete the look.

3 Explain what products you used and how they helped to achieve the look.

4 Take a photograph (perhaps with your mobile) of the finished effect.

ASSESSMENT OF KNOWLEDGE AND UNDERSTANDING

A selection of different types of questions to check your men's styling knowledge.

Q1 The common name for drying hair with just the hands is called _____ drying.
Fill in the blank

Q2 Humidity in the atmosphere will cause a finished style to drop.
True or false

Q3 Which of the following are finishing products?
Multi selection

Mousse	☐ 1
Wax	☐ 2
Gel	☐ 3
Setting lotion	☐ 4
Hairspray	☐ 5
Conditioner	☐ 6

Q4   The keratin bonds of stretched hair are said to be in the beta state.   True or false

Q5   Which of the following is the odd one out?   Multi choice

Vented brush   ○ a

Denman brush   ○ b

Round brush   ○ c

Paddle brush   ○ d

Q6   Finger-drying is similar to scrunch-drying.   True or false

Q7   Which of the following are better sterilized in a UV cabinet rather than in Barbicide™?   Multi selection

Cutting comb   ☐ 1

Conditioning comb   ☐ 2

A Denman brush   ☐ 3

A vented brush   ☐ 4

Plastic sectioning clips   ☐ 5

Metal sectioning clips   ☐ 6

Q8   A _____ is an attachment for a blow-dryer which reduces the hot hair blast.   Fill in the blank

Q9   Which item of equipment is best for smoothing and flattening frizzy, unruly hair?   Multi choice

Curling tongs   ○ a

Ceramic straighteners   ○ b

Crimping irons   ○ c

Blow-dryer   ○ d

Q10   Hair should be rough-dried before styling.   True or false

10 Setting and dressing hair

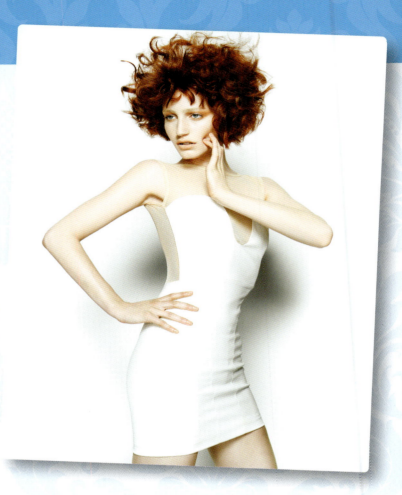

LEARNING OBJECTIVES

◆ Be able to prepare yourself and work efficiently and safely at all times

◆ Understand how to maintain standards of personal health and hygiene

◆ Be able to use a range of techniques, products and styling tools

◆ Confirm the techniques and style requirements with the client

◆ Maintain an even tension when plaiting or twisting sections of hair

◆ Ensure that plaits or twists move in the desired direction

◆ Secure the ends of the plait or twist design securely

◆ Be able to apply suitable products to help form or control the desired effect

KEY TERMS

alpha keratin	brick wind	hair-ups	scalp plaits
back-brushing	brush out	hydrogen bonds	traction alopecia
back-combing	clockspring curl	ornamentation	vertical roll
barrel curl	cornrow	pincurls	
beta keratin	double brushing	restructurants	
braiding band	flat clips	salt bonds	

Unit title

GH11 Set and dress the hair

GH13 Plait and twist hair

Information covered in this chapter

◆ The types of products used when styling hair and how they work

◆ The types of equipment used when styling hair and how they are used

◆ How to set and dress hair into a style

◆ How to plait and twist hair into a style

◆ A variety of styling techniques that you will use for both setting and dressing

◆ The basic science of the physical changes that take place during setting as well as the effect that heat and humidity have on the hair

◆ How to remove plaits and twists from hair

◆ The advice you should give to clients in order to maintain their own hair

INTRODUCTION

In recent years, the art of setting and dressing has been difficult for students to grasp. They didn't want to do it because it seemed *old fashioned* and boring; the clients that were available for training didn't really stretch the imagination or the technical abilities of the learner either. However, do not dismiss this important and vital skill set out of hand; the techniques used within setting and dressing underpin virtually all the other hairstyling skills and drills. This chapter combines *two* units to show you the techniques of folding, shaping, smoothing, fixing, curling, plaiting and twisting. Learn now, at the beginning, and a lot of the difficulties that your colleagues in training will have later in their career will be a 'walk in the park' for you.

Maintain effective and safe methods of working when setting, dressing and plaiting hair

Although Unit G20 covers many of the general aspects that you need to know about health, safety and hygiene within the salon environment, each technical procedure you carry out has particular things that are relevant to health and safety. Styling and dressing hair are always carried out at the styling units and therefore the main health and safety concerns should relate to the client's comfort, positioning and protection as well as your posture, accessibility and care.

To avoid unnecessary duplication, many of the things that you need to know about relating to preparation and health and safety are covered elsewhere in this book. For more information on these aspects, see the referenced pages below.

- ◆ *Preparing, protecting and positioning the client (pages 140–141, 166)*
- ◆ *Preparing and positioning the equipment ready for use (pages 20 & 268–269)*
- ◆ *Working safely and preventing infections (pages 16 & 270–271)*
- ◆ *Reducing risks – good salon safety and salon equipment (pages 6–16)*
- ◆ *Personal health and hygiene (pages 16–18)*
- ◆ *Reducing risks – contact dermatitis (pages 13–14)*
- ◆ *Reducing risks – handling chemicals (pages 13–14)*
- ◆ *Reducing risks – working with electricity (page 15)*

BEST PRACTICE

Always look after your brushes, combs and other tools. Make sure they are washed, dried and hygienically clean before you start your work.

TOP TIP

Why work with semi-dry hair?
During cutting and styling services it enables the natural tendencies of the hair to be seen. This is extremely important as the hair's wave, movement and hair growth patterns are all being considered as the style is developed.

Preparing the tools and equipment for setting and dressing hair

Make sure that you have prepared the area. Get everything that you need together beforehand, this includes the equipment that you need, as well as the products. You should have your trolley prepared with all the materials you will need. Rollers for setting should have been previously prepared by thorough washing and combs, brushes, sectioning clips, etc. should be all cleaned, sterilized and made ready for use.

For more information on cleaning, sterilization and general hygiene see Chapter 1, Unit G20.

BEST PRACTICE

Make sure that you always:

✓ Wash your hands before attending to any clients

✓ Wear the minimum of jewellery that can dangle or tangle in the client's hair

✓ Wear comfortable (flatter) footwear when on the salon floor

✓ Be aware of bad breath – use breath fresheners if you do have a problem

✓ Take a shower daily before going to work

✓ Make sure your workwear is clean and fresh every day

✓ Think how you want to be seen by others – is the image you portray one you are proud of?

✓ Minimize the risk of cross-infection to your colleagues and clients

Tools and equipment

Equipment	Used for	Effects achieved	Precautions	Cleaning
Setting rollers 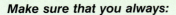	Wet or dry setting hair	Provide a long-lasting effect on wet/damp hair or softer results on dry hair	Poor quality rollers have moulding flaws, and these can catch on the client's hair during removal. Damaged rollers should be thrown away	Washed with hot soapy water and scrubbed clean, then dried and put back in trolleys/trays in sized order ready for future use
Velcro rollers	Dry setting only	Provide a soft and not as durable curl effect as wet setting rollers	Self-clinging rollers tend to lock onto finer hair types. Be careful when removing as they will not only pull the hair but damage it too	Washed with hot soapy water and scrubbed clean, then dried and put back in trolleys/trays in sized order ready for future use
Heated rollers	Dry setting only	Provide a soft but longer-lasting, more durable effect than Velcro rollers	These are very hot when they are first put into the client's hair. Use cotton neck-wool as an insulating base between the bottom of the curler and the client's scalp	Washed with hot soapy water and scrubbed clean, then dried and put back on to their appropriate heating stems ready for future use

Equipment	Used for	Effects achieved	Precautions	Cleaning
Heated tongs BaBylissPRO	Dry curling only. Used for adding more movement during comb-out	Provide a long-lasting effect on dry hair	Electrical item: Remember to check the condition of the lead before use. Very hot when in use: be careful not to burn the client or yourself	Spray cleaner and dried thoroughly after. Remove hairstyling product build-up from the curling surfaces
Tail or pin comb E A Ellison & Co Ltd	Sectioning hair into workable sizes dependent on the setting, plaiting or twisting technique used	They will provide tension when combing through sections and help to manage the hair	The point ends of tail combs can be metal or plastic, but both types are sharp. Be careful in sectioning or combing that you don't scratch the client's scalp	Washed in hot soapy water then kept in Barbicide™ until needed. When needed for setting they should be rinsed and dried first
Straight combs E A Ellison & Co Ltd	Dressing out hair; enabling the hair to be back-combed and smoothed	They will provide tension when combing through sections and help to manage the hair	Be careful during combing or back-combing that you don't scratch the client's scalp	Washed in hot soapy water then kept in Barbicide™ until needed. When needed for setting they should be rinsed and dried first
Flat brushes Image courtesy of Denman	Flat, paddle-type brushes are used initially on wet hair to work setting agents through and to detangle	Used during dressing to remove roller/setting marks, smooth or shape the hair or introduce back-brushing into the hair	Be careful not to brush too vigorously as it can make hair static or be painful to the client	Washed in hot soapy water and scrubbed clean to remove hair and particles. They should be dried thoroughly and put away for future use
Grips and hair pins Images courtesy of HairTools Ltd (www.hairtools.co.uk)	Fixing hair into position as part of the finished hairstyle	Hair-ups, partial hair-up/back effects	Grips and pins are metal with sharp points; care should be used when putting them in and when removing them to avoid tugging and snatching the hair	Washed and dried and put into trolleys or trays

Equipment		Used for	Effects achieved	Precautions	Cleaning
Pin clips		Wet or dry setting hair	Provide a narrow curl stem that can be positioned either flat against the skin or standing away	Pin clips tend to have fairly strong durable springs. These can pull the hair if not careful	Washed with hot soapy water and scrubbed clean, then dried and put back in trolleys/ trays

Other equipment and the effects on different lengths of hair:

Equipment	Short hair	Medium-length layered	Medium to long, one-length	Long layers
Lift pick comb	Dressing/back-combing	Dressing/back-combing	Dressing/back-combing	Dressing/back-combing
'Jumbo' wide-tooth combs	Conditioning, detangling and dressing	Conditioning, detangling and dressing	Conditioning, detangling and dressing	Conditioning, detangling and dressing
Denman Classic styling brush	General brushing, pre-dressing and blow-drying straight	General brushing, pre-dressing and blow-drying straight	General brushing, blow-drying straight	General brushing, blow-drying straight
Vented brush	Disentangling and blow-drying straight	Disentangling and blow-drying straight	Disentangling, pre-dressing and blow-drying straight	Disentangling, pre-dressing and blow-drying straight
Paddle brush	General brushing, disentangling and pre-dressing	General brushing, disentangling and pre-dressing	General brushing, disentangling	General brushing, disentangling and pre-dressing
Radial brushes	Blow-drying with firm wave, volume or curl	Blow-drying with firm wave, volume or curl	Blow-drying with firm wave	Blow-drying with firm wave, volume or curl
Diffuser	Scrunch-drying with movement or texture	Scrunch-drying with movement or texture		Scrunch-drying with movement or texture

More information about brushes is covered in Unit GH10 Style and finish hair, pages 164–191.

TOP TIP

Root direction will determine hair flow within a style.

TOP TIP

Scrunch-drying is a way of drying hair more naturally with a diffuser. It uses the natural body or movement within the hair to create tousled and casual effects.

BEST PRACTICE

Portable appliance testing (PAT)

All items of electrical equipment have to be tested and certified fit for use by a competent person. The items are tested, labelled and recorded and a compiled list is made available for inspection.

Brushes Brushes come in a wide variety and they are vitally important. Each has different applications and uses. Good-quality, general-purpose brushes should have flexible and comfortable bristles. The handles should be designed to fit comfortably in the hand enabling you to get a good grip. The typical salon brushes like this are either vented, to allow good airflow when drying hair, or similar to Denman brushes, which have cushioned removable teeth.

ACTIVITY

Collect information on the range of different styling products available in the salon. Now set out a table to describe:

1. each product by name

2. how it is used

3. what it does

4. which hair type it is for.

Styling products

There is an ever-growing range of styling and finishing products available to the profession. As this has been the major growth area, careful market research and product development have ensured that each one is specifically designed to do a particular job. As a result the huge range is confusing and is driven by successful advertising and brand awareness. If you look closely at each manufacturer's range you will find that the brand leaders all have similar and competing products. The more these numbers of similar products increase, the more confused the purchaser becomes. At this stage the only factor that can help someone to make a choice between one product and another is a reputable and recognizable name.

ACTIVITY

Tools and equipment

Write down what each of the items listed below is used for and how it is maintained.

Tool	What is it used for?	How is it maintained?
Pin clips		
Tail comb		
Velcro roller		
Paddle brush		
Hair grips		
Lift pick comb		

Styling products contain fixatives to hold and support the hair in its shape. Apart from hold, they often have other agents and additives within the products that can retain or resist moisture, provide protective sunscreens, add shine and lustre or add definition and shape.

◆ *Setting lotions* – such as mousses protect the hair from excessive heat. They increase the time that the hair is held in shape and the volume and/or movement created, all whilst being exposed to the blast from the dryer's nozzle. They can be in a variety of different strengths for differing hair types and holds.

◆ *Finishing products* – are products that enhance the hair by adding shine or gloss and improve handling and control by removing static, fluffiness or frizziness from the hair. Certain finishing products like waxes will define the movement in hair, giving texture or spikiness that could not otherwise be achieved.

◆ *Heat protection* – many products provide protection from heat styling. Regular use of straightening irons could damage the hair so there are a number of products that can be applied to eliminate any long-term effects. Other products provide protection from harsh UVA in sunlight in a variety of 'leave-in' treatments that can be used at any time. They are put on before exposure to harsh sunlight and can be removed by washing. This is particularly useful for clients who have coloured hair, as the lightening effects of sunlight will quickly remove colour. Other products have the ability to resist or remove the effects of minerals on the hair such as chlorine from swimming pools. This is particularly useful as blonde hair that is regularly subjected to chlorine tends to look green!

BEST PRACTICE

Always follow the manufacturers' instructions for using setting and dressing products within the salon.

TOP TIP

Moisture is the enemy of any finished set; it weakens the hold and therefore how long the overall effect will last.

More information on styling products can be found in Unit GH10 Style and finish hair, pages 164–191.

ACTIVITY

Equipment and their uses

When would you use the different styling equipment on different lengths of hair?

	Short hair	Medium-length hair	Long hair
Denman brush			
Vented brush			
Tail comb			
Setting rollers			
Velcro rollers			
Heated rollers			

Setting hair

Consultation

Consultation is an essential part of every hairdressing process; you will always need to find out information before you start.

For more, in-depth and specific information about consultation see Unit G7 Advise and consult with clients, pages 100–136.

If you have already reviewed this information or covered it previously within your training, here is a quick checklist to cover the applicable aspects for setting and dressing hair.

Consultation checklist before setting hair

✓ What is the texture, type, tendency and condition of the hair like?

✓ How much hair is there, how long is the hair?

✓ Are there any limiting factors or adverse hair or scalp conditions?

✓ What type of effect does the client want?

✓ Does the hair type/texture/tendency/amount and length support the client's ideas?

✓ What tools and equipment do you need?

✓ What lifestyle limitations are there?

✓ How much time will it take?

✓ How much will it cost?

✓ What sorts of products do you need to use to achieve the effect?

✓ Will the client benefit from buying and using these products at home too?

✓ Agree and confirm the desired effects and costs before you start

The principles of heat styling

Setting (and blow-drying) is a method of forming wet or damp hair into shape and then fixing it, with the aid of heat, to create a finished look. These methods of styling and dressing hair are temporary and the looks can be either classic or fashionable. You can make hair straighter, curlier, fuller, flatter or wavier.

Setting involves placing and positioning wet hair into selected positions, and fixing the movement in to it, while it is dried into shape. You may roll the hair round curlers, secure it with clips or pins, or simply use your fingers. Once dry, you complete the process by dressing the hair with brushes and combs.

The hair should never be excessively heated otherwise permanent damage will result, so always keep an eye on the time that the client is seated under the dryer so that they don't get too hot or that longer-term damage doesn't occur.

Before removing the rollers allow them to cool down in position after taking out of the dryer. The cooling allows the hair set to fix into position as hot hair can 'relax' back to its previous state. (Remember it's the same as using a cool shot when blow-drying, this helps to fix the curl in after using a round brush.)

The dressing part involves the manipulation of the hair in a planned and controlled way. It starts with the removal of the setting marks by brushing and then continues as the hair is combed out. The level of finish achieved during the comb-out relies upon the dexterity and skill of the stylist.

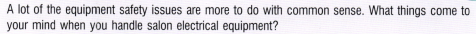

ACTIVITY

Using electrical equipment

A lot of the equipment safety issues are more to do with common sense. What things come to your mind when you handle salon electrical equipment?

List at least six safety precautions that should be considered when handling electrical equipment.

1.
2.
3.
4.
5.
6.

Before styling checklist

  ✓   Prepare the client by carefully making sure that they are comfortable

  ✓   Remove any damp towels and hairclippings, then replace with a fresh, dry one

  ✓   Will the hair benefit from any styling products?

  ✓   Are there any other limiting factors that need to be considered: e.g. physical features, growth patterns or hair density?

  ✓   Agree with the client exactly what is to be done

During styling checklist

  ✓   Is the heat from the dryer comfortable?

  ✓   Is the body or volume OK?

  ✓   Is the parting in the right place?

  ✓   Is the finished hair shape/style OK? If not, what aspect needs to be changed?

The effects of humidity on the hair

As with other techniques, setting produces only a temporary change in hair structure (and this is covered below). The fixed or set effect is soon lost if/when moisture is absorbed or introduced to the hair. You have probably already discovered this yourself: if, after having your hair done, you take a bath in a steamy bathroom, what happens to the hairstyle?

Moisture is all around us though and, in more extremes of humidity, it is seen as mist and fog. To help prevent style deterioration from happening, a wide variety of setting aids are available to slow down the 'collapsing' process and therefore hold the shape longer.

Different effects can be produced by different techniques:

◆ *increasing volume* – adding height, width and fullness, by lifting and positioning 'on base' when rollering or curling

◆ *decreasing volume* – producing a close, smooth, contained or flat style by pincurl stem direction, or by dragged or angled rollering 'off base'

◆ *movement* – varying line waves and curls by using differently sized rollers, **pincurls** or finger-waving.

Relaxed hair effects can be produced by wrapping hair or by using large rollers. Different techniques are used for hair of different lengths:

◆ *Longer hair* (below the shoulders) requires large rollers, or alternating large and small rollers, depending on the amount of movement required.

◆ *Shorter hair* (above the shoulders) requires smaller rollers to achieve movement for full or sleek effects.

◆ *Hair of one length* is ideal for smooth, bob effects.

◆ *Hair of layered lengths* is ideal for full, bouncy, curly effects achieved by, say, barrel or clockspring curls.

Different techniques can also be used to improve the appearance of hair of different textures:

◆ Fine, lifeless hair can be given increased body and movement. Lank hair can be given increased volume and movement.

◆ Coarse thick hair requires firmer control.

◆ Very curly hair can be made smoother and its direction changed.

Setting hair techniques

Curling techniques Curls are series of shapes or movements in the hair. They may occur naturally, or be created by hairdressing – this could be chemically by perming or physically by setting. Curls add 'bounce' or lift to the hair, and determine the direction in which the hair lies.

Each curl has a root, a stem, a body and a point. The curl base – the foundation shape produced between parted sections of hair – may be oblong, square or triangular. The shape depends on the size of the curl, the stem direction and the curl type. Different curl types produce different movements.

You can choose the shape, size and direction of the individual curls: your choice will affect how satisfying the finished effect is and how long it lasts. The type of curl you choose depends on the style you're aiming for – a high, lifted movement needs a raised curl stem; a low, smooth shape needs a flat curl. You may need to use a combination of curl types and curling methods to achieve the desired style – for example, you might lift the hair on top of the head using large rollers, but keep the sides flatter using pincurls.

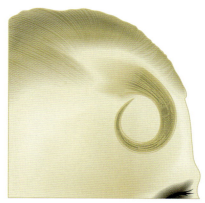

Curl parts

Rollering hair There are various sizes and shapes of roller. In using rollers you need to decide on the size and shape, how you will curl the hair on to them and the position in which you will attach them to the base:

◆ Small rollers produce tight curls, giving hair more movement. Large rollers produce loose curls, making hair wavy as opposed to curly.

◆ Rollers pinned on or above their bases so that the roots are upright, produce more volume than rollers placed below their bases.

◆ The direction of the hair wound on the roller will affect the final style.

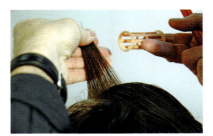
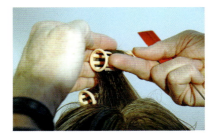

Winding a roller

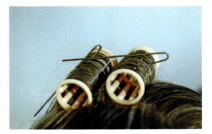
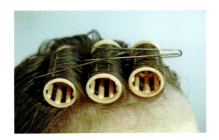

Securing rollers

TOP TIP

Evenly-tensioned curls produce even movements. Twisted curl stems or ones where the tension sags produce movement that is difficult to style.

STEP-BY-STEP: DRY SET (HEATED ROLLERS)

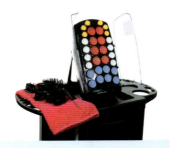
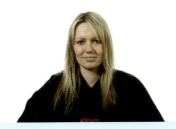
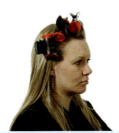

1 Heated rollers provide a softer option for contemporary set effects that cannot be achieved by blow-drying or wet setting.
Prepare your trolley with brushes, combs and the roller sizes that you want to use

2 Prepare your client with a clean fresh gown

3 Start by placing the rollers into the hair from the front

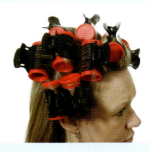

4 As you progress through the set, check with the client that the rollers aren't too hot.

If they are uncomfortable you can use pieces of neck wool as an insulator between the bottom of the roller and the scalp

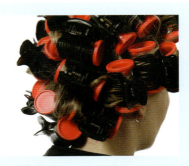

5 Leave the rollers in until all the rollers have cooled down

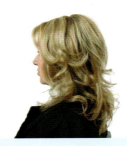

6 Then carefully remove the rollers, starting at the bottom and not the top

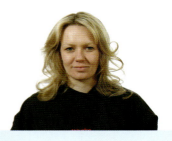

7 Work through with your fingers without brushing to create the looser natural, dressed effect

STEP-BY-STEP: WET SET ROLLERING

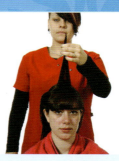

1 Wet setting can achieve similar effects to that of heated rollers.

In this wet set, '**brick wind**', large curlers are used to produce a contemporary, long lasting effect.

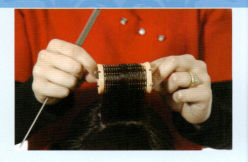

2 The first roller is placed centrally behind a full fringe area.

Care has been taken to ensure that the section taken is no wider or deeper than the roller's footprint

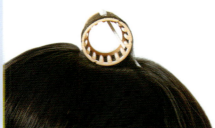

3 Side view – showing root lift and correct plastic pinning

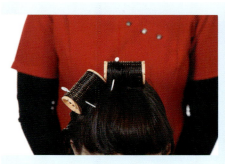

4 Another roller is wound adjacent to the first

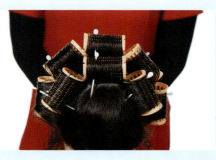

5 More rollers are placed to create a brick-work effect.

This will eliminate roller marks and stop the hair parting in the wrong position

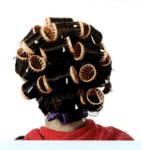

6 The hair set before putting under the dryer.

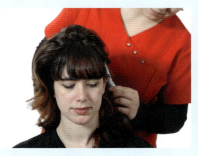

7 For a natural effect, more care is taken during combing out, so that the curls aren't unduly stretched.

A light brushing with a wide-toothed brush

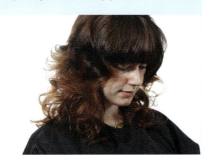

8 The final effect

Pincurling Pincurling is the technique of winding hair into a series of curls or flat waves which are pinned in place with pin clips while drying. The two most common types of curl produced in this way are the barrel curl and the clockspring.

- ◆ The **barrel curl** has an open centre and produces a soft effect. When formed, each loop is the same size as the previous one. It produces an even wave shape and may be used for reverse curling, which forms waves in modern hairstyles. In this, one row of pincurls lies in one direction, the next in the opposite direction. When dry and dressed, this produces a wave shape. When used in just the perimeter outline of a short hairstyle they can control the shape and stop the ends (that could otherwise be set on rollers) from buckling.

- ◆ The **clockspring curl** has a closed centre and produces a tight, springy effect. When formed, each loop is slightly smaller than the previous one. It produces an uneven wave shape throughout its length. It can be suitable for hair that is difficult to hold in place.

TOP TIP

If you are not sure which size roller to use, go for the smaller. If necessary you can brush out and stretch too tightly curled hair later.

Loosely curled hair will drop more readily, so you may not achieve the style you were aiming for.

TOP TIP

Common rollering problems

✓ Rollers not secured properly on base, either dragged or flattened, will not produce lift and volume in the final style.

✓ Too large a hair section will produce reduced movement in the final effect.

✓ Too small a hair section will produce increased movement or curl in the final effect.

✓ Longer hair requires larger rollers unless tighter effects are wanted.

✓ Poorly positioned hair over-falling the sides of the roller will have reduced/impaired movement in the final effect.

✓ Incorrectly wound hair around the roller will create 'fish hook' ends.

✓ Twisted hair around the roller will distort the final movement of the style.

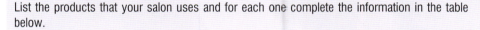

ACTIVITY

Styling and finishing products

List the products that your salon uses and for each one complete the information in the table below.

Product name	How is it used?	What hair type is it for?	Benefits to the hair

STEP-BY-STEP: PINCURLING – (BARREL CURL AND STAND-UP BARREL CURL)

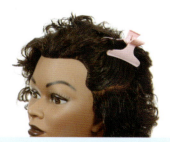

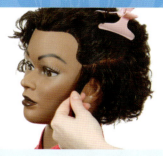

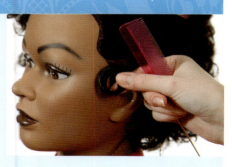

1 Pin curling is often thought to be difficult although like anything else, it's about preparation and placement.

Pin curls should be started at the bottom and then work upwards, working on areas already completed

2 After sectioning off a horizontal row, subdivide the section into a square-based stem.

Comb again to smooth it

3 Now take the curl around and hold the points between your finger and thumb

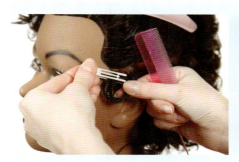 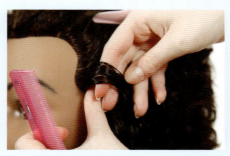 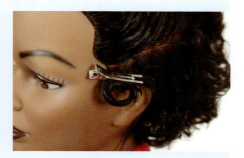

4 Taking a pin clip, now place the clip on the opposite side to where you would take another pin curl.

Repeat steps 2, 3, and 4 for as many as you want

5 Another form of pin curl is the 'stand-up' pin curl. This forms small barrel curls which add movement and lift

6 Take another square section and this time, turn it around your finger

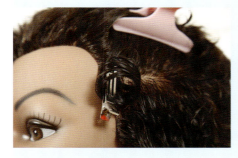 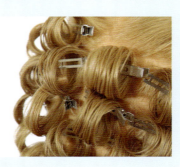

7 This is secured at the bottom of the base with a clip

8 Several 'stand-up' barrel curls

CourseMate video: Pin Curling

TOP TIP

Common pincurl faults

- ✓ Tangled hair is difficult to control. Comb well before starting.
- ✓ If the base is too large curling will be difficult.
- ✓ If you hold the curl stem in one direction but place it in another the curl will be misshapen and lift.
- ✓ If you don't turn your hand far enough it will be difficult to form concentric loops.

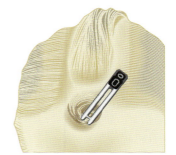

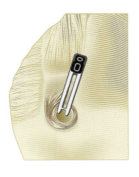

Curl body directions A flat curl may turn either clockwise or anti-clockwise. The clockwise curl has a body that moves around to the right and the anti-clockwise a body that moves around to the left. Reverse curls are rows of alternating clockwise and anti-clockwise pincurls; these will produce a finish that has continuous 's' waves, similar to the effect of finger-waves throughout the style. Stand-up pincurls, like rollers, have a body that lifts away from the scalp.

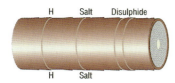

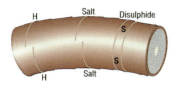

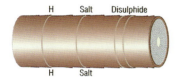

Step-by-step: Drying the set

Wet setting is normally dried under a fixed or portable hood dryer. You need to do the following:

1 Make sure that the client is comfortable.

2 Set the dryer to a temperature that suits the client. Most dryers have an adjustment for the client so that if the dryer becomes too hot they can turn it down themselves.

3 Set the timer for drying. You should allow around 15 minutes for short fine hair, and up to 45 minutes for long thick hair. The average is around 25–30 minutes.

4 Always check the client from time to time during the process.

5 After drying has finished, remove the hood dryer and let the hair cool down for a short while.

6 Then check to see if the hair is dry by carefully removing one roller from the crown area, one from the nape and one from the front; if they are all dry carry on carefully removing all the pins and rollers, leaving the set curl carefully in its position without dragging or distorting the formed curl.

The physical changes taking place in the hair   Hair in good condition is flexible and elastic. As hair is curled or waved, it is bent under tension into curved shapes. The hair is stretched on the outer side of the curve and compressed on the inner side. If it is dried in this new position, the curl will be retained. This happens because when hair is set the **hydrogen bonds** and **salt bonds** between the keratin chains of the hair are broken. The linking system is moved into a new temporary position. (The stronger disulphide links remain unbroken.)

Hair, however, is *hygroscopic*, it is able to absorb and retain moisture. It does so by capillary action: water spreads through minute spaces in the hair structure, like ink spreading in blotting paper. Wet hair expands and contracts more than dry hair does, because water acts as a lubricant and allows the link structure to be repositioned more easily. So the amount of moisture in hair affects the curl's durability. As the hair picks up moisture the rearranged beta keratin chains loosen or relax into their previous alpha keratin shape and position. This is why the humidity – the moisture content of air – determines how long the curled shape is retained.

The condition and the porosity of hair affect its elasticity. If the cuticle is damaged, or open, the hair will retain little moisture, because of normal evaporation. The hair will therefore have poor elasticity. If too much tension is applied when curling hair of this type it may become limp, overstretched and lacking in spring. Very dry hair is likely to break.

TOP TIP

Alpha and beta keratin

The keratin bonds of unstretched hair are in alpha keratin state and the keratin bonds of stretched hair are in beta keratin state. This is the basis of cohesive or temporary setting.

TOP TIP

If too much heat is applied to the hair it will sustain permanent, unrepairable damage.

ACTIVITY

How are the following items made safe and hygienic and prepared for salon use?

1. Heated curling tongs
2. Crimpers
3. Ceramic straighteners
4. Hot brushes
5. Heated rollers
6. Hand dryers

Dressing hair – *(brushing out)*

BEST PRACTICE

Always let the hair cool before removing all the rollers. Hot hair may seem dry when you first check it, but when it cools it may actually be damp.

Dressing (*i.e. The* **brush out**) is the process of achieving finish to previously set hair. Setting gives movement to hair in the form of curls or waves. Dressing blends and binds these movements into an overall flowing shape, the style you set out to achieve. It produces an overall form that flows, lightening the head and face and removing dull, flat or odd shapes.

Dressing uses brushing and combing techniques, and dressing aids such as hairspray to keep the hair in place. If you have constructed the set carefully and accurately only the minimum of dressing will be required.

Step-by-step: brushing out

Brushing out blends the waves or curls, removes the partings or set marks left at the curl bases during rollering and gets rid of any stiffness caused by setting aids.

1 One way of achieving the finished dressing is with a brush and your hand. The thicker the hair, the stiffer the brush bristles need to be. Choose a brush that will flow through the hair comfortably.

2 Apply the brush to the hair ends. Use firm but gentle strokes.

3 Work up the head, starting from the back of the neck.

4 Brush through the waves or curls you have set, gradually moulding the hair into shape.

5 As you brush, pat the hair with your hand to guide the hair into shape. Remember, though, that overdressing and over-handling can ruin the set.

Double brushing The technique of **double brushing** uses two brushes, applied one after the other in a rolling action; this will remove setting marks better and quicker than a single brushing technique.

Back-brushing **Back-brushing** is a technique used to give more height and volume to hair. By brushing backwards from the points to the roots, you roughen the cuticle of the hair. Hairs will now tangle slightly and bind together to hold a fuller shape. The amount of hair back-brushed determines the fullness of the finished style.

Tapered hair, with shorter lengths distributed throughout, is more easily pushed back by brushing. Most textures of hair can be back-brushed; because it adds bulk, the technique is especially useful with fine hair.

Step-by-step: back-brushing

1 Hold a section of hair out from the head; for maximum lift, hold the section straight out from the head and apply the back-brushing close to the roots.

2 Place the brush on the top of the held section at an angle slightly dipping in to the held section of hair.

3 Now, with a slight turn outwards with the wrist, turn and push down a small amount of hair towards the scalp.

4 Repeat this in a few adjacent sections of hair

5 Smooth out the longer lengths in the direction required, covering the tangled back-brushed hair beneath.

Back-combing This technique is similar to back-brushing above; however, in this situation a comb is used rather than a brush to turn back the shorter hairs within a section to provide greater support and volume. Back-combing is applied deeper toward the scalp than back-brushing and therefore provides a stronger result.

TOP TIP

The more the hair is back-brushed the greater the volume and support will be.

back-combing

TOP TIP

Back-combing is applied to the underside of the hair section. Don't let the comb penetrate too deeply otherwise the final dressing and smoothing out will remove the support you have put in.

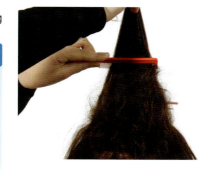

ACTIVITY

Answer these questions in your portfolio:

1. What difference would there be from setting with rollers on base as opposed to off base?

2. What type of effect do you get from clockspring pincurls?

3. What type of effect do you get from barrel curls?

4. Why do you need to brush the hair first when combing out?

5. What is the difference between back-combing and back-brushing?

Use the styling mirror As you work keep using the mirror to check the shape that you are creating. If you find that the outer contour is misshaped or lacking volume, don't be afraid to go back to resection and back-brush/comb again.

When you have finished the look hold a back mirror at an angle to maximize what the client can see of their hairstyle.

All these styling aspects create the basis for creating a variety of effects. The next part of this chapter looks at how this is applied to long hair dressings.

See Unit GH10 Style and finish hair: GH10.4 Finish hair pages 164–191.

For more information about heated styling equipment see pages 185–187.

Electrical accessories health and safety checklist

- ✓ Don't get too close to the client's head with hot styling equipment
- ✓ Don't leave the styling equipment on one area of hair for more than a few moments
- ✓ Don't use damaged equipment under any circumstances
- ✓ Do replace the styling tools into their holder at the workstation when not in use
- ✓ Do check the filters on the back of hand dryers to make sure that they are not blocked (this will cause the dryer to overheat and possibly ignite)
- ✓ Do look out for trailing flexes across the floor or around the back of styling chairs
- ✓ Do let tools cool down before putting them back into storage
- ✓ Do check for deterioration in flexes or equipment damage

ACTIVITY

In your portfolio explain each of the following:

1. alpha keratin

2. beta keratin

3. why hair should be allowed to cool before it is brushed out

4. the effects of humidity on hair

5. the effects of excessive heat upon the hair

6. what advice on hair maintenance you could give to the client.

Dressing and styling longer hair

Many people find working with longer hair or doing non-routine services quite daunting, but they needn't be. The main reason why someone finds any part of hairdressing difficult is because they are not doing that particular aspect or discipline regularly.

The most important things to remember with long **hair-ups** are:

◆ assessing whether a particular look or effect is going to suit the client

◆ agreeing the effect before you start

◆ having a plan of what you are trying to achieve

◆ building enough structure to support the look.

It may seem like this list states the obvious, but each one is vital and this is why:

Assess the style's suitability

This is the first aspect that you should consider. In most cases, non-routine hairdos are for special situations. It's not a quick, casual throw-up that the client does to get their hair out of the way. They come to the salon for the things that they can't achieve themselves: that's what hairstyles for special occasions are.

The problem from a suitability point of view is, how will the client know if they are going to like their hair up if they seldom have it styled that way? For people who don't normally wear their hair in plaits, pleats or twists, there are always underlying reasons and these could be:

◆ their hair is too thick

◆ they don't like the shape of their ears

◆ they feel that 'head-hugging' shapes make them more conspicuous

◆ it makes their nose look bigger

◆ they prefer their hair to have volume so they don't like it scraped back

◆ their hair isn't really long enough.

The table below provides a quick look up for the physical limiting/influencing factors

Physical features – style suitability

	Physical features							
	Head shapes							
Hairstyle	Oval	Round	Heart	Triangular	Square	Protruding ears	Prominent nose	Short neck
Vertical roll/pleat	✓	with height to compensate	✓	with height to compensate	with height and width to compensate	volume at the sides to cover	volume at the sides	needs to be sleek
Barrel curls	✓	✓	✓	✓	✓	volume at the sides to cover (not triangular)	volume at the sides	needs to be sleek
Low knot or chignon	✓	✓ with height	✓	✗	with height	volume at sides except triangular	✗	✗
High knot	✓	✓	✓	✓	✓	volume at sides except triangular	✗	needs to be sleek
Plaits	✓	✓ with height	✓	✓	✗	volume at sides except triangular	✓	needs to be sleek
Twists and cornrows	✓	✓ with height	✓	✓	✓ use designs that involve curves and not straight lines/linear effects	volume at sides except triangular	✓	needs to be sleek

✗ = not appropriate

Agree the effect before you start When you have selected a suitable look you need to find examples of how this would look on the client. Visualization and, more importantly, self-visualization from the client's point of view is very difficult, and that's why they want your advice. You need to try to rearrange the hair loosely, so they can get an idea of the weight distribution, height and width. If you can convey to them roughly what it will look like when their face is exposed, and they like what they see, you are halfway there. It will save lots of time later and save you having to unpick everything that you have done.

Have a plan – get organized If the client likes the effect in principle then you can set out a plan of how you will achieve it. You need to work out where you need to start, the midpoint in the styling and what the final touches will be. The starting point will be a position that you will be unlikely to get at and change later on, so it's a bit like making a cake.

- You start with a recipe – the style you want to create.
- You gather the ingredients – all the pins, grips, bands and accessories.
- Get out tools – get all the equipment you need together.
- Start preparing the mix – start the process.
- Place in the oven – mould and spray.
- Take out and ice the cake – finish off with the decoration/accessories.

Building a base structure for vertical rolls/pleats Some styles need support; they cannot last and stay in without it. It needs to be secure as well as creative in its effect, but it can only be secure if you use back-combing, grips, bands, etc. Do not be afraid to back-comb the hair. It may look as if the whole thing is getting too big, but don't forget you can take out as much as you like when you smooth the dressing. Back-combing provides you with a solid base that you can grip without the fear of the grips dropping out. As you become more experienced in handling long hair, you will find that you won't need to use much spray in the styling stage, but only later in the finishing off.

The other main tool for giving structure and support is grips. Kirby grips have one leg with a serrated profile; this helps them to stay in the hair much better.

Wherever possible ensure that you interlock (criss-cross) your grips, whether the patterning is in a straight line (e.g. in supporting and fixing a pleat) or whether it is placed in a complete interlocking circlet (e.g. in hair dressed in knots, chignons or any other centrally-positioned dressings).

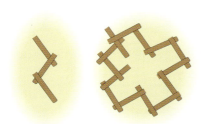

Interlocking grips

Vertical roll (French pleat) The vertical roll is a formal classic dressing that suits many special occasions. The hair can be enhanced further by the additions of accessories or fresh flowers. If you review the planning stages for putting hair up you will see under 'building the support' that back-combing is an essential aspect for creating a solid foundation. This should be your starting point for the step-by-step procedure.

STEP-BY-STEP: VERTICAL ROLL (FRENCH PLEAT)

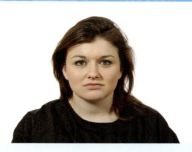

1 Before
Prepare the hair by brushing through smooth – you may have to consider straightening first if the hair is too curly

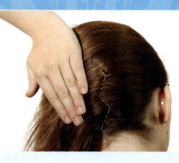

2 Place a vertical row of interlocking grips from the lower hairline to a position just below the crown.
Double row the interlocking grips if needs be

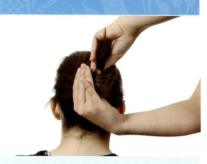

3 Smooth the hair across from the other side and hold with your hand pointing downwards and hair held in the palm of your hand

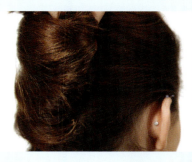

4 Turn inwards to form the pleat

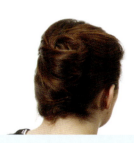

5 Now secure the side of the pleat with fine pins

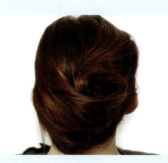

6 Finished effect

ACTIVITY

Setting techniques

The list below covers a range of setting techniques, what are they for and when are they used?

Technique	What does it do?	When is it used?
Back-brushing		
Back-combing		
Barrel curls		
Off-base setting		
On-base setting		

CourseMate video: French Pleat

STEP-BY-STEP: ASYMMETRIC CHIGNON

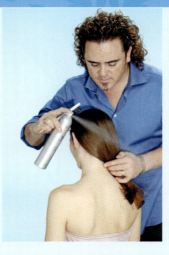

1 Brush through well and smooth down the side opposite to where the chignon will be.

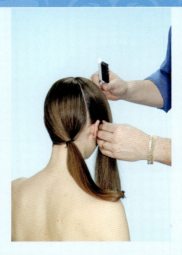

2 Divide the hair down to the ear. Fix one section with a band low to the hairline at the nape behind the ear.

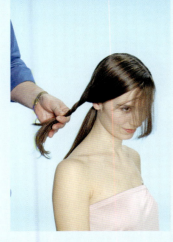

3 Twist the remainder down to meet the hair secured with the band.

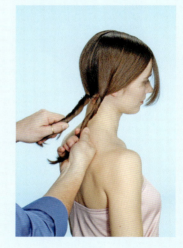

4 Now twist the hair in the covered band too.

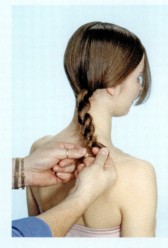

5 Twist this section underneath the other and continue through to the ends with both sections.

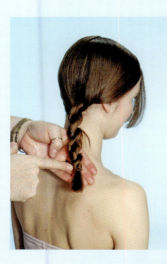

6 Secure the sections together with a band at the ends.

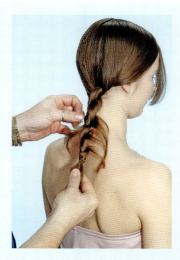

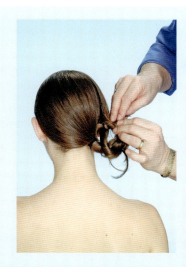

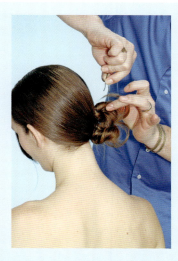

7 Now feather the effect by pulling out some loose ends.

8 Loop around and fix in position.

9 Continue to twist and secure with grips.

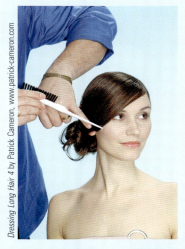

Dressing Long Hair 4 by Patrick Cameron, www.patrick-cameron.com

10 Finally smooth out the front area and fix down into position.

Plaiting and twisting hair

Plaiting hair

Plaiting is a method of intertwining three or more strands of hair to create a variety of woven hairstyles. When this work is done for specific occasions, it is often accompanied by **ornamentation**: fresh flowers, glass or plastic beads, coloured silks and added hair are also popular.

The numerous options for plaited effects are determined by the following factors:

◆ number of plaits or twists used

◆ positioning of the plait or twist across the scalp or around the head

◆ the way in which the plaits are made (under or over)

◆ any ornamentation/decoration or added hair applied.

TOP TIP

The tension used in plaiting can exert exceptional pressure on the hair follicle and scalp-type plaits/cornrows create more vulnerability than free-hanging plaits. In extreme cases hair loss may be caused by this continued pulling action; areas of hair become thin and even baldness may be the result!

This condition is called *traction alopecia* and is particularly obvious at the temples of younger girls with long hair who regularly wear their hair up for school, sport or dancing.

'Plaits' usually refers to a free-hanging stem(s) of hair that is left to show hair length. This length can be natural or can be extended by adding hair during the plaiting process; an example is the 'French' 'Rope' or 'Fish Tail' plait.

STEP-BY-STEP: ROPE PLAITING

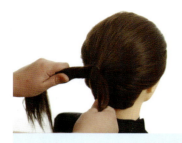

1 Fix the hair centrally at the back in a pony with a covered band

Then divide the pony into two equal parts

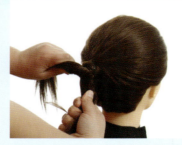

2 Both stems should be twisted in a clockwise direction

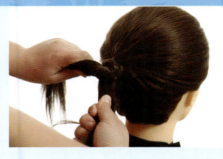

3 And then wound around each other

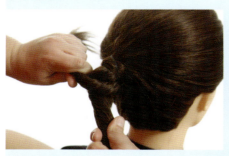
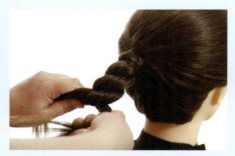
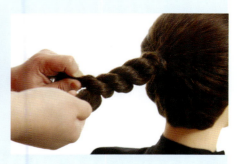

4 Continue twisting and then winding around each other down the length of the pony tail

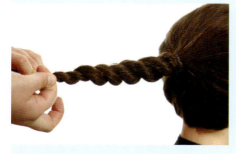

5 Use a **braiding band** to bond the ends together

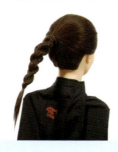

6 Finished effect

CourseMate video: Rope Plait

STEP-BY-STEP: THREE-STEM 'FRENCH' PLAITING

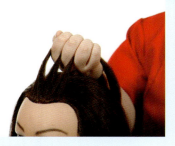

1 Divide the hair at the front into three equal stems

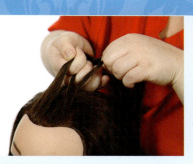

2 Hold them with one stem in one hand and two in the other,

then pass one of the outer stems across and into the centre

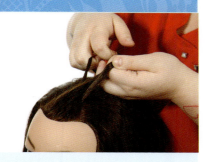

3 Do the same on the other side

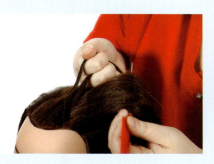

4 With the first part done, you now take an extra section on one side and join it in with the outer stem

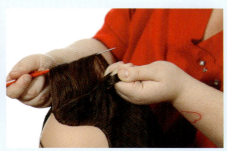

5 Do the same on the other side

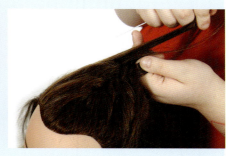

6 Continue the sequences 4 and 5 taking in a new section of hair from the hairline each time

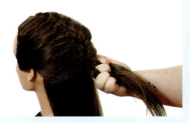

7 Your French plait will now form

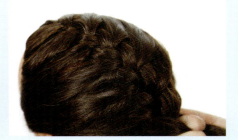

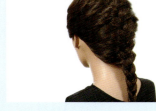

8 The finished effect

CourseMate video: French Plait

STEP-BY-STEP: FISHTAIL PLAITING

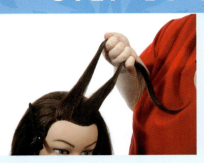

1 A fishtail plait differs from all the other plaiting techniques as it involves four stems and not three.

Start by separating the hair into two stems

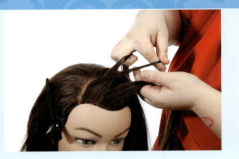

2 Whilst holding each stem in each hand, sub divide each one, taking the outer, narrower stem and passing it across the other and into the centre

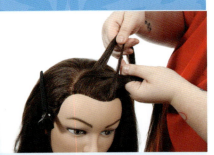

3 Do the same with the other side – sub-divide and pass the outer over and into the centre

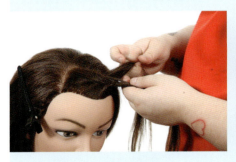

4 Repeat this movement and work down the hair length

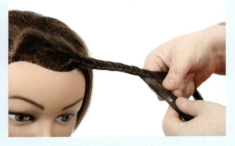

5 The fishtail now forms

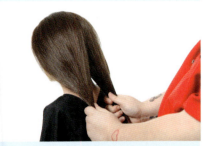

6 Now repeat the same sequence when done at the back of the hair

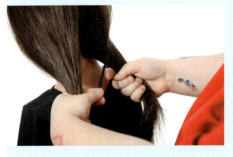

7 While holding each stem in each hand, sub-divide each one, taking the outer, narrower stem and passing it across the other and into the centre.

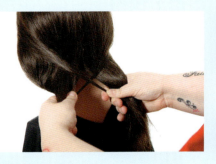

8 Do the same with the other side – sub divide and pass the outer over and into the centre.

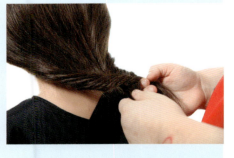

9 Repeat this movement and work down the hair length.

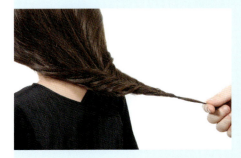

10 Finished effect

CourseMate video: Fish Tail Plait

Longer-lasting plaits and twists

Introduction Another popular effect is the **cornrow**. The cornrow is a type of three-stem plait that is secured close to the scalp to create head-hugging patterned designs.

'Cane rows', otherwise known as 'cornrows', are a technique that originated in Africa. Their ethnic origins have been a unique way of displaying hair art and design and have often incorporated complex patterns that historically indicated status or tribal connection. In fact, as this art form has been passed down by subsequent generations for thousands of years, it is quite probable that the very first hairdressers worked on these elaborate techniques, as it is unlikely that people could do these themselves.

Cornrows create design patterns across the scalp by working along predefined channels of hair. These channels are secured to the scalp by interlocking each of the three subdivided stems as the plaiting technique progresses.

TOP TIP

Hair products designed especially for these services are often very different to the everyday styling products you would use in other styling services. Use these products in line with manufacturers' instructions and be careful not to overload the hair during the styling process.

When the product has been applied to the hair it will be difficult to remove it without re-washing!

Short or even layered hair can be made to look longer still if hair is added, via extensions, during the process. The added hair is plaited into the style along each of the sections that create the plaited effect.

When cornrows have been applied to the hair the effect can last for up to six weeks or more before they should be removed. Advice should be given on handling and maintaining the hair although regular shampooing can still be carefully achieved.

Preparation for cornrows and twists Unlike loose plaits designed to last for just a day or so; the closer, tighter technique of plaiting lasts up to several weeks. Because of this you need to make sure that you cover all the aspects of durability, maintenance and expected results with the client from the outset. This type of work takes a lot longer than basic loose plaits, so make sure that you also give the client a good idea of the costs involved.

A thorough consultation for this type of work is essential. All of these intricately designed effects take a lot of time and you need to have a clear idea of what you are trying to achieve before you start. Plaiting and twisting involves some additional tension on the hair and this can put the client's hair roots under considerable excess stress. Our clients want their hair designs to be neat, controlled and easy to manage and to last for as long as possible. Because of this, it is very easy to cause **traction alopecia**.

As we noted earlier, traction alopecia is caused by the excessive and continuous strain put on the roots by hairstyled effects such as plaits and twists. You need to make sure that you ask the client throughout the service that the work that you are doing is comfortable and not pulling at different areas across the scalp.

You need to be able to recognize during consultation any previous signs of traction alopecia. The first indications of traction alopecia can be seen around the front hairline, often around the temples. This shows as an area of thinned or missing hair and if the condition is recent, it will be sore and tender.

Before any plaiting, twisting or weaved effects can be applied to the hair, you need to assess the suitability of this form of styling for the client.

Other factors affecting the service of plaited or twisted hairstyles

The following list provides you with a quick checklist of things that you should consider in addition to the normal consultation covered previously in this chapter

- ✓ Style terminology
- ✓ Style suitability
- ✓ Hair condition
- ✓ Hair length
- ✓ Removal of previous plaits or braids.

TOP TIP

Traction alopecia is a problem caused by hair tensioning. Hair is capable of sustaining its own weight and, within reason, a certain amount of mechanical wear and tear, such as brushing, combing and detangling knots. Any added hair is an extra weight or mass upon the hair roots and where extensions have been attached to small areas of the hair, thinning or baldness can occur!

Style terminology

This is an important aspect for client consultation. It is all too easy for the client to understand a technical term as meaning one thing, while you know it to mean something completely different. This communication aspect may seem rather basic, but it is still the single main reason why clients end up being dissatisfied with a service. It is always better to get down to basics; try to refrain from using clever technical terms. It might be appropriate with your colleagues as you speak the same language. But often the terms used by clients (wrongly) are words picked up from magazines, TV and other people, such as friends or work colleagues. Different people have different ways of saying things; a cornrow to one person could mean a Senegalese twist to another.

ACTIVITY

Create a portfolio of work

Finding ways to describe effects to clients is very difficult. You may have a clear idea of what you are trying to achieve, but can you convey that to your client before you start?

Complex work takes a lot of time and you can save yourself from dealing with a surprised, shocked or dissatisfied client by collecting a portfolio of elaborate work. When you see examples of different or complex effects, make sure that you keep them for a visual aid that you can use in consultation.

What will take you five minutes to cut and paste into a style book could save you a lot of time if you finish and have to start again.

These complex ways of styling hair involve a lot of work and take a lot of time. In most cases they would take considerable time to unravel and redress. So make sure that you both have a clear idea of what you are trying to achieve. Use visual aids; examples of pictures communicate effects that often cannot be put easily into words.

Style suitability

This is an important aspect of consultation. Any work that you are planning to do should be really thought through beforehand. If you were to do a full head of **scalp plaits**, would they suit the client's head and face shape? It may look elaborate when it's finished, it may impress other people, but you do need to ask yourself whether the style enhances the client and is an improvement on what they looked like before. All of this type of work takes a lot of time and when it's done well, the final effects are long-lasting too.

For more information on style suitability see Unit G7 Advise and consult with clients, pages 100–136.

Hair condition Test the hair for poor elasticity, look for damage or over-porous hair. Hair that is weakened for any reason is a contra-indication for plaiting or twisting. If the client is definitely intent on having some form of plait or twisted hair design work, think about recommending a course of **restructurants** or hair strengtheners beforehand.

Hair texture Hair texture is also a major consideration: if the hair is curly it will need smoothing or straightening first, so that the hair is easier to handle and to improve the final look of the designed work. Remember, hair curl patterns can vary across the scalp; some areas such as the lower nape may be tighter than other areas, so make sure that you check the hair and scalp all over.

Hair length This is an obvious consideration. Make sure that the hair is long enough to produce the effect that you want to achieve. If not, would the hair benefit from added hair extensions?

TOP TIP

Previous plaiting is difficult to remove. Make sure that you are careful and patient when you disentangle the hair. When plaits are removed you may also find that the scalp sheds a lot of dead skin cells. This is quite normal and shouldn't be mistaken for something more sinister. Scalp plaits can be washed, but the wearer seldom rubs them too much as they don't want to spoil the effects. This means that dead cells are locked in and cannot be shed in the normal way, over time. This is easily remedied when you cleanse and condition the hair thoroughly.

Removal of previous plaiting If the client needs their previous design work removed you should dissuade them from having a new set of plaits or twists put in straight away.

Extra care should always be taken when removing the old plaits, as the scalp may be quite tender, sensitive or even sore. Over time, products can build up around the scalp and this can bond the hair together making detangling quite difficult. In any event you will need patience and care to disentangle or unravel the hair, so that it is not weakened, broken or damaged any further.

Shampoo and condition the hair The hair must be shampooed and conditioned thoroughly before any plaiting or twisting service is done. You need to make sure that any traces of product – moisturizers, gels, serums and oils – are removed from the hair first.

Drying into shape Both plaiting and twisting techniques tend to make the hair appear shorter, as with plaits, much of this length is used laterally (across and around the head) as decoration. So you would need to blow-dry the hair first, to make the most of its overall length. This is necessary anyway, as the hair needs to be dried and made smoother before any other work can take place. After blow-drying, the hair and scalp can be prepared with hair oils or dressings. Any moisturizing will be beneficial to the hair, making it more elastic, improving its brittleness and making it more pliable.

Cornrows Cornrows are a type of scalp plait that creates linear designs across the head. They will last anything from one week to a couple of months; although with washing and general wear and tear they tend to look a little untidy after a couple of weeks. Cane rows create design patterns across the scalp by working along pre-defined channels of hair. These channels are secured to the scalp by interlocking each of the subdivided stems as the plaiting technique progresses.

Short or even layered hair can be made to look longer still by adding hair extensions to the client's hair during the process. The added hair is plaited into the style along each of the sections that create the braided effect.

Advice should be given on handling and maintaining the hair, although regular shampooing can still be carefully achieved. This type of work is ideal for natural hair as it can be worn with or without added hair extensions, even making short hair look long. They are easily removed, although the smaller the plait stems and sections the more difficult and fiddly it becomes.

STEP-BY-STEP: CORNROWING

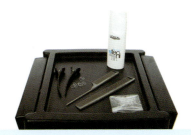

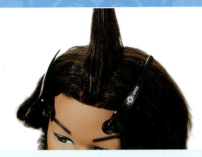

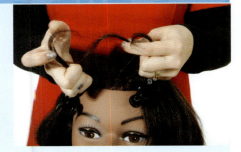

1 Prepare your trolley with:

1 Flat sectioning clips
2 A tail comb
3 A straight cutting comb
4 Braiding bands
5 Suitable styling products

2 Decide on the linear design that you want to create first, as this will have an impact on where you start.

Section off a channel of hair – the length of the scalp plait required. Section all the other hair out of the way with **flat clips**

3 Take a small section from the front and divide into three stems.

Cross-over the left and right stems, under the central one.

Move the outer left stem, over the central stem, now bring the right outer stem in and over the central stem

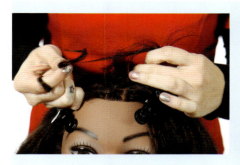

4 To progress along the scalp – pick up a small section and incorporate it into the left stem and again – Move the outer left stem, over the central stem, now bring the right outer stem in and over the central stem

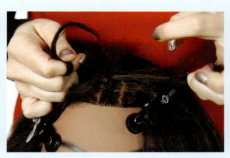

5 Repeat step 4 until you have worked along the scalp to the desired point

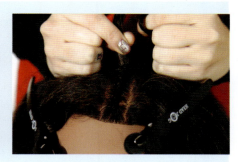

6 Remember to keep the plait taught with an even tension to avoid 'bagging'

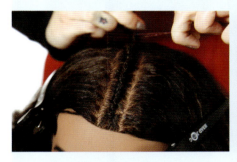

7 When you have reached the end of the plait, secure the remainder with a braiding band

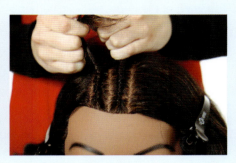

8 Complete the other cornrows in the same way

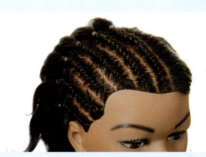

9 Final effect

TOP TIP

Added hair/extensions

There are many ways that you can incorporate added hair into a hairstyle:

1   It can be worked into the style during plaiting.
2   It can be knotted onto a single stem of a plait and form other stems of the plait as you work through the hair.
3   It can be twisted around natural hair and secured at the ends by tying with thread.

Method for adding hair into the cornrow The method for adding or extending the hair is similar to the above except that narrow strands of hair extensions are taken and added to take the place of the two outer sections, i.e. it is looped across the client's natural hair to create the first and third stem of the braid. Then as each time the outer braid introduces part of the client's hair, the added hair is secured down to the scalp.

Added hair or extension hair can be made from a variety of materials that can be natural or synthetic. They come in a variety of different textures, types and colours and can be added to the client's natural hair for a variety of different styling reasons. Subtle, harmonizing tones and textures can be added to make the client's own hair appear longer than it is. Conversely, bright fashion colour extensions can be added to create dramatic, contrasting effects.

Single plaits

Single plaits are a popular method of styling for men or women. They can be done on natural or chemically processed hair although the effects are more dramatic on longer hair. This doesn't mean that people with shorter hair can't have plaits; they are obvious candidates for extensions and added hair. Single plaits are quite durable and typically they will last for up to three months, but, like cane rows, their appearance deteriorates after a few weeks. The ends of the plaits should be secured with professional rubber bands.

Method for single plaits

1 Wash, condition and pre-dry the hair straight.

2 Starting at the nape, section the hair horizontally and secure the remainder.

3 Subdivide the horizontal section into small 1cm by 1cm square sections and separate into three equal stems.

4 Hold the first section between the middle and third finger of the left hand and the next, middle section between the index finger and thumb. Now take the last or third section between the middle and third finger of the right hand.

5 Continue to cross the outer stem on the left, over the centre stem, and then pass the outer stem on the right over what is now the centre stem.

6 Repeat this down to the ends of the hair and secure with a professional band.

7 Move to the next square section of hair and repeat steps 4–6.

8 Continue this by working up the back of the head, then to the lower sides and again up to the top of the head.

If added hair extensions are required, do the above steps 1 and 2 then at:

3 Subdivide the horizontal section into smaller square sections, then attach extension hair to each of the stems of the client's hair and plait as normal as a three-stem plait above.

Twisting techniques

Twists are an alternative to plaited styles; they will last for up to a month before they become untidy. Unlike plaits they don't involve any interlocking of hair, so they usually require an application of pomade or light styling gel to bond the hair while the twists are being formed.

Remember to use products sparingly though, as it would be easy to apply too much product, which would make the hair feel greasy or dirty and then it would have to be washed again.

Twisting is achieved by using the fingers or a comb to twist the hair into strands. This can be done in linear patterns along the scalp such as flat twists, or off the scalp as with single twists or two stem twists.

Method for creating a flat twist
Flat twists have a similar appearance at a distance to cornrows, but when you look more closely you can see that the hair isn't

interlocked in the same way. The durability of the effects depends upon the type of hair, but as a rule of thumb, twists don't last as long as cornrows. But on a positive note they don't take anything like the same amount of time to put in as tight, three-stem scalp plaits.

STEP-BY-STEP: TWISTING

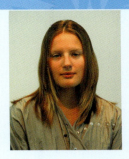

1 Shampoo, condition and dry the hair roughly into shape.

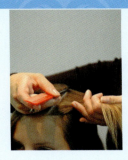

2 After brushing the hair to remove any tangles, start the style at the front by dividing the hair with a tail-comb.

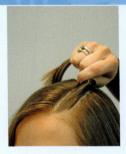

3 Twist the section of hair firmly but not too tightly back towards the crown area.

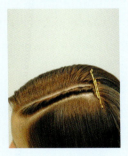

4 Grip the twisted section into place before starting the next channel.

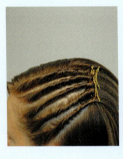

5 Continue with the same technique on each of the channels.

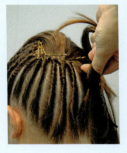

6 Twist the sections at the back from the nape up to the crown in the same way.

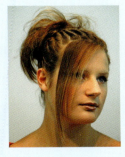

7 Leave a section at the front to soften the hairline profile. Lightly back-comb the remaining hair to finish.

Method for creating single twists

1 Wash, condition and towel-dry the hair.

2 Divide the hair into four quadrants and secure with sectioning clips.

3 Section off horizontally at the nape and secure the remainder out of the way.

4   Subdivide the horizontal sections into smaller areas of just a few millimetres across. (The smaller the sections the tidier the twist will look.)

5   Apply the gel or pomade throughout the length of the twist stem.

6   Place a tailcomb into the stem close to the root and start to turn in either a continuous clockwise (or anti-clockwise) movement. Work down the section of hair to the end.

7   Continue on to the next twist in the horizontal section and repeat steps 5 and 6.

8   Continue working up the head.

9   When all of the twists have been completed, arrange them neatly in the direction of the desired style and place under a dryer for 20–30 minutes.

10   When completely dry, apply product; either a spray fixative or serum to complete the look.

Method for creating two-stem twists

1   Wash, condition and towel-dry the hair.

2   Divide the hair into four quadrants and secure with sectioning clips.

3   Section off horizontally at the nape and secure the remainder out of the way.

4   Subdivide the horizontal sections into smaller areas of just a few millimetres across. (The smaller the sections the tidier the twist will look.)

5   Apply the gel or pomade throughout the length of the twist stem.

6   Subdivide the single stem, making two stems and start twisting left over right (or vice versa) and continue through the length of the hair.

7   Continue on to the next twist in the horizontal section and repeat steps 5 and 6.

8   Continue working up the head.

9   When all of the twists have been completed, arrange them neatly in the direction of the desired style and place under a dryer for 20–30 minutes.

10   When completely dry, apply product – either a spray fixative or serum – to complete the look.

TOP TIP

If hair is left in a plaited or twisted style for too long, the quality and condition of the hair can deteriorate. Here is a list of the potential effects:

◆ dryness and brittleness – the hair lacks moisture
◆ hair damage or breakage
◆ traction alopecia from constant root tension
◆ hair knotting or matted and impossible to remove without cutting
◆ scalp dryness and flaking.

Senegalese twists Senegalese twists are a scalp twist effect; they consist of stems of hair that are always twisted in the same direction with hair crossing over and creating a rope effect.

1   Wash, condition and pre-dry the hair smooth.

2   Section out a channel of hair with a tail comb to create the direction and the design required.

3   Using the fingers, start close to the root, take a small section of hair and twist it in a clockwise movement.

4   As you work along the channel pick up and work in more sections of hair to create the scalp twist effect.

5   When the channel of twisted hair is finished, secure until all of the others are finished.

6   The free ends of the twists can be interlocked together, and then after they have been dried under a dryer the effect can be thermally styled to complete the total effect.

Provide aftercare advice

Good service is supported through good advice and recommendation. The work that you do in the salon needs to be cared for at home by the client too. What would be the point of creating something if the client doesn't know how to achieve and/or maintain the same effects at home?

Home and aftercare checklist

✓   Talk through the style as you work; that way the client sees how you handle different aspects of the look.

✓   Show and recommend the products/equipment that you use so that the client gets the right things to enable them to get the same effects.

✓   Explain how routine styling with tongs or straighteners can have negative effects.

✓   Demonstrate the techniques that you use so they can achieve that salon hair look too.

✓   When you have put the client's hair up, or provided a plaited or twisted effect, give them advice on how to take the style down/remove the plaits or twists.

Talk through the style as you work

It's very difficult to do two things at the same time and you have probably found this yourself at work. Have you noticed how a senior stylist chats with the client whilst they are working? On the other hand, have you noticed the difference when a junior stylist is trying to do a similar technical piece of work? It seems to go very quiet!

The client probably notices this too; that's because a less confident stylist will always divert their attentions to the job in hand.

It's far easier to talk about the things that you are doing with the hair than to talk about the client's children at school, who may be taking their exams. Make a point of talking through your technique as you go. The benefits are twofold:

1 it eliminates long periods of silence whilst you are working and, more importantly,

2 it is really useful to the client as they get useful advice on how to recreate a similar effect at home.

So when you use a particular product, why not hand it to them so they can have a closer look. This way they get to see, smell and feel the product too and subconsciously this has a very powerful effect on them. By doing this you are involving the client in what you are doing by giving them a greater experience of the service. They will be able to see a direct link between what you are doing and the effects that you are achieving on their hair, with the added benefit of knowing that buying those particular products will help them to recreate a similar effect.

Explain how routine styling tools can have detrimental effects

Only hair in good condition is easy to maintain. You know how difficult it is to make dry, damaged hair look good. It tends to be lifeless, dull and sits there just like a wig! Your clients can recognize the difference between good and poor condition and given the choice, they will always choose hair that has lustre, shine, flexibility and strength.

With these known facts, you would be doing an injustice to your clients if you didn't warn them of the pitfalls of repeatedly using hot styling equipment, so make a point of asking them if they use them at home too. If they say that they use straighteners or tongs on a daily basis then tell them about the benefits of using heat protection sprays. Remember, the condition of their hair is directly proportional to the amount of heat applied to it. So if they are locked into using these styling tools their hair is going to need all the help it can get.

Demonstrate the techniques that you use
Clients want to be able to recreate the effects that you achieve in the salon and this is your chance to show them how to do it. Clients haven't had the benefit of your training; they don't know the little tricks and techniques that make it seem so simple. Show them how to do things; correct brushing, back-combing, twists or rolls. We have all seen the effects when these are not done properly, so make a point of giving them a few tips on how they can achieve a similar result.

Advise on how to take the style down
Damage occurs when the hair is mistreated and this is a simple fact that we all know. When hair is put up, it tends to use a lot of *scaffolding* in support. All that metal work in pins, grips, ornaments and accessories or even rubber hair bands can have a damaging effect on the hair if they are not handled and removed in the proper way.

Tell your clients where they need to start; most people try to feel around the back and take out the first grip or pin that they come to. That's not the way to do it. You know that if the innermost hair sections are pulled out first then it creates a big knot and then every thing just tangles together. If you were taking it down, you would start at the last area that was secured into place. Tell clients where they should start and the negative, damaging effects on their hair if they just pull the style apart.

Finally, tell your client about the things that they may need help with. If you are doing a bridal hair-up, then it might involve a headdress too. Many brides will wear one through the ceremony and the reception after, but want to remove this at some point later in the evening. If these accessories aren't removed carefully they could pull the whole hairstyle out of shape, therefore explain how they are positioned into the hair and the ways that they can be removed carefully without destroying the hairstyle.

TOP TIP

In shops, people are more likely to buy things that they have handled, so make a point of passing the products that you use to the client so that it initiates interest and discussion.

TOP TIP

The condition of the client's hair is directly proportional to the amount of heat applied to it, i.e. the greater the temperature the worse the hair will be.

SUMMARY

Remember to:

✓ prepare clients correctly for the services you are going to carry out

✓ put on the protective wear available for styling and dressing hair

✓ listen to the client's requirements and discuss suitable courses of action

✓ adhere to the safety factors when working on clients' hair

✓ keep the work areas clean, hygienic and free from hazards

✓ promote the range of services, products and treatments within the salon

✓ clean and sterilize the tools and equipment before they are used

✓ work carefully and methodically through the processes of setting and blow-drying hair

✓ place, position and direct the hair appropriately to achieve the desired effect

✓ tell the client what you are doing, keep them informed.

Knowledge Check

For this project you will need to gather information from a variety of sources.

Collect together photographs, digital images and magazine clippings about styling, blow-drying, setting and dressing techniques.

Include styles for long hair as well as short; for weddings, special occasions and casual wear.

In your portfolio describe:

◆ how the styles were achieved

◆ why each is suitable for its purpose

◆ the equipment (with examples) that was used to create the effects

◆ the products (with examples) used to help hold or define the effects.

ASSESSMENT OF KNOWLEDGE AND UNDERSTANDING

A selection of different types of questions to check your setting and dressing hair knowledge.

Q1 Self-cling rollers are commonly known as _____ rollers.   Fill in the blank

Q2 Humidity in the atmosphere will help to retain set hairstyles.   True or false

Q3 Which of the following dressings are traditionally long 'hair-up' styles?   Multi selection

Plaits	☐ 1
Knots	☐ 2
Weaves	☐ 3
Rolls	☐ 4
Braids	☐ 5
Pleats	☐ 6

Q4 The keratin bonds of stretched hair are said to be in the beta keratin state.   True or false

Q5   Which chemical bonds within the hair are *not* affected during setting?   Multi choice

Hydrogen bonds   O a

Disulphide bonds   O b

Salt bonds   O c

Oxygen bonds   O d

Q6   Heated rollers are a quick way of setting wet or dry hair in to style.   True or false

Q7   Hair set on rollers produces which of the following results and effects?   Multi selection

Increased body at the roots   ☐ 1

No body at the roots   ☐ 2

No movement at the ends   ☐ 3

Straighter effects   ☐ 4

Wavy effects   ☐ 5

Same as blow-dried effects   ☐ 6

Q8   On long hair, a ___ is a vertical fold, placed centrally at the back.   Fill in the blank

Q9   Which item of equipment would smooth and flatten frizzy, unruly hair best?   Multi choice

Curling tongs   O a

Ceramic straighteners   O b

Crimping irons   O c

Blow dryer   O d

Q10   'Hair-ups' are easier to perform on hair that has just been washed, conditioned and dried off.   True or false

11 Adding and extending hair

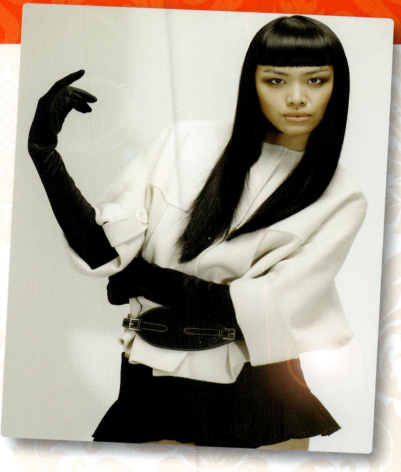

LEARNING OBJECTIVES

◆ Be able to use safe and effective methods of working

◆ Be able to plan and prepare hair attachments

◆ Be able to attach and blend pieces of hair

◆ Be able to remove hair pieces or hair attachments

◆ Be able to provide aftercare advice to clients

◆ Know how to perform tests for hair extensions

◆ Understand the factors that affect the hair, scalp and skin in relation to hair extension services

◆ Know how to prepare a client for hair extensions

◆ Understand how to use different hair attachment systems

◆ Know how to provide aftercare advice for clients

KEY TERM

clip-on extension

contra-indications

hair strengtheners

pre-bonded hot extension
   systems

restructurants

self-adhesive extension

skin sensitivities

traction alopecia

wefts

Unit title

GH15 Attach hair to enhance a style

Information covered in this chapter

◆ The different types of hair attachments and equipment that can be used

◆ How to apply hair extensions

◆ The things that you should look out for before conducting hair extension services

◆ How to safely remove extensions from the hair

◆ The advice you should give to clients for maintaining their hair

INTRODUCTION

Why are extension services so popular? The answer is fairly obvious, people choose hair extensions for a variety of immediate reasons:

◆ to make their hair longer than it already is

◆ to make their hair thicker than it is

◆ to add colours and colour effects to their natural hair.

So in a world where people no longer want to wait for hair to grow, it provides a quick, temporary solution to meet their needs.

The term hair extensions now covers a wide variety of natural and synthetic pre-formed and post-formed hair additions. They can be applied as single pieces that can be woven or bonded to the client's natural hair, as wefts that can be stitched, clipped or stuck to the client's hair, or as added fibres that are introduced to the client's hair, making the hair fuller and longer and providing a long-lasting effect.

Maintain effective and safe methods of working when attaching hair

You will be using two different types of hair extension at Level 2:

1   The first, a **clip-on extension** that is a quick and simple way of adding pre-coloured hair to create a new, generally longer hairstyle effect that will last for an event or an evening out.

2   The second, a **self-adhesive extension** that is pre-coloured with wefts of hair that have a sticky, peel-back strip, on double sided tape. These are positioned so that they stick to the hair, close to the scalp. The effects created will last longer (up to several weeks) but need careful removal by trained people using chemicals that unstick the **wefts** before they move too far away from the scalp as the hair continues to grow out.

Although Unit G20 covers much of the general aspects that you need to know about health, safety and hygiene within the salon environment, each technical hairdressing procedure you do has particular things that are relevant to health and safety.

A full head of hair extensions (even temporary ones) takes quite a long time to apply, so the main health and safety concerns should relate to the client's comfort, their positioning and their protection. Your posture, work accessibility and personal hygiene are equally important.

Therefore, many of the preparations that you should make regarding these issues are covered elsewhere, so in an attempt to reduce duplication and repetition, please note that some essential knowledge components are diverted to other locations.

Client preparation and protection

◆   Preparing, protecting and positioning the client (pages 140–141,166)

◆   Preparing and positioning the equipment ready for use (pages 20, 268–269)

◆   Working safely and preventing infections (pages 16, 270–271)

◆   Reducing risks – good salon safety and salon equipment (pages 6, 16)

◆   Personal health and hygiene (pages 16–18)

◆   Reducing risks – working with electricity (page 15)

Your preparation, protection and working position

See Unit GH10.1 Maintain effective and safe methods of working when styling and finishing hair (page164–194)

See Unit GH20 Make sure your own actions reduce risks to health and safety (pages 4–23)

Service timings

Different extension services take differing lengths of time; you need to be clear in your own mind how long these services take. For example, a partial head of clip-on wefts is going to take less time than a whole head of self-adhesive extensions. So therefore, the cost implications in relation to materials used, cost of labour and profit margin required by the salon will all vary considerably. You need to find out how much your salon charges for each type of service so that you can inform clients about the range of options available to them, prior to any consultation/examination taking place.

How long will it take? To get a rough idea of how long a hair extension service will take, you could time how long it takes to apply one extension then multiply that by the total amount that you will use to create the whole effect.

Synthetic (artificial hair) wefts

Most temporary hair extensions are made of 'man-made' fibres (acrylic and nylon) and need special care and handling. These types of extensions have specific advantages and disadvantages which are highlighted below and in the typical problems table at the end of this chapter.

See Select your material and prepare the hair for extensions on page 256 for more information.

Hair extension type	Advantages	Disadvantages
Clip-on synthetic wefts	Very easy and relatively quick to apply. Colours don't fade; they are pre-coloured in a variety of single or multi-toned effects. Can be shaped and cut easily to suit or achieve the desired effect. Bulk up fine hair, or hair that lacks volume. Can provide a quick, cost-effective solution to people who want longer hair. Can be removed at home with care providing the right advice has been given.	Needs careful handling, tends to get matted very easily. Needs to be brushed regularly when applied to avoid tangling. Avoid heat styling as all synthetic extensions are very susceptible to becoming misshapen or damaged when excess heat is applied. Can cause traction alopecia if incorrectly applied.
Self-adhesive wefts	Last for a long time with care and attention. Provide a cost-effective solution to the need for longer-lasting hair extensions. Far quicker to apply than single, **pre-bonded hot extension systems**. Colours don't fade; they are pre-coloured in a variety of single or multi-toned effects. Can be shaped and cut easily to suit or achieve the desired effect. Bulk up fine hair, or hair that lacks volume.	Need careful home maintenance so advice/products are essential to maintain the look. Need to be removed at the salon by trained staff. Avoid heat styling as all synthetic extensions are very susceptible to becoming misshapen or damaged after excess heat has been applied. Can cause traction alopecia if incorrectly applied.

TOP TIP

If they are looked after, some hair extensions such as clip-ons can be used again, whereas self-adhesive types can only be used once.

Plan and prepare to attach hair

It's not a positive thing to look for reasons why *not* to do something; but with hair extensions you really do have to find out if your client is suitable for the service.

Your client may be very keen to have them, but you need to safeguard the salon's good name and remove the possibility of legal action being taken at some later time, by making sure that you:

- ◆ conduct a thorough consultation with the client
- ◆ correctly identify any contra-indications to the extension service
- ◆ carry out the necessary tests upon the client
- ◆ ask the client the right sorts of questions
- ◆ record the responses that the client makes in answer to your questions
- ◆ clean and prepare the hair.

Consultation

You need to consider many things before you start the process of adding hair. It may be an exciting piece of work for you to do and make a long day much shorter; but remember, that's not the point. It's not worth doing unless it '*ticks all the boxes*' for the client too. Wanting hair extensions is not enough; they have to be suitable for the intended purpose/effect, appropriate to their needs and abilities and achievable in the light of any **contra-indications**.

Style suitability

This is an important aspect of consultation. Any work that you are planning to do should be really thought through beforehand. When you add hair to the client's existing hair it will change the appearance dramatically, by making the roots a lot fuller than they were to start with. You need to make this clear to the client beforehand as it is very difficult for anyone to visualize what the difference will be after the service is finished.

Similarly, if you were to do a full head of hair extensions, will they still suit the client's head and face shape afterwards? It may be a very professional application when it's finished, it may impress many other people, but you do need to ask yourself whether the style enhances the client and is it an improvement on what they looked like before.

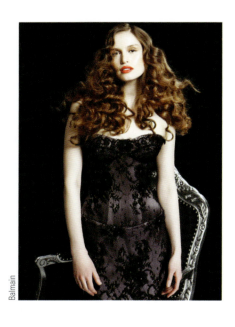

Balmain

Hair condition

Test the hair for elasticity strength and sustainability and look for damage or over-porous hair.

Hair that is weakened for any reason is a contra-indication for hair extensions. If the client is definitely intent on having extensions, think about recommending a course of **restructurants** or **hair strengtheners** beforehand.

Hair tendency

This is also a major consideration: if the hair is curly it may need smoothing or straightening first, but remember when the hair is washed it will revert back to its natural state and this may look very strange if the hair extensions don't match the rest of the natural tendency.

Hair density

The amount of natural hair will affect the choice of extension and the amount needed to provide an overall balanced result.

Hair styling

It is unlikely that new wefts of hair can be applied without any form of styling or cutting after the application. The wefts are not the hairstyle themselves; they are the material that you add in order to create a new style afterwards.

Make this clear to the client from the outset; you will need to adapt the newly applied lengths to suit both the natural fall and abundance of the hair as well as the client.

Cutting into newly applied lengths of hair can be quite shocking to clients as they see this as the core of what they are paying for. You need to be reassuring in the course of action that you take; if you need to do a lot of cutting, explain why.

Face and head shapes

Style suitability is about balance and proportion, so you need to take the client's physical features into consideration during the consultation.

TOP TIP

Any hair extensions work takes a lot of time and when it's done well, the final effects can be long-lasting too.

The basic principles of how these apply is covered in Unit G7 Advise and consult with clients, and a further aesthetic evaluation can be seen in Unit GH11 Physical features – style suitability, on pages 126–128, 170, 227.

The principles applied to hair-ups can be used here although the considerations applicable to hair extensions are more to do with adding width and height.

ACTIVITY

Preparing for hair extensions

Complete this table by filling in the missing information. Review this chapter again if you need to find out more.

Preparation	What do you need to do?	What things do you need to look out for?
Styling tools		
The client		
Yourself		
Clip-on extensions		
Self-adhesive extensions		

> ### TOP TIP
>
> Traction alopecia is a problem caused by hair tensioning.
>
> Hair is capable of sustaining its own weight and, within reason, a certain amount of mechanical wear and tear, such as brushing, combing and detangling knots. Any added hair is an extra weight or mass upon the hair roots and where extensions have been attached to small areas of the hair, thinning or baldness can occur!
>
> You should explain this to the client during your consultation.

Looking for contra-indications to hair extension services

One of the more serious after-effects of wearing hair extensions is **traction alopecia**. This occurs when a constant pressure, resulting from wearing hair tied up or adding weight from hair extensions, is exerted upon the roots of the hair. This can result in hair loss in patches upon the scalp showing as baldness and is particularly obvious in areas of weaker hair such as the temples or hairlines.

If your client hasn't had hair extensions before, they could still suffer with traction alopecia, as this is the result of any hair tensioning styling effect. But make a point of visually inspecting the scalp to look for the signs.

Skin sensitivity

This is another consideration. You should ask the client if they have any sensitivity issues relating to product intolerances or to synthetic materials. Not everyone is comfortable with wearing hair attachments; some people don't like the added weight caused by added hair pieces and headaches can be caused by the constant pressure formed at the roots by wearing extensions. Similarly, the amount of added synthetic material can slow down the ventilation to the scalp, causing the head to get hotter and sweat or simply feel generally uncomfortable. This effect is similar to that of wearing synthetic fabrics over the body; not everyone can do this and many people, given the choice, prefer to wear natural fibres.

Allergies

This is not to be mixed up with **skin sensitivities**. Someone may have a sensitivity to certain things but it doesn't mean that they are allergic to them, the allergic reaction is something quite different and, potentially, far more dangerous. It is unlikely that a client would be allergic to synthetic hair; but it is quite possible that they might be allergic to the chemicals that you would use to maintain the looks or to remove long-lasting hair extensions at some later time.

Again ask the client if they have any known allergies to certain products or chemicals.

Hair and scalp disorders

Look for the obvious signs that something is wrong. Hair loss, general thinning, hair damage, weakened hair, infestations and scalp infections are all contra-indications. If you are not sure, then ask someone in authority with more experience for a second opinion.

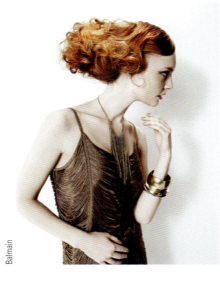
Balmain

Medical advice

If you are unsure of any indicators that you see or hear of, from asking the client questions, then the service must be postponed at least until the client has sought medical advice.

Carry out the necessary tests

Even if you have no reasons so far not to carry out the extensions service, you must still do a few tests before carrying out the service. First of all think about the type of extension service that you are going to offer.

Clip-on hair extensions You need to check the hair's strength and elasticity to make sure that the added weight to the hair doesn't create a pressure and tension that the hair will not be able to sustain and hence cause damage or breakage.

Self-stick extensions In addition to a pull test and an elasticity test you should also do a skin test with the removal chemicals that you will be using in several weeks' time. There is no point in applying the extensions if they cannot safely be removed at some later time.

Asking the client the right questions

You cannot find out enough information about the client by examination alone. In addition to the questions you should ask covering the previous aspects, you need to find out whether the client has had an extensions service before and whether they had any problems with them.

Ask the client how they intend to manage their hair themselves, as if they have had extensions before, they may have covered many of the pitfalls that others tend to find difficult. Most of the difficulties that clients encounter are to do with having more hair than they have been used to before. People don't like to change their habits; the ways in which they use products and equipment have to change if they want to maintain their hair in looking its best and you have an obligation to give them the benefit of your professional opinion.

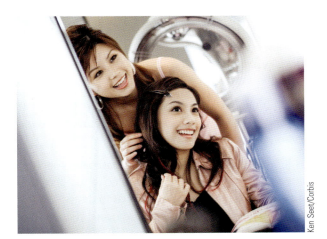

Ken Seet/Corbis

TOP TIP

Too much weight upon the hair will result in traction alopecia, hair damage or breakage!

See Unit G7 Advise and consult with clients for more information about conducting tests and testing (pages 100–136).

Record the client's responses Make sure that you record the responses to the questions that you ask as well as the details of the tests that you perform. Update the client's record card in full and immediately after you have done the test.

Don't leave it until later, you might forget! These records are essential information that will be needed again and help to show that a competent service has been provided at that time.

This would be vitally important if there was a problem at some later stage, particularly if something went wrong and it involved any legal action taken against the salon.

BEST PRACTICE

Record the client's responses to your questions and the comments about how the results of any tests affected their hair and skin.

If you are not sure about the results of any tests that you perform, ask a senior member of staff for their second opinion.

ACTIVITY

Hair tests for extensions

Complete this activity by filling in the missing information in the spaces provided

Type of test	What is the purpose of the test?	How is the test carried out?
Elasticity test		
Pull test		
Skin test		

Prepare the hair for extensions

After conducting your consultation, you need to select the appropriate extensions.

Both clip-on and self-adhesive wefts are available in a range of natural and vivid fashion shades. You will have found out during your consultation what result the client is expecting. Do they want strong colour contrasting effects that will obviously stand out from their own hair, or do they want it to match their natural hair to give a new longer effect? After selecting your colour, you need to work out how much material you will need.

Hair extensions are applied to a point that will create a horseshoe section around the head at the temples. If you continue further up than this they will stick out from the head too much and show.

So, generally speaking for a complete head of self-adhering extensions you would need three or four wefts on both sides and five to seven at the back. This, making a total of around 11–15, would be enough although some thicker densities could take even more. As clip-on extensions can be more bulky because of the comb/clip attachments you may need fewer as they will stick out at the sides.

Before continuing with the application you should wash, condition and dry the hair into style. This is particularly important for longer-lasting extensions as this could be the last time the scalp would get a good rubbing to remove dead skin cells for some time.

When hair extensions have been left in for some time it is quite normal to see dandruff forming at or near the scalp. This is because it is very difficult to remove the shedding layers of the epidermis when the extensions attachments are so close to the scalp. This is easily removed by washing after the extensions have been removed. (Explain this to the client so that any shocks later are avoided and they know that this is a normal expectation for this type of service.)

BEST PRACTICE

Handle the synthetic wefts of hair with care, they can become easily matted or tangled; always hold them by the bonded end, allowing the free hair ends to fall naturally. Comb or brush carefully to keep them smooth.

BEST PRACTICE

Always follow the manufacturer's instructions for preparing, handling and applying hair extensions to hair.

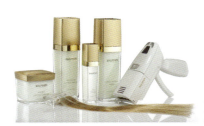

ACTIVITY

Practise the techniques

You will not be able to jump straight in and complete a full head of self-adhesive extensions without having seen how they work and can be adapted to different hair types and lengths.

Get used to working with extensions before carrying out the service on your clients; practise the tensioning and application on modelling blocks beforehand. This will get you up to speed with the placement, timings and dressing of the hair, well before trying it out live!

Attach and blend pieces of hair

Step-by-step: Technique for adding clip-on extensions

1 Starting at the lower nape, section off the hair into neat areas, securing the lengths out of the way.

2 Back-comb the section near the root to provide an area for the clip-on extension to bond to. Apply a little hairspray to help fix the hair.

3 Select your extension, making sure that the hair is free from tangles and that the snap-in clips are open and ready to use.

4 Clip-on the extension along the weft and into the back-combed section of hair. Snap the clips closed to lock into place.

5 Continue the steps 2–4 around the head until you reach a point near to the temple area.

6 Drop the upper section over the extensions and style to create the finished effect.

TOP TIP

Hair extensions will often need some form of trimming or styling too, so practise this part of the service after you have applied them.

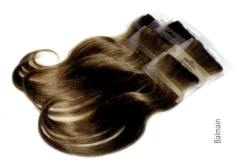

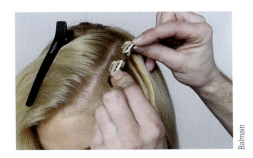

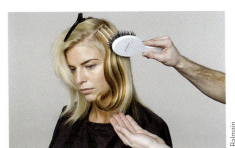

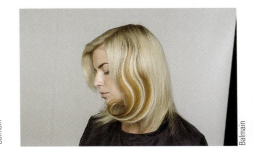

STEP-BY-STEP: ADDING SELF-ADHESIVE HAIR EXTENSIONS

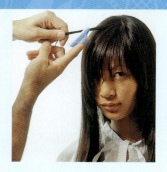

1 Preparing the natural hair. Taper the hair using thinning scissors to soften the edges and use a finger razor to flat taper the fringe area and remove any straight blunt cut lines so that the fibre will blend with the natural hair.

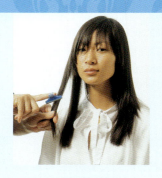

2 Preparing the natural hair.

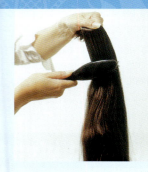

3 Mega-mixing the extension hair colours together.

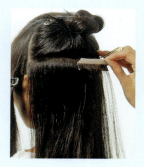

4 The wefts are applied. The practitioner uses a hair parting tool on her finger to help take straight clean sections of hair. The weft is measured to the same width as the hair section and cut to size using an old pair of hairdressing scissors.

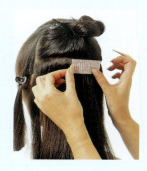

5 Apply the weft directly onto the natural hair.

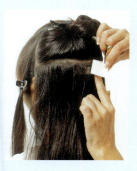

6 Applying the extension hair.

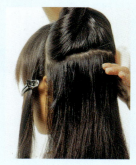

7 Take a fine section of natural hair (about ¼ cm) above the tape and drop it down over the tape, pressing the natural hair to the topside of the tape to ensure that the weft is secure and that the tape is undetectable. Follow the same procedure in steps 2, 3 and 4, before placing the titian highlights into areas 5 and 6.

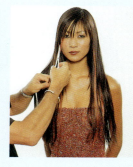

8 The titian fibre is applied by cutting 1cm square sections of the tape and placing it visually.

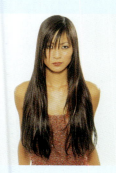

9 Final effect

Special note: Be careful to maintain an even tension when you take down each section of hair and place it onto the self-adhering strip. You can only position the weft once, as when it has adhered to the hair, you won't be able to remove and reposition it again!

A successful extension service must position the wefts as close to the roots as possible, any slack areas will cause the effect to either fail prematurely or to become unmanageable for the client at home.

Caution: If you use heated styling equipment to finish the effect, make sure that you don't apply any excessive heat to the hair extensions. They will distort, get matted and unmanageable or melt!

Final shaping and styling

The reason why clients have extensions is because they want their hair to appear longer and/or thicker; but sometimes the effect created by the extensions is then out of balance with the remainder of their own hair and needs further work.

So after applying the extensions and finish to the hair you should show the client the effect to see if it compares with what they expected.

In nine cases out of ten the client will be thrilled at the quick results of added length and the job is done. However, there will be the odd occasion where the added length seems disproportionate with the rest of the client's hair, or they have stray ends that need tidying up. In either event, you need to do some freehand cutting or trimming to finish the effect.

> **TOP TIP**
>
> You can't cut hair extensions into layered effects very easily as the sections are difficult to hold. If you do need to cut the added hair afterwards, always finish off the effects by freehand cutting.

> **TOP TIP**
>
> Before you do any cutting after the extensions have been applied, show the client the different types of perimeter shapes that can be achieved, so that they can choose between solid or shattered outline effects.

See Unit GH12 Cut hair using basic techniques, for more information.

ACTIVITY

Revision questions

Each hairdressing service has its own particular aspects that need care and thought. The questions below will help you to focus upon the things that you need to know about attaching hair ends that need tidying up. In either event, you need to do some freehand cutting or trimming to finish the effect.

1. Why do you need to do a consultation beforehand?
2. What sorts of things would be contra-indications to this service?
3. Why does tension and positioning make a big difference to the attachment techniques?
4. Why do you need to do a skin test for attaching self-adhesive extensions?
5. What has traction alopecia got to do with hair extensions?
6. What sorts of advice should you give the client?
7. What things can you do with natural hair that you can't with artificial/synthetic hair?

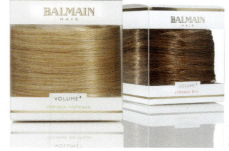

Balmain

Remove pieces of hair

Clip-on extensions

Clip-on hair extensions can, with care, be removed by the client themselves. So you need to show them how they are attached and how the clips snap into position. Explain to them how they should be removed carefully and how this will prevent any lasting damage to their hair.

Self-adhesive extensions

The amount of time that hair extensions last is difficult to estimate. The durability of the effect is always directly proportionate to the handling and care that the client provides themself. So with this in mind a client can be told that they can expect them to last up to a certain point; then after this they must be removed so that they don't become too difficult to manage or cause any longer-lasting damage to the hair.

Unlike clip-on extensions, the self-adhesive type need to be removed professionally, with a revisit to the salon.

You need to make this clear to the client right from the start. At the point where the hair with the attached extension has grown more than 1cm away from the root area (which is approximately four weeks) the hair will start to become harder to manage. It will be more difficult to shampoo as rubbing will work the edges of the extension away from the hair. Brushing/combing will be more problematic as the hair will keep snagging and tangling on the bristles or teeth. At the point when this starts to happen, the extensions must be removed; even if a new set is to be applied.

Self-adhesive extensions use special chemical sprays or solutions to dissolve the bond attaching them to the hair. When this is applied/sprayed on to the self-cling tape it quickly reduces the adhesion and therefore releases the weft from the hair. The removed weft can then be inspected to see if it is worth keeping or whether it should be thrown away.

ACTIVITY

Create a style portfolio

The effects that are created by the addition of hair extensions aren't necessarily obvious to the untrained eye. Therefore you would be better off using visual aids that show hair with extensions rather than not.

Your clients would like to see effects that can be created for them and the most obvious way that you can do this is by developing a portfolio of the work and effects that your salon can do and provide as a service.

Start by collecting a number of pictures that show this type of work. You can then, over time, add to this by taking pictures of work that you have completed in the salon.

The self-adhesive strips can be removed from the weft in the same way that the extension is removed from the hair and, depending on its quality, the weft can be washed, re-conditioned and retained for future use, or discarded. If the weft is to be reused, new, double-sided self-adhesive tapes will need to be applied after the wefts have been dried.

STEP-BY-STEP: REMOVING SELF-ADHERING EXTENSIONS FROM DRY HAIR

Hair by Theresa Bullock, photography by Ozzie Rizzo

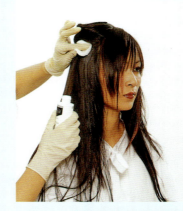

1 Pour a small amount of the removal solution onto a cotton wool pad. Wipe the top side of the tape near the root area then lift the tape weft and wipe the underside of the weft.

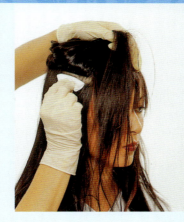

2 Allow the removal solution to penetrate for 30 seconds to one minute.

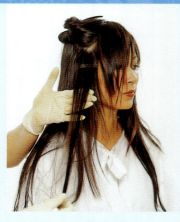

3 Hold the end of the extension hair contained in the tape and gently pull it away from the hair and scalp. The weft comes away easily from the natural hair in a matter of seconds.

Finally

The hair and scalp should be shampooed and conditioned thoroughly and carefully to remove any dead skin cells or product build-up. It can then be dried in preparation for other salon services.

Provide aftercare advice

The durability and the quality of your client's new hair extensions are dependent upon the information and advice that you provide to the client. If clients aren't given the right or sufficient information on how they can handle their hair afterwards then the effect won't be very successful or won't last very long.

Typical problems with artificial/synthetic hair extensions

Problem	Advice to give
Hair extensions tend to tangle or get knotted easily	Suggest suitable products and tools that will help to make grooming and brushing easier.
	Explain that the longer lengths should always be combed from points to roots. Long hair and particularly synthetic hair needs to be disentangled by working and freeing-up from the ends back through the lengths towards the bonded area of the weft with a wide-tooth comb rather than a brush.
Hair lengths tend to get matted when they are shampooed	Suggest conditioning products that are designed to work on synthetic/artificial hair. Sometimes the conditioners for acrylic hair are best applied before the hair is wetted; this reduces the locking and matting result caused by the action of rubbing during shampooing.
	Suggest that the hair is shampooed in a different way along the lengths by a smoothing action, rather than rubbing at the scalp.

Problem	Advice to give
Longer lengths get matted or knotted during sleep/overnight	People who are more restless during sleep may find that the rubbing action of the hair on the pillow makes the extensions lock together overnight. Suggest tying the hair in a ponytail with a soft fabric ribbon; this reduces the movement and the effects caused by chafing on the pillow. Alternatively, if the hair is very long, you can advise wrapping the hair in a silken scarf. This holds the lengths together and stops any chance of knotting.
Hair gets in the way at work or in sport	Clients who are used to shorter hair will not be familiar with the problems associated with long hair. Explain the benefits of wearing hair up as opposed to down during work/sport as this may have a more professional or beneficial effect.
Limited styling options after extensions have been applied	When artificial extensions have been applied to the hair, the options available to the client for future styling/finishing in other ways are limited. Synthetic hair does not respond well to hot styling, the hair can't be moulded or shaped in the same ways that you would style natural hair. You must make the client aware of this from the outset. Any excess heat applied to the hair will cause it to distort, matt together or melt. When this occurs, the only course of action is to cut the damaged lengths off, or to remove them altogether! This can be avoided as long as you point out the problems before the client leaves the salon.

Home-aftercare checklist

✓ Talk through the style as you work; that way the client sees how you handle different aspects of the look.

✓ Show and recommend the products/equipment that you use so that the client gets the right things to enable them to achieve the same effects.

✓ Explain how routine styling with blow-dryers, heated tongs or straighteners can have detrimental effects on hair extensions.

✓ Demonstrate the techniques that you use so they can achieve that salon hair look too.

✓ If you use clip-on extensions give the client the advice on how to take the extensions out safely without causing damage to the hair.

✓ Tell the client how long the extensions are likely to last.

For more information about the advice to give clients about aftercare see Unit G7 Advise and consult with clients.

SUMMARY

Remember to:

✓ prepare clients correctly for the services you are going to carry out

✓ put on the protective wear available for attaching hair

✓ listen to the client's requirements and discuss suitable styling options

✓ adhere to the safety factors when working on clients' hair

✓ keep the work areas clean, hygienic and free from hazards

✓ promote the range of services, products and treatments within the salon

✓ clean and sterilize the tools and equipment before they are used

✓ work carefully and methodically through the processes of attaching hair

✓ place, position and tension the hair correctly when attaching extensions

✓ tell the client what you are doing, keep them informed.

Knowledge Check

For this project you will need to gather information from different sources.

Collect photos, digital images or magazine cuttings for different hair extension types. Include different looks for both longer and shorter hair for the following occasions:

A. weddings

B. parties

C. general going out.

In your portfolio describe:

◆ how the styles were achieved

◆ why each is suitable for its purpose

◆ the type of extension that was used to create each effect.

ASSESSMENT OF KNOWLEDGE AND UNDERSTANDING

A selection of different types of questions to check your knowledge about extensions

Q1 Hair extensions can either be natural hair or _____ made fibres. Fill in the blank

Q2 Synthetic/artificial hair can be styled with tongs and straightening irons. True or false

Q3 What sorts of attachment are used for temporary hair extensions? Multi selection

Hot bonding	☐	1
Cold bonding	☐	2
Clips	☐	3
Self-adhesive strips	☐	4
Glue	☐	5
Cement	☐	6

Q4   Hot bonded extensions are permanent.   True or false

Q5   Which type of extension is suitable for a single event or 24 hours?   Multi choice

Clip-on extension	○ a
Glued-on extension	○ b
Plaited extension	○ c
Self-adhesive extension	○ d

Q6   Clip-on extensions are a quick way of making hair appear fuller/longer than it is.   True or false

Q7   To what positions are hair extensions normally affixed so that they can blend with the client's own hair?   Multi selection

On the ends of the hair	☐ 1
Near the roots of the hair	☐ 2
At the crown of the head	☐ 3
Over the top of the head	☐ 4
In areas lower than the temples	☐ 5
In areas lower than the ears	☐ 6

Q8   Hair extensions are pre-bonded _____ of either natural or artificial hair.   Fill in the blank

Q9   Which item of equipment would smooth and flatten frizzy, unruly hair before attaching hair extensions?   Multi choice

Curling tongs	○ a
Ceramic straighteners	○ b
Crimping irons	○ c
Blow-dryer	○ d

Q10   Hair extensions cannot be worn up after they have been attached to the hair.   True or false

12 Cutting hair

LEARNING OBJECTIVES

◆ Be able to maintain safe methods of working

◆ Be able to cut hair to achieve a variety of looks

◆ Know how to work safely, effectively and hygienically

◆ Understand the factors that can affect the service

◆ Understand one length, graduation, reverse graduation and uniform layering cutting techniques

◆ Understand the aftercare advice that you should provide to clients

KEY TERMS

autoclave

Barbicide™

clipper over comb

club cutting

cowlick

cross-check

double crown

freehand cutting

hair growth patterns

nape whorl

sharps

point cutting

re-shape

re-style

reverse graduation

scissor over comb

UV cabinet

widow's peak

Unit title

GH12 Cut hair using basic techniques

Information covered in this chapter

◆ The tools and equipment used during cutting, and how they are maintained

◆ The factors that influence hair cutting options

◆ The factors that control cutting accuracy and quality

◆ One length, graduation, reverse graduation and uniform layering cutting techniques

◆ The aftercare advice that you should give

INTRODUCTION

Cutting at Level 2 requires the student to learn four basic cutting methods and the final, perimeter outlines that they create.

The basic cuts are:

1 One length cut

2 Uniform layering

3 Graduation

4 Reverse graduation

When you have mastered the basics, you will be able to combine these techniques to create all sorts of hairstyles for your clients. It may take some time for you to 'grasp' these essential factors, but when you have, the limits are boundless.

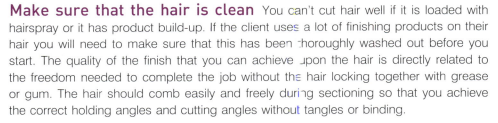

Maintain effective and safe methods of working when cutting hair

Preparation and maintenance

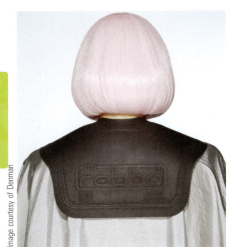

Image courtesy of Denman

Preparing the client Your salon has its own policy and codes of practice for preparing clients and you must observe these. Some things are general common sense and courtesy, whereas others are client or salon specific. But at the very least your salon will have a procedure for gowning and protecting the client from spillages or hair clippings, methods for preparing tools and equipment and the expectations for personal standards in relation to technical ability and hygiene.

You may be an experienced operator but don't forget the basics.

Above all you do need to remember the client's personal comfort and safety throughout the salon visit, i.e. cover the client with a clean, laundered gown and place a cutting collar around the shoulders.

Make sure that the gown is on properly and fastened around the neck. It should cover and protect their clothes and come up high enough to cover collars and necklines. Don't make the fastening too tight, but it should be close enough at least to protect the client's clothes and stop hair clippings from going down their neck which is both uncomfortable whilst they are in the salon and irritating if they are returning to work or doing things for the rest of the day.

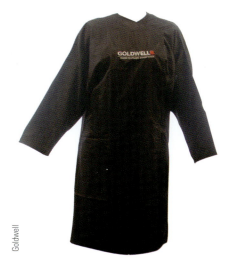

Goldwell

Make sure that the hair is clean You can't cut hair well if it is loaded with hairspray or it has product build-up. If the client uses a lot of finishing products on their hair you will need to make sure that this has been thoroughly washed out before you start. The quality of the finish that you can achieve upon the hair is directly related to the freedom needed to complete the job without the hair locking together with grease or gum. The hair should comb easily and freely during sectioning so that you achieve the correct holding angles and cutting angles without tangles or binding.

Check the client's hair after washing too. If the hair hasn't been rinsed thoroughly and still has lather or conditioner in it, you won't be able to see the natural fall of the hair and this could cause you to miss significant factors.

Adjust the working position and height Client positioning has a lot to do with your safety too. If a client is slouched in the chair, they are a danger not only to themselves but to you too as they will put unnecessary pressure on the spine and you will not be able to stand up properly, causing fatigue or risk of injury from poor posture.

Client comfort should extend to the point where it makes the salon visit a welcome and pleasurable experience. They shouldn't clutter the floor around the styling chair with bags, magazines and shopping. Anything that can safely be stored away should be: it is not only a distraction, it's a safety hazard too.

Salon chairs are designed with comfort and safety in mind; your client should be seated with their back flat against the back of the chair, their legs uncrossed and the chair at a height at which it is comfortable for you to work. You need to be able to get to all parts of the head, so the chair's height should be adjusted to suit the particular height of the client. Don't be afraid of asking the client to sit up: it is in their best interest too!

Position in relation to mirror

The positioning of the client in front of the mirror is very important. The angle of the head should be perpendicular to the mirror and the seated position or the line and balance of the haircut will be effected.

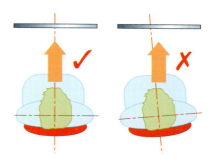

Many salon workstations have built-in foot rests and there are good reasons for this. The foot rest:

1 is there to improve the comfort for the seated client at any cutting height

2 helps balance the client and encourages them to sit squarely in front of the mirror

3 tries to discourage the client from sitting cross-legged

4 promotes better posture by making the client sit back properly with their back flat against the back of the chair.

All of the above factors are critical for you and the client in ensuring their comfort throughout, and that you are not hindered in doing your task. For example, if your client sits with crossed legs, it will alter the horizontal plane of their shoulders and this will make your job of trying to get even and level baselines more difficult.

Rough-dry the hair so that you work only with damp hair throughout the cut.

Dry off the client's hair so that they are not sitting with saturated hair, it is uncomfortable for them as wet hair soon feels cold even if it doesn't drip onto the gown and their clothes. During cutting, having the hair pre-dried allows the natural tendencies, movements and growth directions of the hair to be seen. This is extremely important for cutting, as the wave movement and hair growth patterns are all being considered as the style develops.

Your personal hygiene Personal hygiene can't be stressed enough; it is vitally important for anyone working in personal services.

Preparing the tools and equipment Get your own scissors, clippers, combs and sectioning clips ready beforehand; that doesn't mean as the client arrives in the chair from the basin! You must be prepared; your tools and equipment must be hygienically clean, sterilized and safe to use. You would have needed to have removed your combs from the **Barbicide**™ or **UV cabinet** before use. Items in the Barbicide™ jar would be rinsed and dried and put near to your workstation. All cutting tools would need to be checked and maintained on a daily basis.

Plastic and rubber cutting accessories

◆ Never use dirty or damaged tools. Germs can breed in the crevices and corners and can cross-infect other clients.

◆ Clean or wipe all tools before disinfecting or sterilizing.

◆ Cutting collars should be washed and dried before use.

Other metal cutting tools

◆ Some disinfectants can corrode metal and blunt edges. Check the manufacturer's instructions before using them.

◆ If corrosion or rusting occurs the equipment is rendered unsafe. Always make sure that this doesn't happen.

◆ Take special care when cleaning and lubricating scissors.

◆ All electrical repairs should be carried out by professional people. Do not attempt to undertake them yourself.

TOP TIP

Always dry the client's hair well to remove the excess water before cutting, blow-drying or finger-drying.

For more information on this topic see Unit G20 'Make sure your actions reduce risks to health and safety'.

ACTIVITY

What is your salon's policy for the disposal of sharps?

Contact your local council offices' environmental health department for more information.

HEALTH & SAFETY

Disposal of sharp items

Used razor blades and similar items should be placed into a safe container ('sharps box'). When the container is full it can be disposed of correctly. This type of salon waste should be kept away from general salon waste as special disposal arrangements may be provided by your local authority.

TOP TIP

Hair science: did you know

We all carry large numbers of micro-organisms inside us, on our skin and in our hair. These organisms, such as bacteria, fungi and viruses, are too small to be seen with the naked eye. Bacteria and fungi can be seen through a microscope, but viruses are too small even for that.

Many micro-organisms are quite harmless, but some can cause disease. Those that are harmful to people are called pathogens. Flu and cold sores for example are caused by a virus, thrush and athletes foot by a fungus and bronchitis often by bacteria. Conditions like these, which can be transmitted from one person to another, are said to be infectious.

The body is naturally resistant to infection; it can fight most pathogens using its inbuilt immunity system, so it is possible to be infected with pathogenic organisms without contracting the disease. When you have a disease, the symptoms are the visible signs that something is wrong. They are the results of the infection and of the reactions of the body to that infection. Symptoms help you to recognize the disease.

Infectious diseases should always be treated by a doctor. Non-infectious conditions and defects can be treated with products available from the chemist.

Preventing infection

A warm, humid salon can offer a perfect home for disease-carrying bacteria. If they can find food in the form of dust and dirt, they may reproduce rapidly. Good ventilation, however, provides a circulating air current that will help to prevent their growth. This is why it is important to keep the salon clean, dry and well aired at all times. This includes clothing, work areas, tools and all equipment. Every salon uses some form of sterilizing device as a means of providing hygienically safe work implements.

Sterilization means the complete eradication of living organisms. Different devices use different sterilization methods, which may be based on the use of heat, radiation or chemicals.

Ultraviolet radiation Ultraviolet radiation cabinets may be utilized to store previously sterilized/disinfected tools and equipment.

Chemical sterilization/disinfectants Chemical sterilizers should be handled only with suitable personal protective equipment, as many of the solutions used are hazardous to health and should not come into contact with the skin. The most effective form of salon disinfectant is achieved by the total immersion of the contaminated implements into a jar of fluid such as Barbicide™.

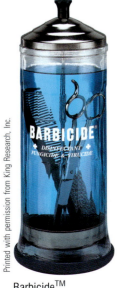

Barbicide™

Autoclave The **autoclave** provides a very efficient way of sterilizing using heat. It is particularly good for metal tools, although the high temperatures are not suitable for plastics such as brushes and combs. Items placed in the autoclave take around 20 minutes to sterilize (check with manufacturer's instructions for variations).

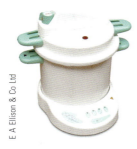

E A Ellison & Co Ltd

Autoclave

Your working position and posture

The client's position and height from the floor have a direct effect on your posture too. You must be able to work in a position where you do not have to bend 'doubled up' to do your work. Cutting involves a lot of arm and hand movements and you need to be able to get your hands and fingers into positions where you can cut the hair unencumbered, without bad posture:

1 You should adjust the seated client's chair height to a position where you can work upright without having to over reach on the top sections of their head.

2 You should clear trolleys or equipment out of the way so that you get good all-round access (300°) around the client.

Hairdressing, as you already know, involves a lot of standing and because of this you need to be comfortable in your work. You should always adopt a comfortable but safe work position and sometimes comfortable and safe are not necessarily the same thing.

Working efficiently, safely and effectively

Working efficiently and maximizing your time are essential, so making the most of the resources available should occur naturally. Always treat the salon's materials in the same way that you would look after your own equipment; always try to minimize waste, being careful of how much product you use.

Salon cleanliness is of paramount importance – the work area should be clean and free from clutter or waste items. Any used materials should be disposed of and not left out on the side; failure to do so (a) is unprofessional and (b) presents a health hazard to others.

For more information about good posture see Unit GH10 pages 166–167.

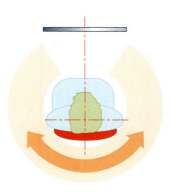

You need to work in an orderly environment; you should have the materials that you need at hand and the equipment that you want to use in position and ready for action. This is a good exercise in self-organization and shows others that you are a true professional.

Keep an eye on the clock; you must remember that you need to be working to time and that means providing the service in a commercially acceptable time.

TOP TIP

Look out for ways and things that can make your client's visit more comfortable and pleasurable. This is the first step in providing a better customer service.

ACTIVITY

Every salon has their own way of doing things. Write down in your portfolio under the following headings your salon's code of practice in respect to:

◆ meeting and greeting clients
◆ gowning
◆ maintaining tools and equipment
◆ hygiene and preventing the spread of infection or infestation
◆ expected timings and duration for a one-length hair cut, cutting hair with uniform layers, a short graduation, a long hair graduation.

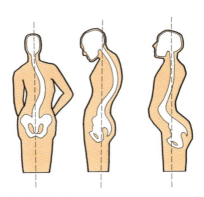

Postural faults

Consultation

Effective communication with the client, as in any service, is an essential part of cutting hair. Consultation is not just a process that takes place before a service; it is a continual process of reconfirming *what* is taking place *whilst* it is taking place. So, during your discussions, you must determine what the client wants and weigh this against the limiting factors that will influence what you need to do.

You need to understand your client fully and be able to negotiate and seek agreement with them throughout the service.

Be sure to listen to your client's requests. Many mistakes can be avoided if you achieve a clear understanding of what the client is asking for.

The haircutting style that you choose with your client should take into account each of the following points about the client's:

◆ face and head shape

◆ physical features and body shape, size and proportion

◆ hair quality, abundance, growth and distribution

◆ age, lifestyle and suitability

◆ purpose

◆ ability or time to recreate the effect themselves.

You may have already completed Unit G7 in Chapter 6 which covers consulting with the client. Read the chapter again to refresh your knowledge and find the relevant parts important to cutting.

Head and face shapes The proportions, balance and distribution of the hairstyle will be a frame for the head and face. Therefore you need to examine the head and face carefully. If you look at the outline of your client's face, you will see that it's round, oval, square, heart-shaped, oblong or triangular. Only an oval face suits all hairstyles, so all the others listed present some form of styling limitations; in other words they become an influencing factor in the choices for styling.

General styling limitations

Physical feature	How best to work with it
Square and oblong facial shapes	are accentuated by hair that is smoothed, scraped back or sleek at the sides and top. The lines and angles are made less conspicuous by fullness and softer movement.
Round faces	are made more conspicuous if the side and front perimeter (the longest outline hair) lengths are short or finish near to the widest part of the face. This is made worse if width is added at these positions too. Generally this facial shape is complemented by length beyond the chin and/or height on the top.
Square angular features, jaw, forehead, etc.	are improved with softer perimeter shapes, so avoid solid, linear effects around the face. Shattered edges and texturizing will help to mask these features.
Flatter heads at the back	are improved by graduation, creating contour and shape that is missing from having a flatter occipital bone.

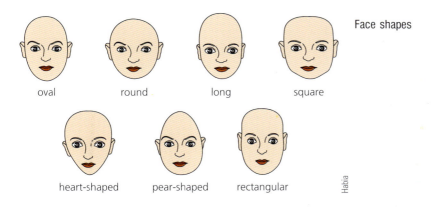

Face shapes

oval   round   long   square

heart-shaped   pear-shaped   rectangular

Habia

Hair growth patterns

Working with the natural fall of the hair   Hair doesn't just grow out of the scalp and downwards; it would be very easy to deal with if it did. Unfortunately, people's hair grows in all sorts of ways and you need to consider this and the impacts that it will have on your haircut.

Some **hair growth patterns** provide useful aspects to work with and can enhance what you are trying to do. Here are some helpful ones:

◆ A client with a low front hairline will naturally have hair that falls as a fringe. Don't ignore this as a fringe is a good choice for this client: it hides their narrow forehead.

◆ Some nape hair growth tends to grow inwards towards the centre of the neck and not straight down. Now this is not really noticeable on long hair, but if it is cut short and tightly graduated on to the neck, you can make a feature of this as the finished effect will always look really neat and tidy even if after washing, it doesn't always get blow-dried.

◆ Natural partings should always be noticed. If a client with longer hair tends to have a definite split in hair directions around the parting at the front, then you can safely suggest shorter styles as options too. The hair around the face, even if it is cut shorter, will always lie well as it won't fall across the face when it is finished. (Needless to say, if you ignore a strong natural parting and try to create a new one somewhere else, it just won't work.)

Other growth patterns to look out for

Double crown	The client with a **double crown** will benefit from leaving sufficient length in the hair to over-fall the whole area. If it is cut too short, the hair will stick up and will not lie flat.	
Nape whorl	A **nape whorl** can occur at either or both sides of the nape. It can make the hair difficult to cut into a straight neckline or tight 'head-hugging' graduations. Often the hair naturally forms a V-shape. Tapered neckline shapes may be more suitable, but sometimes the hair is best left long so that the weight of the hair over-falls the nape whorl directions.	
Cowlick	A **cowlick** appears at the hairline at the front of the head. It makes cutting a straight fringe difficult, particularly on fine hair, because the hair often forms a natural parting. The strong movement can often be improved by moving the parting over so that the weight over-falls the growth pattern. Sometimes a fringe can be achieved by leaving the layers longer so that they weigh down the hair.	
Widow's peak	The **widow's peak** growth pattern appears at the centre of the front hairline. The hair grows upward and forward, forming a strong peak. It is often better to cut the hair into styles that are dressed back from the face, as any 'light fringes' will be likely to separate and stick up.	

Reason for hairstyle

The reason or purpose for the hairstyle is a big factor in deciding what is suitable or otherwise.

A style suitable for a special occasion will differ from one that is selected for work. The requirements for competition or show work are quite different from those for general daily wear. But versatility needs to be considered for everyone: people want styles that they can dress up or down. Modern hairdressing has parallels with modern lives: both are about flexibility and choice. People like options, so build this into your plans. The majority of clients need hairstyles that are easy-to-manage and that can be dressed up with styling products or accessories for social events. Versatility is definitely the key: while people like simple, easy-to-manage effects, they also like the opportunity to look different now and again.

Some jobs have special conditions about hair lengths and styles; for example, people working in the armed services or police have to wear their hair above the collar while at work. Men have easily accommodated this by using clippers for very short styles. Women have either had to have short, layered styles or hair that is long enough to wear up and out of the way.

TOP TIP

The success of any hairstyle is based on the information that you get during the consultation. Be thorough: an extra five minutes spent discussing the final effect could make all the difference!

How hair quality, quantity and distribution, affect styling

Good hair condition is essential for great hairstyling. It doesn't matter how much work has gone into the thought and design of a hairstyle, if the hair is in poor condition to start with, it still will be after. Some aspects cannot be altered by cutting alone; for instance, if the hair is dry, dull and porous when the client enters the salon, it still will be when they leave.

Regular salon clients in the UK – the ones you tend to see more often than the others – tend to have something in common: difficult hair.

It can be difficult for a number of reasons; it can be fine or unmanageable, lank and lacking volume or just not responsive to styling without force. Thin, sparsely distributed hair is always a problem: if there isn't enough hair to get coverage over the scalp, then there is not a lot you can do about it. One thing that you should remember though is not to put too much texturizing into it; this will only make the problem more noticeable. Fine hair presents many problems too. Very fine hair is affected by dampness and quickly loses its shape. This type of hair always benefits from moisture repelling styling products so get your client used to using them.

Dry, frizzy hair can also be a problem, as the more heat styling it receives, the more moisture is lost and the less it responds to staying in shape – in other words, the harder it is to style. The problem just keeps going on like a merry-go-round. Dry, unruly thick hair needs to be tamed and most clients with this problem would like their hair to look smoother and shinier. Again, this is a conditioning issue and you need to attack the problem before tackling the style. Sometimes this type of hair benefits from finishing products so put them on as you finish and define the hairstyle.

Very tight curly hair can be difficult to cut too. Is it possible to smooth or straighten out the hair first so that you can see more clearly, what you have to work with?

Cutting wavy hair presents some problems, but not if it is looked at carefully before it's wet. Avoid cutting across the crests of the waves; you can't change the natural movement in the hair so try to work with it.

Straight hair, particularly if it is fine textured, can be difficult to cut. Cutting marks or lines can easily form if the cutting sections and angles are not right. Make sure that you only take small sections of hair and remember to **cross-check** after, at 90° to the angle in which you first cut, to avoid this happening to you.

Hair tends to grow at a steady regular rate of about 1.25cm per month, so you need to consider this as a factor for how long a hairstyle will last. For example, a one-length classic bob may look really good if it is cut so that it creates a continuous line just above the shoulders. But how long will it last like that? When it gets to the point of touching the shoulders, the clean sharp line to which it was originally cut will now be broken up by falling in front and behind the shoulder line. Always consider the impact that a small amount cut off will make and more importantly how long a style will last.

ACTIVITY

Hair growth patterns

Hair growth patterns do have an impact on the way that hair can be styled. For each of the listed growth patterns below, write down in what ways this will influence your cutting options.

Hair growth pattern	Effect on styling
Widow's peak	
Nape whorl	
Double crown	
Cowlick	

Style suitability Style suitability refers to the effect of the hair shape on the face, and on the features of the head and body. A hairstyle is, quite simply, suitable when it 'looks right'. But this is a difficult or certainly a subjective thing to quantify.

Aesthetically and artistically speaking, the client's hair will 'look right' when the hairstyle does one of two things. It either harmonizes (i.e. fits the shape of the face and head) and is therefore a backdrop to an overall image, or contrasts (i.e. accentuates features of the face and head) creating a prominent frame for the overall image.

Age As much as you would like to demonstrate your creative ability on everyone who walks through the salon door, bear in mind that some styles are inappropriate for certain clients. Beyond the physical aspects of style design, age does create some barriers to suitability.

Younger children (7- to 11-year-olds) are better suited to simpler hairstyles that don't require too much maintenance. More often than not, and certainly from a hair health and hygiene point of view, they are better off with shorter hairstyles. The next age banding (12 to 16 year olds) want to have fashionable looks and many want colours too!

However, as under 16's are classified as minors, the paying parent and educational establishments often have the last say as to the suitability of their hair style.

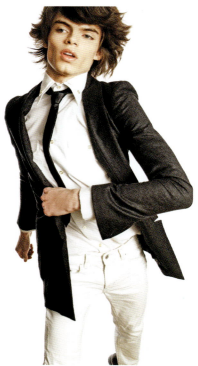

Young men and women can get away with anything, but fashion will always dictate, and, more often than not, even if there are reasons for not doing a particular style, they will insist on it. This group can enjoy more extreme and dramatic effects and what's more they can get away with it. There are more styles applicable to this age group (16- to 25- year-olds) than to any other. This is because of social cultures and the diversity of music and TV; these people are influenced by the music they buy, the celebrities they follow on TV and the people they mix with.

Professional men and women tend to go for watered-down versions of young fashion. Thinking about this in another way: in the clothing fashion world the designs that are seen on catwalks in Paris, London and New York are always the catalysts and precursors for what the high street shops will sell. Dozens of the haute couture fashion houses demonstrate their season's offerings at the pre-season shows. But not all designs are picked up by the buyers of commercial high street fashion chains; they usually go for the lesser extremes. People want to appear to be trendy and in touch, but not look ridiculous.

Older clients require greater consideration. Often the signs of ageing in the skin show quite clearly and therefore they must influence the way in which you select only appropriate and suitable effects.

TOP TIP

It is also important you are aware of EU Directives regarding permanent colours on minors. For more information on Guidance on Use of Hair Colour on and by People Under 16 Years Old visit **www.habia.org.uk**

ACTIVITY

Facial shapes

For consultation purposes, as hairdressers, we tend to group clients into categories that follow a range of basic facial shapes.

From the list below, what styling options or limitations does each one provide?

Facial shape	Styling options/limitations
Round	
Oval	
Square	
Oblong	
Heart	
Triangular	

Cutting tools

Scissors Scissors are and will always be the most important piece of hairdressing equipment that you will ever own. Your future income, popularity and success will rely upon this relatively inexpensive item. If you look after them, you will be surprised how long a single pair will last. Scissors can be used on either wet or dry hair and vary greatly in their design, size and price. There isn't any single way of choosing the correct pair for you; however, there are a number of aspects that you should consider. Scissors should never be too heavy or too long to control; heavy scissors become cumbersome in regular use and if they are too long you may not be able to manipulate them properly

BEST PRACTICE

Take care with your scissors; they are precision instruments that will be easily damaged if they are dropped.

for precision, angular work. Long blades are really good for cutting solid baselines on longer hair, but a real nuisance for precise work around hairlines and behind ears!

To judge a pair of scissors' balance and length, put your fingers in the handles as if you were about to use them. When the scissors are held correctly the pivotal point should just extend beyond the first finger. This allows the blades to open easily and means that the thumb is in an ideal position to work them.

The more expensive scissors will often have one single blade that has small serrations throughout the length. This is really beneficial as this lower blade has cutting grips that stop the hair from being pushed away by the closing blades. Sharpening of this type of scissor blade is not recommended though, as this factory finish will be removed immediately, leaving the scissor with a flat surface.

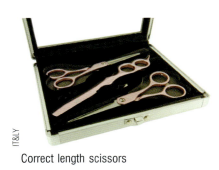

IT&LY

Correct length scissors

Cutting comb
Get into the habit of only using good-quality cutting combs. You will find that by spending only a little more you will get so much more out of them.

The design of a cutting comb for hairdressing is different to that of barbering. The hairdressing cutting comb is parallel throughout its length whereas the barbering comb is tapered. There are two sorts of cutting comb. The first and by far the most popular have two sets of teeth, one end to the middle is fine and close together the other end is wider and further apart. This provides more control with finer sections on fine hair and wider sections on coarser hair. The second type of cutting comb has uniform teeth throughout the length of the comb.

The length of cutting combs varies greatly. Again, what's best for you depends on the size of your hands and what you can manage and manipulate quite easily. The normal length of a cutting comb is around 15cm but long ones are now very popular and provide a better guide when cutting freehand baselines.

The quality of combs and the materials they are made from varies greatly. The best-quality combs are made from plastics that have the following properties:

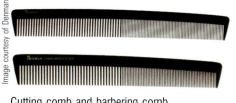

Image courtesy of Denman

Cutting comb and barbering comb

◆ They are very strong but flexible; the teeth do not chip or break in regular use.

◆ They remain straight after regular use.

◆ They are constructed by injection moulding and do not have sharp or poorly formed edges (as opposed to combs that are made from pressings and have flawed seams and tend to scratch the client's ears and scalp).

◆ They are resistant to chemicals, making them ideal for cleaning, sterilization and colouring (as they will not stain).

◆ They have anti-static finishes that help to control finer hair when dry cutting, reducing the hair's tendency to become fly away.

Thinning scissors
Thinning scissors can be used on dry or wet hair and can have either one or both blades with serrated teeth. These cutting surfaces will remove bulk or density from the hair depending on the way in which they are used. This has two useful applications for cutting:

1 the tips or last quarter of finely serrated/castellated scissors provide a quick way for texturizing the perimeter edges of hairstyles;

2 the whole blades can be used for removing weight (tapering or thinning) from sections of hair but closer to the head.

BEST PRACTICE

Use good-quality combs

The comfort of good-quality combs and in particular cutting combs is the most important factor.

Your professionalism will be apparent from the comb that you use. There is nothing worse than using cutting combs on clients when each time you take a section you scrape and scratch the client's scalp! You will also find that, in regular use, if you persist in using cheap combs your hands will become sore as the teeth will scratch you when you pass the comb into your hand on every section that you take!

Maintaining the tools and equipment

	Tools	Method of cleaning/ sterilization
Image courtesy of Denman	Neck brush	Wash in hot soapy water and place in ultraviolet cabinet for ten minutes
IT&LY	Sectioning clips	Wash in hot soapy water and immerse in Barbicide™ jar for 30 minutes
Image courtesy of Denman	Cutting comb	Wash in hot soapy water and immerse in Barbicide™ jar for 30 minutes
IT&LY	Scissors	Brush away hair fragments from pivot area and blades with a colouring brush. Carefully wipe the blades with sterile wipes and then place them in an open position in the ultra violet cabinet for 15 minutes each side.
IT&LY	Thinning scissors	Brush away hair fragments from pivot area and blades with a colouring brush. Carefully wipe the blades with sterile wipes and then place them in an open position in the ultra violet cabinet for 15 minutes each side.

HEALTH & SAFETY

Never keep scissors in your pockets: it is unhygienic but, more importantly, it is a dangerous thing to do.

BEST PRACTICE

When new scissors are bought they come in a protective case, get into the habit of keeping them in it. This will make them easy to identify when there are plenty of other pairs about and will also provide useful protection when they are carried around.

Thinning scissors with both blades serrated will remove hair more quickly than those with serrations on just one side, and this is more noticeable on scissors that have broader castellations or 'notches' in them as opposed to fine teeth.

Neck brushes, water sprays and sectioning clips

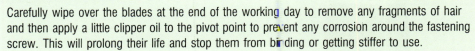

Neck brushes are used to remove loose hair clippings from around the neck and face. Get used to passing the neck brush to your client when you are cutting dry hair as the small fragments are irritating when they fall onto the face. Neck brushes usually have soft synthetic bristles and these are easily washed and dried before they are sterilized in a UV cabinet.

BEST PRACTICE

Maintain your scissors

Carefully wipe over the blades at the end of the working day to remove any fragments of hair and then apply a little clipper oil to the pivot point to prevent any corrosion around the fastening screw. This will prolong their life and stop them from binding or getting stiffer to use.

Water sprays are used for damping down dry or dried hair to assist you in controlling the haircut. Stale water is unhygienic, so make sure that the water is emptied out and refilled on a daily basis.

Sectioning clips are usually made from plastic or thin alloys. They are used to divide the hair and keep bulk out of the way whilst you work on other areas. They are sterilized by immersing them into Barbicide™ solution for the manufacturer's recommended length of time.

ACTIVITY

Wet and dry

There are advantages and disadvantages for cutting both wet and dry hair. Write down your reasons in the table below.

Cutting wet hair

Advantages	Disadvantages

Cutting dry hair

Advantages	Disadvantages

ACTIVITY

(With the electric clippers removed from the power supply or rechargeable clippers 'run down'.)

Knowing how to remove, replace and maintain the clipper blades is an essential part of hairdressing. Get your supervisor to show you how the lower blade-retaining screws are undone and removed. This will give you access to both cutting blades and the area below the armature (the vibrating arm that works them) for cleaning purposes.

When you have dismantled the blades get used to checking for signs of corrosion. If a rusted area exists it will look like blackened areas around the blade edges. If blades have been allowed to get to this stage they should be replaced by new ones as their ability to cut cleanly without friction has been greatly reduced.

With the blades stripped down, you can now use clipper oil to lubricate the two blades, wiping any excess away. Now you can replace the blades (the right way up) and partially re-tighten the retaining screws. Finally, readjust the alignment of the blades and tighten the screws. Check the alignment once more: the lower cutting blade should extend around 3 mm further than the upper cutting blade with the clippers adjusted fully forwards to the shortest cutting length.

Hand them back to your supervisor so that your maintenance can be checked.

Cutting checklist

- ✓ Prepare your tools and equipment making sure that everything you need is close at hand.

- ✓ Make sure that the client is protected.

- ✓ Always gain agreement before attempting anything new or different.

- ✓ Make sure you consider the reasons and the purpose for the style.

- ✓ Look for style limitations, hair problems or physical features.

- ✓ Avoid technical jargon or style names. If jargon is used, by you or the client, always clarify in simple terms what it means to avoid confusion.

- ✓ Don't just do the style if you think that it's wrong. If there are reasons why you think it will be unsuitable, you will be doing the client a big favour in the longer term if you tackle the issue straight away.

- ✓ Always give the client some advice on how to handle the style themselves.

Cut hair to achieve a variety of looks

Cutting and styling hair

Accurate sectioning With everything else done, the only thing that you need to consider is how you go about tackling all that hair. Very short hair doesn't really pose any problem but sectioning isn't just for those with very long hair; any hair not being worked on needs to be sectioned up and out of the way.

In order for you to be able to manage sizeable amounts of hair at any one time, you must organize and plan the haircut. The planning bit becomes automatic; it's the few moments that you spend thinking:

- How do I go about this?
- Where do I start?
- What is the finish going to be like?

So, if the planning is automatic it's the organization bit that you have to address. Quite simply, being organized is about working in a methodical way. It is the way in which you routinely start at one point; divide all the rest of the hair out of the way, finish that bit, and then take down the next part to work on, and so on. Each part or section that you work on should be small enough for you to cope with, without losing your way and continuing on blindly! It seems a strange term to use, but 'blindly' is exactly the right word. If the sections are too deep or too wide you will not be able to see the cutting guide that you need to work to. Accurate sectioning guarantees that every cut mesh is addressed to the same length every time.

Cut hair with natural fall Cutting with the natural fall of the hair is extremely important. Looking for the directions of growth within the hair is an essential part of consultation as it is within the execution of the haircut. If you work with the natural fall, i.e. partings, nape hair growth, double crowns, etc. you will be compensating for these anomalies and be able to produce an easier to manage result. If however, you ignore these factors, you and your client will have a hard job trying to style it.

As previously covered in preparation, always try to wash the hair, even if it is only a hair cut. This way when you dry the hair off, you will be able to see the natural fall far easier and be able to work with it.

TOP TIP

Cutting baselines/perimeter outlines

A baseline is a cut section of hair, which is used as a cutting guide for following sections of hair. There may be one or more baselines cut: for example, a graduated nape baseline may be cut; another may be cut into the middle of the hair at the back of the head. Other baselines may be cut at the sides and the front of the head. The baselines will determine the perimeter of the hairstyle, or part of the style, and may take different shapes according to the effects required.

Symmetrical: The baseline for evenly balanced hair shapes in which the hair is equally divided on both sides of the head. Examples are hairstyles with central partings or with the hair swept backwards or forwards.

Asymmetrical: The baseline to be used where the hair is unevenly balanced, for example where there is a side parting and a larger volume of hair on one side of the head, or where the hair is swept off the face at one side with fullness of volume on the other.

Concave: The baseline may be cut curving inwards or downwards. The nape baseline, for example, may curve downwards.

Convex: The baseline may be cut curving upwards and outwards – the nape baseline, for instance, may be cut curving upwards.

Straight: The baseline may be cut straight across, for example where you wish to produce a hard, square effect.

Controlling the shape There are three aspects of cutting that you must get right on every haircut:

1 *The holding angle* – the angle at which the hair is held out from the head.

2 *The cutting angle* – the angle at which the scissors, razor, etc. cut the hair.

3 *The holding tension* – the even pressure applied to sections of hair when it is held ready for cutting.

That doesn't seem much to guarantee success, but it does take a lot of practise and concentration. Even if you start well in the haircut you cannot afford to lose it in the closing stages.

Cutting lines or perimeter lines are the outline shape created when layered hair is held directly out with tension (perpendicular) from the head. The curves and the angle in relation to the head, determines the shape of the cut style. The main ones are:

◆ the contour of the shape from top to bottom

◆ the contour of the shape around the head, side to side.

Cutting guidelines are prepared sections of hair that control the uniform quality of the haircut. When the cutting guide is taken and first cut, it is to this length and shape that all the other following sections relate. In preparing this cutting guide you need to take all the client's physical features and attributes into consideration, i.e. eyes, eyebrows, nose, bone structure, head shape, neck length, hairlines, etc.

Creating guidelines The guideline is the initial cutting line that is created as a sort of template for all the subsequent sections that are taken.

As a general rule the simpler or more basic the hairstyle the fewer the guidelines there will be. On the other hand, the more complex the hairstyle, the more guidelines will be involved.

So at Level 2 the styles that need to be done involve fewer guidelines:

◆ uniform layered haircut has one

◆ a basic graduation has two

◆ and one-length hair cuts have one.

A uniform layered haircut has layers of equal length all around the head, so the first cutting guideline dictates the overall length for the rest of the haircut.

For easier control of a haircut, they are always started at the back; this way the bulk of the hair is tackled and checked before moving on to the sides and top. So after dividing the hair vertically and evenly down the back, take a horizontal section at both sides about 2cm above the hairline and secure with sectioning clips out of the way. Cut this baseline to the length that you need to and after checking, take down the next section 2cm above and secure the remainder.

(a) Uniform layers

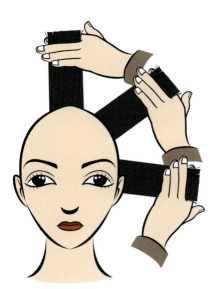

(b) Graduation

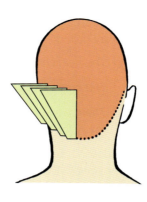

At the point beneath the vertical division in the hair, take and hold a vertical section as shown in figure (a) without twisting and with an even tension. Cut this perpendicularly (at a vertical angle) to the head. (The client's head should be horizontal and not chin down or head back.)

With the guideline cut, you take the next section; parallel to the guideline; with the same even tension, so that you can see the lengths of the previously cut guideline through the held mesh. Cut this to the same length as the guideline. Continue this throughout each section until the complete horizontal area has been cut. Then take down another 2cm on either side and repeat the process, slowly working up the back to the crown.

With the back done, you take a horizontal section above the ears; through to the front, cut your perimeter baseline and follow the guideline through from behind the ear working towards the front hairline. Repeat up to the top and cut the other side in the same way.

Finish the haircut over the top working forwards from the known guidelines at the top. Finally, trim the front hairline perimeter shape to complete the hairline profile shape and cross-check to see that the sides, back and top are all in balance.

The graduated haircut uses a similar guideline process to that of uniform layering; the only difference is that the hair is held out at an angle from the head as opposed to perpendicular. The steeper the angle is held away from the head, the lower the bulk line will be and the greater the weight distribution for the overlying lengths. On the other hand, the shallower the angle of the cut, the higher the bulk line will be and the less weight distribution for the overlying lengths.

Cross-checking the cut Possibly at different points during the cut, but certainly after the cut, you will need to re-check what you have already done. This is done by taking and holding sections at an angle which is at right angles (90°) to the original cut sections. (In other words if you originally cut the hair in vertical meshes, your cross-check will be done with horizontal meshes.)

Cross-checking provides a final technique for checking the continuity and accuracy of the haircut. Where you find an imbalance in weight, or extra length that still needs to be

For more information on cutting guidelines on uniform layers or graduation see the step-by-steps later in this chapter.

removed, it provides you with the opportunity to remove it in order to create the perfect finish.

Dealing with cutting problems

A lack of attention during the cut or a missed detail or aspect during the consultation can lead to cutting mistakes. The variety of mistakes is too varied to cover, but normally result in an imbalance in weight proportions or a difference in perimeter lengths.

If, on finishing a symmetrical cut, you feel that one side seems to be slightly longer than the other, you need to stop before taking anything off the apparently longer side. If it is obviously longer and the client has commented too, you need to put your comb and scissors down and re-check through the fingers.

Standing behind the client you take a small piece of hair from the same position on the head at either side with your forefingers and thumbs. Then slowly slide your fingers down either side until you get to the ends. Looking at the length through the mirror, see if the ends terminate at the same lengths either side; if they do, the cut is fine. Often a cut can seem wrong and the more you look at it the worse it seems. By putting the scissors and comb down you break the fixation and blind panic, and have a chance to review it again calmly, with your hands empty. (Most hairdressers make the fatal mistake of immediately taking some off the apparently longer side; only to find that the other side then seems wrong and then as they continue, each side gets shorter and shorter!) If, however, there is a difference in both lengths then you now have the chance to redress the balance.

Clients are particularly attached to their fringes (pardon the pun); if a fringe is taken too short the client generally feels very conspicuous. So how can you replace hair that is already too short? Well you can't replace the hair but you can lessen the effect by reducing a solid fringe line by slightly **point cutting** to 'break up' the density and reveal a little skin of the forehead through.

What really bothers people is the stark contrast between the solid line created by the fringe against the skin; this focuses even more attention on the area. Therefore the solution is to reduce this contrast by softening this demarcation line between the two areas. (This technique of reducing obvious mistakes can be used throughout the perimeter of hairstyles, as it works in most cases.)

Finally, another popular cutting fault is caused by an imbalance of weight in layering on one side to the other. Again if you get to a cross-check situation and find that the layer pattern on one side seems different to the other side; stop.

You need to find out if it is due to:

◆ one side being longer than the other, or

◆ a greater reduction in weight by texturizing on one side rather than the other.

If it is length then you can easily re-cut the longer side to match. But if it is due to weight reduction, you will see a 'collapse' in the overall style shape on the side that has had the greater amount of texturizing. You can then remedy the fault by further texturizing the hair from the thicker side.

Cutting and styling techniques

Club cutting This is the method of cutting hair bluntly straight across. It systematically cuts all the hair, at an angle parallel to the first and middle finger, to the same length. It is the most popular technique and often forms the basis or first part of a haircut, before other techniques are used.

Club cutting is used in both a uniform layered cut and one-length cut. As the most popular and easily controlled form of cutting, it is the one technique that optimizes the amount of hair at the points and is therefore used for maintaining or creating bulk and volume.

The majority of clients visiting salons within the UK have finer to normal hair textures so this technique is ideal for them as most people with finer hair types like to make their hair fuller or more bodied.

As previously covered in this chapter, cutting with the correct tension is an essential part of achieving an accurate finished result. In club cutting the hair is held out away from the head and the fingers form a guiding line, beyond which the cut is made. This basic principle is replicated throughout the cut, providing a progressive and systematic approach to creating the effect.

Cutting faults will occur:

◆ if you don't maintain the correct tension throughout the cut

◆ if you twist the cutting meshes whilst you are holding and cutting them

◆ if you over-direct the hair, allowing parts of the cut meshes to be longer than needs be.

Incorrect holding/cutting techniques for club cutting

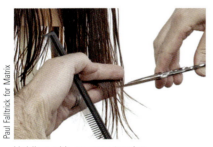

Holding with an even tension

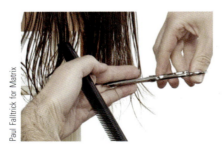

Cutting with the scissor blades parallel to the fingers

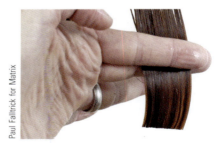

A completed 'club cut' section

Freehand cutting **Freehand cutting** is mainly used on straighter hair for creating the baseline perimeter shape. The technique is used on straighter hair because curlier hair needs more control, through holding and tensioning.

As the name suggests, freehand cutting relies upon one hand holding and combing the hair into position, and the other controlling the scissors to make the cut. More often than not, when cutting longer, one-length hair, the comb is used to create the guide for making the cut.

This technique is more widely used in cutting fringes though. Adults with fringes are particularly cautious about what the exact finished length should be. Therefore it is easier to comb the length into position and create a profile shape that both suits the client and follows or covers the eyebrows. This would be guesswork if the hair were held between the fingers and cut because the width of your fingers would obscure the exact length and position you are trying to cut.

Therefore, the freehand cut is made with the scissors very close to the skin or body, as this gives you a clearer idea of what needs to be cut off to achieve the exact length required by the client. Obviously, you need to be particularly careful in cutting your profiles as it would be easy to snip an eyebrow or an ear! One thing that you can do to minimize any risk to the client is to use your comb behind the hair you want to cut, as this has a couple of benefits.

◆ The comb can be held parallel to the angle of the scissor blades, giving you a useful back-up guideline.

◆ The comb keeps eyebrows, ears and lined or 'sagging', skin back away from the cutting edges/points of the scissors.

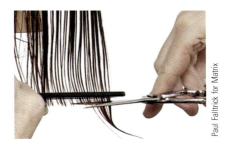 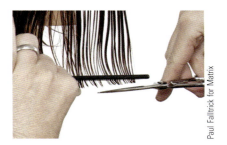 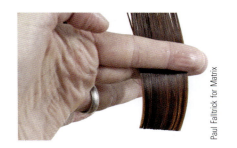

Paul Falltrick for Matrix

Scissor over comb This technique has been traditionally a barbering technique. In recent years there has been a move in hairdressing generally towards easier-to-manage hairstyles, so therefore this technique is widely used in hairdressing for cutting short styles on both men and women.

ACTIVITY

Planning your work

Any service that you provide to the client needs to be thought about before you start. This planning is essential for achieving a successful result, so in this activity, complete the table below to create a checklist of things that you should consider before carrying out the service.

Checklist for cutting

1.

2.

3.

4.

5.

6.

Scissor over comb cutting is ideal for producing

A. Tapered layering shapes with close-cut, 'fade-out' perimeters (faded or graduated perimeters have no set baselines; they rely upon the hairline profile and are graduated out from that into the rest of the hairstyle).

B. Uniform layered shapes with layers of equal lengths.

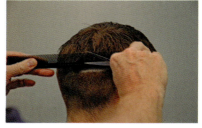

Correct angle for scissor over comb

Graduation/Reverse graduation

The technique is used with either wet or dry hair and uses the comb as a guide to hold the hair and maintain an even lift or tension away from the head, whilst you cut.

Scissor over comb is ideal for very short hair that cannot be held between your fingers, it is best started at the lower nape area providing that the hair isn't too long. The hair is lifted away from the head and the comb mirrors the contour of the back of the head so that the upper edge is tilted away and not towards the back of the head. If the angle of the comb leans towards the head your finished cut length will gradually get shorter as you work upwards.

The image below shows the correct sectioning position.

Reverse graduation   **Graduation**

BEST PRACTICE

The most important factor in cutting hair

Very few people can do two things at the same time! You will have to learn very quickly that you need to hold a conversation with the client without losing your way and concentration on the haircut. This is the biggest single cause of poor quality hairdressing! (If you cannot do this yet, tell your client that you need the time to focus on the task ahead. Believe it or not, they won't mind.)

Thinning Thinning is a technique which can be done with scissors or a razor and can be used for reducing or tapering bulk from thicker hair without reducing the overall length. It is also used as a way of texturizing the edges of hairstyles to remove solid lines from profile shapes to create more softer, faded or 'shattered' effects.

When thinning is done to remove bulk and weight in short or long layered hair, the hair sections should be held in vertical meshes and the thinners should be introduced to the hair at an angle so that the longest parts of the thinned hair are nearer to the base lines or perimeter. This helps the hair to remain smoother without 'bunching' when it is dried. (When longer thinned hair over lies shorter thinned hair an unflattering result occurs; producing width with fluffy, unruly edges.)

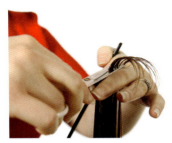

(a) Club cutting

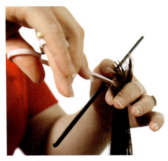

(b) Point cutting

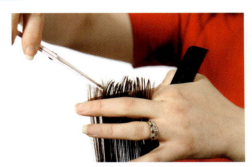

(c) Chipping

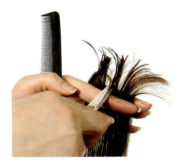

(d) Deep pointing

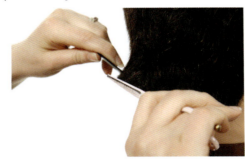

(e) Scissors over comb

Checklist – Before the cut

- ✓ Prepare the client and your working area.
- ✓ Discuss the client's styling options.
- ✓ Use visual aids to help show ideas and themes.
- ✓ Examine the hair – its type, length, quality, quantity and condition.
- ✓ Look for factors that influence the choice of style and cutting methods.
- ✓ After your analysis, agree or negotiate with the client the suitable courses of action to take.
- ✓ Try to show the hair length to be removed.
- ✓ Discuss the time that will be taken and the price that you will charge.
- ✓ Choose the right tools and techniques for achieving the effects.

Checklist – During the cut

- ✓ After shampooing and towel-drying, dry off the hair so that any previously unseen hair tendencies or growth patterns can be seen.
- ✓ Try to keep the hair damp but not saturated, so that any newly added technical features can easily be seen.
- ✓ Take care with your precision or accuracy by checking each angle at which the hair is taken and held from the head.
- ✓ Create your baselines and guideline cuts first, so that there is a continuity within the section patterning.
- ✓ When preparing baselines and guide sections, make sure that you attend to the features of your client's face and head. Use these as guides for accurate directions in the cut lines.
- ✓ Remember always that the first cuts you make often determine the finished shape of the style.

BEST PRACTICE

Far more customers are dissatisfied as a result of the stylist not listening and taking too much off than because of poor or inaccurate haircuts.

Checklist – After the cut

- ✓ Cross-check each of the sections of the side, nape, top and front for accuracy and finish.
- ✓ Check the balance, density, texture and features of the haircut.
- ✓ Position, place and mould the hair where necessary to see the shape clearly.
- ✓ When all the loose hair clippings have been removed and the client is prepared and comfortable, continue to blow-dry, set and finish the style.

STEP-BY-STEP: ONE-LENGTH HAIRCUT

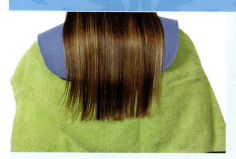

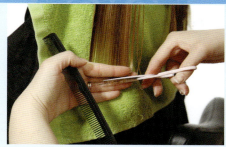

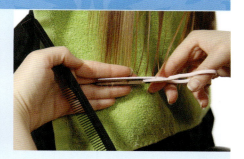

1 Very long one-length hair can be very difficult to cut.

People that have one-length long hair often have quite a lot of damage and this needs to be looked for before you start.

One of the main areas is the underlying lengths around the nape. These can often get caught in clothes and over time will start to break.

CHECK FIRST to see if there is any missing hair, it may prevent you from cutting too much off!!

2 If the hair is quite thin, you may not need to section so far down as the nape. In this situation you could take your first section below the occipital and secure the remainder out of the way.

Start in the centre of the back and work outwards to the shoulders.

3 Check your balance, before taking down another section. Then use the previously cut guideline to act as a template for this section.

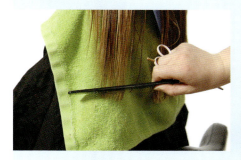

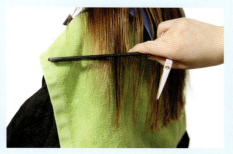

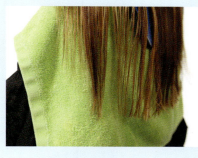

4 Check with the client if they want the same amount off all around, if there is an area that is still growing down, ask them if they want it trimmed or not.

Don't just go ahead and think that they need it cut.

5 When you move around to the sides, section off the lower hair and comb down the length to see where it fits with the back.

Damaged hair will look frayed or tapered, if you are permitted to tidy the ends up, carefully trim the profile shape.

6 Take down subsequent sections and trim the same length.

CourseMate video: Long Length Cut

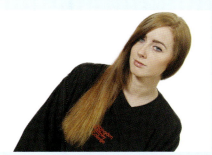

7 You can check your final balance and shape when the hair is dry.

STEP-BY-STEP: UNIFORM LAYERS

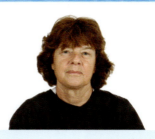

1 A uniform layered haircut is cut to the same length all over. When it is done on short hair, it creates a 'head hugging' shape.

Gown and prepare your client.

Check hairlines and growth patterns before you start.

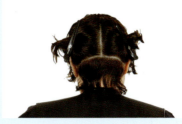

2 Start at the back, section off an area so that you can work without hair falling in the way.

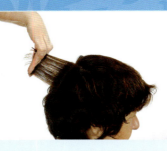

3 Take a central, vertical section to create your guideline and cut your first section.

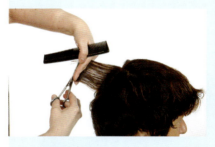

4 Continue the same layer pattern length to either side.

Tidy up the perimeter shape now and it will save time later on.

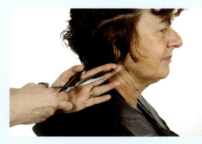

5 Moving up further, take another central section and cut it to the same length as the guideline below.

Again, extend this to both sides of the head.

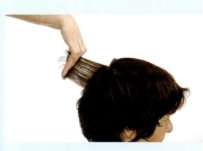

6 If, on short hair, you intend to take it around the ears, you need to do this before cutting your layered length.

Remember to hold the ears out of the way.

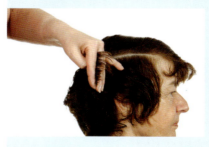

7 Now blend the side length to the same previously cut hair at the back.

Work forward to the front hairline.

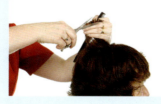

8 With the back and sides done, you now need to connect the side and back length into the top area.

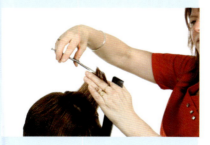

9 Working forwards, make sure that your lengths are even by cross-checking, i.e. holding the hair in the opposite plane to which it was cut.

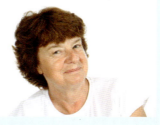

10 The final effect.

CourseMate video: Uniform Layer

STEP-BY-STEP: SHORT GRADUATED LAYERING (NAPE AND NECK)

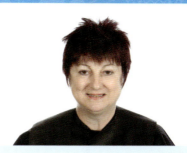

1 Before

Prepare your client with a clean fresh gown and a cutting collar to stop fragments of hair going down the client's neck. Make sure you check the growth patterns before you start.

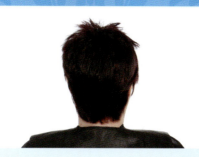

2 Haircuts are easier if started at the back because it enables you to ensure that the balance is correct whether it is perimeter length, or layer patterning.

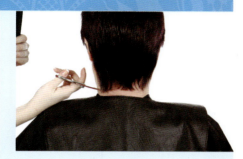

3 Tidy the perimeter shape first.

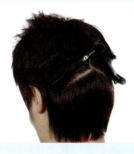

4 Section off the back so that you have a clear area to work with.

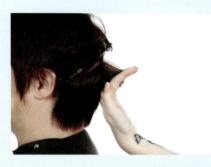

5 A graduation is where the lower perimeter length hair is shorter than the overlying, upper and inner length hair.

The cutting angle is held like this.

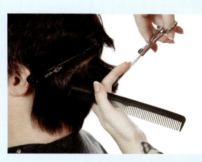

6 Take a section of hair from the centre, hold it vertically and create your cutting guideline.

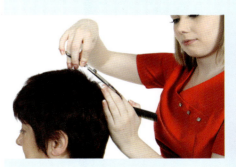

7 Follow the guideline out to either side and the graduated part is complete. Now determine the overall length for the top and cut this guideline over the crown.

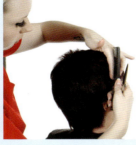

8 Follow the graduated lines from the back into either side and work forwards.

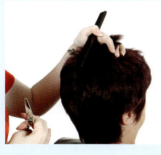

9 The length cut at the crown should now be continued forwards to the fringe area.

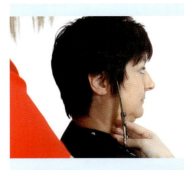

10 Profile the perimeter edges around the sides taking care around the ears.
Follow this length to finish the fringe.

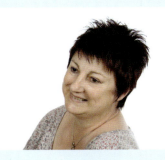

11 Finished effect.

CourseMate video: Graduated Layer

STEP-BY-STEP: LONG REVERSE GRADUATED LAYERING

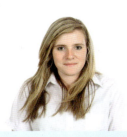

1 A reverse graduation is probably the most difficult to grasp at Level 2. It is all too easy to take too much hair away (especially on longer hair) and leave the hair with little density.

Prepare your client with a clean fresh gown and a cutting collar to stop fragments of hair going down the client's neck.

Make sure you check the growth patterns before you start.

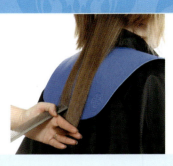

2 Haircuts are easier if started at the back because it enables you to ensure that the balance is correct, whether it is perimeter length or layer patterning.

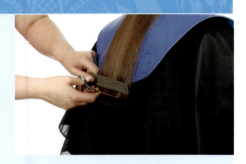

3 After sectioning off the lower nape section of the hair, start at the centre and create you first guideline.

Cut the perimeter to the same length and do the same with subsequent sections, up to the occipital.

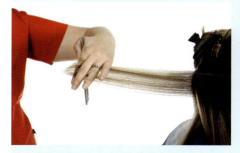

4 The first reverse graduation guideline is taken at the occipital bone area and is held out away from the head.

The reverse graduation cut creates a cut line that is longer towards the perimeter length and runs to a shorter length towards the crown.

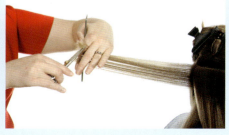

5 Use this reverse graduation cut line to create your guideline.

Continue this at either side.

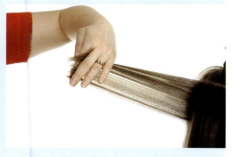

6 On the next section towards the crown we can clearly see the guideline and the hair that needs cutting to continue the style line.

Cut this through to the crown and at either side.

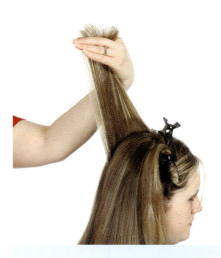

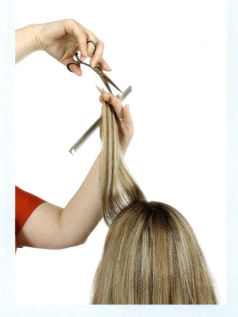

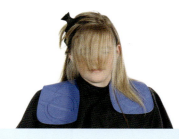

7 With the back done, you now need to hold and cut the hair over the top.

8 You can see from the guideline that has been created that the angle inverts downwards towards the parting.

Use this inversion as your guideline towards the parting at both sides of the head.

9 With the reverse graduation completed, you now need to profile the fringe and sides.

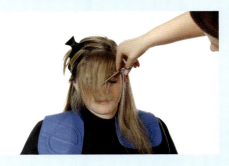

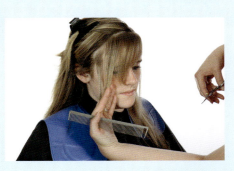

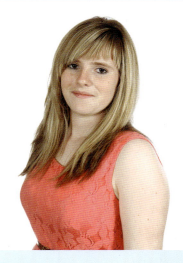

10 When hair is worn in a side parting, you have to create a fringe somewhere, and this is the most daunting aspect of the haircut.

Take time to choose your shortest point and take the plunge. Start at this point and graduate downwards and into the side length.

11 Finally, check the balance and tidy where needed.

12 Final effect.

CourseMate video: Reverse Graduation Cut

Fringes

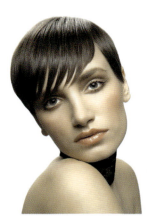
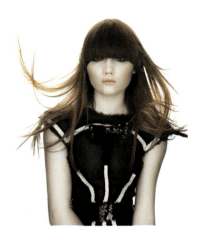
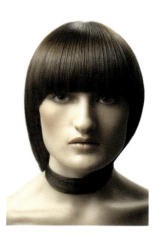
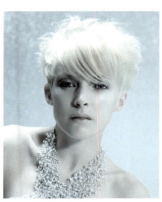

Provide aftercare advice

Good service is supported through good advice and recommendation. The work that you do in the salon needs to be cared for at home by the client too. What would be the point of creating something if the client doesn't know how to achieve and maintain the same effects at home?

Style durability

Hair grows at a steady rate of around 1.25cm per month so at the six to eight week point the hair will be considerably longer than when it was first cut. If the hair is thick and coarse the first thing that the client will notice is an increase in the width of the hairstyle on both sides. Similarly, if a client has a shoulder-length cut, then it will now be beyond the shoulders and separating in front and behind. In other words whatever the client selected for a style at the beginning, it will now have taken on a different look.

Make a point of outlining the benefits of having a regular cut; give your client an idea of how long the style will last and, ideally, because you know how long that will be, get them to re-book their style reshape before they leave the salon. People who don't make appointments before they leave the salon often tend to drift beyond the normal interval times. Then, when they do realize that their hair needs doing, they find that they can't get an appointment at a time that suits them. So by the time you get to work on it again the hair really needs a sort out.

Home and aftercare checklist

- ✓ Talk through the style as you work; that way the client sees how you handle different aspects of the look.

- ✓ Show and recommend the products/equipment that you use so that the client gets the right things to enable them to get the same effects.

- ✓ Tell the client how long the style can be expected to last and when they need to return.

- ✓ Show them how they can achieve that salon hair look too.

Talk through the style as you work Make a point of talking through your styling techniques as you go as:

A. it eliminates long periods of silence whilst you are working and, more importantly,

B. it is really useful to the client as they get useful advice on how to recreate a similar effect at home.

Show and recommend the products/equipment that you use As you talk about the ways in which you have styled the hair, make a point of talking through the products that you have used as well.

This way they will be able to see a direct link between the effects that you are achieving on their hair, with the added benefits of buying those particular products that will help them to recreate a similar effect.

Explain how routine styling tools can have detrimental effects
Only hair in good condition is easy to maintain. You know how difficult it is to make dry, damaged hair look good. With these known facts, you would be doing an injustice to your clients if you didn't warn them of the pitfalls of repeatedly using hot styling equipment, so make a point in asking them if they use them at home too. If they say that they use straighteners or tongs on a daily basis then tell them about the benefits of using heat protection sprays.

Demonstrate the techniques that you use Clients want to be able to recreate the effects that you achieve in the salon and this is your chance to show them how to do it. Clients haven't had the benefit of your training; they don't know the little tricks and techniques that make it seem so simple. Show them how to do things; correct combing, blow-drying or positioning of brushes. We have all seen the effects when these are not done properly, so make a point of giving them a few tips on how they can achieve a similar result themselves and how long they can expect it to last.

ACTIVITY

Home care advice

Good home aftercare advice is about giving the client the correct advice on looking after their hair. This will include advice on:

- ◆ products
- ◆ tools and equipment
- ◆ future salon services.

1. What advice should you give regarding products?

2. What advice do you need to provide regarding tools and equipment?

3. What advice could you provide regarding future salon services/treatments?

SUMMARY

Remember to:

- ✓ prepare clients correctly for the services you are going to carry out

- ✓ put on the protective wear available for styling and dressing hair

- ✓ listen to the client's requirements and discuss suitable courses of action

- ✓ remember the safety factors when working on clients' hair

- ✓ keep the work areas clean, hygienic and free from hazards

- ✓ promote the range of services, products and treatments within the salon

- ✓ clean and sterilize the tools and equipment before they are used

- ✓ work carefully and methodically through the cutting processes

- ✓ place, position and direct the hair appropriately to achieve the desired effect

- ✓ tell the client what you are doing, keep them informed.

Knowledge Check

For this project you will need to gather information from a variety of sources.

Close observation of your senior colleagues whilst they work is an invaluable means of learning. At first, cutting hair can be slow and difficult, but with practise this soon changes.

To gather together information on cutting and styling you will need to visit hairdressing demonstrations, exhibitions and competitions. Using photography and video recording is ideal. Practising first cuts, or experimenting with the various techniques, can be carried out on modelling blocks, slip-ons and models.

You need to record as much as you can, including the following:

1. Carefully list the movements and techniques that you see and outline the effects produced. Try to capture the positions of the sections taken, the angles of cut, the direction of cutting lines, etc.

2. Outline the plan of the cut and list the important factors to consider.

3. How do the different growth patterns affect your cutting? Describe these and try to illustrate them in your notes.

4. Try to describe the different cutting procedures and refer particularly to the different parts of the head – the fringe, sides, nape, top and back. Explain how these parts are blended or fit together.

Investigate other sources of haircutting information: magazines, DVDs, TV. The information you collect could include these items:

- ◆ how to choose suitable cutting tools

- ◆ the effects produced by the different tools

- ◆ how metal cutting tools are maintained and cleaned

- ◆ how to select the right tool for the effect required

- ◆ the difference between wet and dry cutting, and the tools used for each

- ◆ how tools should be used safely.

ASSESSMENT OF KNOWLEDGE AND UNDERSTANDING

A selection of different types of questions to check your cutting hair knowledge.

Q1 Accuracy is achieved by ___ and cutting the hair at the correct angle. Fill in the blank

Q2 Scissors should be sterilized in Barbicide™. True or false

Q3 Select from the following list those that are *not* texturizing techniques: Multi selection

Club cutting ☐ 1
Graduation ☐ 2
Slice cutting ☐ 3
Layering ☐ 4
Point cutting ☐ 5
Chipping ☐ 6

Q4 Symmetrical shapes produce equally balanced hairstyles. True or false

Q5 Which of the following is not a cutting term? Multi choice

Cross-checking ○ a
Thinning ○ b
Freehand ○ c
Freestyle ○ d

Q6 Precision cutting is dependent upon cutting angles and even tension. True or false

Q7 Which of the following hair growth patterns will affect the natural fall and way that a fringe lies after it is cut? Multi selection

Nape whorl ☐ 1
Double crown ☐ 2
Widow's peak ☐ 3
Low hairline ☐ 4
Cowlick ☐ 5
High hairline ☐ 6

Q8 A _____ is the perimeter shape produced by cutting. Fill in the blank

Q9 Which of the following cuts would easily describe a disconnection? Multi choice

Graduation in a long hairstyle ○ a
Reverse graduation in a long hairstyle ○ b
A fringe in a shoulder-length bob style ○ c
Texturizing in a short cropped style ○ d

Q10 Clubbing is a technique of cutting that maximizes the hair density. True or false

13 Cutting men's hair

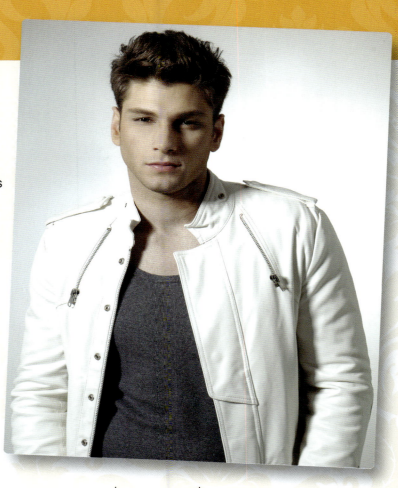

LEARNING OBJECTIVES

◆ Be able to maintain safe methods of working

◆ Be able to cut hair to achieve a variety of men's barbering effects

◆ Know how to work safely, effectively and hygienically

◆ Understand the factors that can affect the barbering service

◆ Understand freehand, scissor over comb and clippering techniques

◆ Understand the aftercare advice that you should provide to clients

KEY TERMS

attachments	cross-check	scissor over comb
autoclave	fading	shaper
Barbicide™	male pattern baldness	sharps box
blend area	open (cut-throat) razor	sideburns
clippers	razor	UV cabinets

GB3 Cut hair using basic barbering techniques

Information covered in this chapter

- ◆ The tools and equipment used during cutting and barbering
- ◆ The preparations that you should make prior to cutting
- ◆ The factors that influence hair cutting decisions
- ◆ Basic cutting and barbering techniques
- ◆ The aftercare advice that you should give clients

INTRODUCTION

Men and women share the same hair types, hair textures, hair tendencies and colours, so what are the differences? Traditionally the differences were more to do with length, but now even those differences are less defined. With different trends encouraging women to sport shorter hair and men often wearing their's longer, the barber of today has to cover an increasingly large array of hairstyles for men.

Basic barbering

Basic barbering involves the traditional aspects of club cutting, **scissor over comb** work, cutting using electric **clippers** and clipper grade **attachments**. In addition to these, you will be using a range of techniques that *cross over* to ladies' hairdressing, such as club cutting, freehand and thinning. This chapter takes you through the aspects of contemporary barbering under the following topics:

- preparation and maintenance
- client consultation
- identifying the influencing factors that affect style choice
- cutting techniques and accuracy
- good customer care.

TOP TIP

Cutting men's hair (as with many other services) uses many of the principles of cutting women's hair. Review other chapters in this book for more information.

BEST PRACTICE

A finished hairstyle always looks better if it is cut wet. Try to get your clients to book for a wet cut at the very least:

- It will be easier for you to create new effects.
- They will be able to see a better, more professional result.
- You will generate a better professional service with your clients.
- You will break the habits of men expecting a quick, cheap haircut.
- It is more hygienic for everyone concerned.

Be able to maintain effective and safe methods of working when cutting hair

The preparatory outcome for this unit is very similar to other technical services although there are variations that relate to:

- specific differences for doing male and female clients
- the individual salon policy where you work
- the differences in the tools and equipment used.

As client protection is the first aspect that you must consider, a quick reference for cutting dry or wet is listed on the following page along with the essential knowledge components.

Protecting the client

Most barbers will gown their clients before the consultation, but some may choose to do it later. Whatever the salon policy, the client must be protected before a dry cut is started or, if the service is a wet cut, then before the client is shampooed.

For dry cutting

Use a clean fresh cutting gown and put it on your client while he is sitting at the styling location. Make sure that the back is fastened and that any open, free edges are closed together, keeping any loose clippings away from the client's clothes. Place a cutting collar around his neck to ensure that any bumps or lumps in his clothing don't present any false, physical baselines for the haircut and that the collar edges fit snugly against the neck, so that there are no irritating hair fragments that will leave the client itching until he gets home.

For wet cutting

Do the same as above but, when your client is at the basin, place a clean fresh towel around his shoulders before positioning him back carefully and comfortably. Make sure that the basin supports the client's neck properly and that the flanged edges of the basin nestle comfortably on to the client's shoulders, which are protected from any spills or seepage by a clean fresh towel.

See Unit GH8 on pages 140–141 for more information.

It is essential that you work safely when cutting hair and in order for you to demonstrate this you need to:

◆ organize all the equipment that you are going to use; gowns, towels, combs, scissors, razor and clippers, etc.

◆ check that they are ready for use, e.g. new blades for the **razor**, freshly laundered towels and gowns, washed cutting collars, cleaned and sterilized combs, brushes, clipper blades and scissors

◆ put them at the work station and ready for use

◆ ensure that the client is comfortable and in a position where you can work safely.

More information can be found elsewhere, but here is a quick reference guide to other parts in this book covering the essential information.

Topic	Related information	See page
Client preparation and protection	Unit GH12 Cut hair using basic techniques	268
Working position and height	Unit GH12 Cut hair using basic techniques	268
Preparing tools and equipment	Unit GH12 Cut hair using basic techniques	269
Working efficiently, safely and effectively	Unit GH12 Cut hair using basic techniques	271
Personal hygiene	Unit GH12 Cut hair using basic techniques	269

HEALTH & SAFETY

Disposal of sharp items

Used razor blades and similar items should be placed into a safe container (**sharps box**). When the container is full it can be disposed of. This type of salon waste should be kept away from general salon waste as special disposal arrangements may be provided by your local authority.

ACTIVITY

Every salon has their own way of doing things. Write down in your portfolio under the following headings what your salon's code of practice is in respect to:

- meeting and greeting clients
- gowning
- maintaining tools and equipment
- disposal of sharps
- hygiene and preventing the spread of infection or infestation
- expected standards of service.

Disposal of waste and sharps

Most of the waste produced in a barber's shop is harmless, and as long as it has been placed in a strong polythene bin liner and tied at the top, it can be disposed of as general commercial rubbish. However, there are some items that should be handled with care.

Barbers also use a lot of chemicals and many of these such as shampoos, conditioners and styling products, are not necessarily potential hazards. In fact much of the other chemical waste created by salons ends up being rinsed down the sinks too and unless this form of disposal has local by-laws ruling against it, then these chemicals shouldn't present a disposal hazard either.

But sharp items such as disposable razor blades do need to be handled with extreme care. Used sharps must be disposed of carefully to prevent any injury or cross-infection. They should be put in the sharps box and sealed properly before refuse collection.

Prevent infection

Infection and disease occurs by two obvious methods within the salon/barber's shop environment. It is:

- either brought in by a 'carrier' visiting the salon who then cross-infects other people within the salon
- or the result of poor hygiene and cleanliness within the salon.

Most of the preparatory aspects covered in this chapter aim to keep the standards of hygiene within your working environment very high.

But there would be little point in maintaining the healthy environment unless you checked your clients for signs of infections or infestations during your consultation, as warm, humid salon conditions can offer a perfect home for disease-carrying bacteria. If they can find food in the form of dust and dirt, they may reproduce rapidly.

Good ventilation, however, provides a circulating air current that will help to prevent their growth. This is why it is important to keep the work area clean, dry and well aired at all times. This includes clothing, work areas, tools and all equipment. Sterilization provides the most effective way of providing hygienically safe work implements in salons. Sterilization means the complete eradication of living organisms.

ACTIVITY

What is your salon's policy for the use of razors and the disposal of sharp items?

Different types of equipment use different sterilization methods, which may be based on the use of heat, radiation or chemicals.

Ultraviolet radiation UV cabinets may be utilized to store previously sterilized disinfected tools and equipment.

Chemical sterilization/disinfectant Chemical sterilizers should be handled only with suitable personal protective equipment, as many of the solutions used are hazardous to health and should not come into contact with the skin. The most effective form of salon disinfection is achieved by the total immersion of the contaminated implements into a jar of fluid such as Barbicide™.

Autoclaves The autoclave provides a very efficient way of sterilizing using heat. It is particularly good for metal tools although the high temperatures are not suitable for plastics, such as brushes and combs. Items placed in the autoclave take around 20 minutes to sterilize. (Check with manufacturer instructions for variations.)

Further information on working position and safety can be found on pages 268 and 271 Unit GH12.

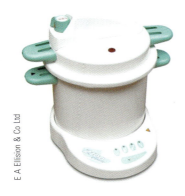

E A Ellision & Co Ltd

Autoclave

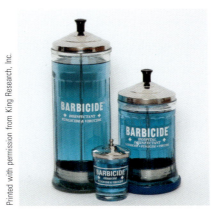

Printed with permission from King Research, Inc.

Barbicide™

ACTIVITY

Wet and dry

There are advantages and disadvantages for cutting both wet and dry hair. Write down your reasons in the table below.

Cutting wet hair

Advantages   Disadvantages

Cutting dry hair

Advantages   Disadvantages

Preparation checklist

✓ Make sure that the styling section and chair is clean, safe and ready to receive clients.

✓ Make sure that the seat is lowered, providing easier access for the clients whether they be young, old or with physical conditions.

✓ Make sure that the client is well protected with a clean fresh gown and a close-fitting cutting collar.

✓ Make sure that you have your tools prepared and close at hand.

✓ Find out what the client wants. Men can often be more difficult during consultation as they are often reluctant to use a technical term that they are not sure about or even express themselves clearly to people they don't know (see the section on consultation below).

✓ Style books/files provide lots of male looks to help the consultation process.

✓ Make sure you comb or brush the hair thoroughly before you start to remove tangles; see if all product can be removed and check for growth patterns.

✓ Assess the styling limitations – hair and skin problems or physical features.

✓ Avoid technical jargon or style names; if you do use them, always clarify in simple terms what you mean to avoid confusion; this will help to educate your clients for the future.

✓ Don't just do the style if you think that it's wrong. If there are reasons why you think it will be unsuitable, you will be doing the client a big favour in the longer term if you tackle the issue straight away.

✓ Always give them some advice on how to maintain their hairstyle; men often need products to help them achieve similar effects themselves. Make sure you show them how they can use and apply any new product at home to maintain their own hair/skin condition or styling effect.

✓ Give them an idea of how long it will last and remember to re-book their next appointment before they leave. Alternatively, if they prefer just to pop in on the off-chance, tell them when they should expect to revisit.

Client consultation

Finding out what the client wants Finding out what the client wants is essential if you are going to achieve a satisfactory result, but don't forget the factors such as practicality, suitability and the client's ability to do their own hair.

The final effects will be influenced by other considerations too:

◆ the amount of hair

◆ the distribution of the hair over the scalp

◆ the texture of the hair

◆ the condition of the hair and scalp

◆ the tendency of the hair, i.e. the amount of wave or curl.

For more information on consultation see Unit G7 Advise and consult with clients pages 100–136.

Unless you do take all these factors into consideration, you could have an unhappy, disgruntled client on your hands.

Brush or comb the hair before you start You must try to get as much information about the client's hair before you start, even if they are only having a dry cut. Part of this may seem obvious; it's the questions that you ask the client regarding what they want. But that's not the only way you find out what's needed. You need to brush or comb the hair in different directions to see if the hair and scalp has:

◆ *Growth patterns* – that limit or influence the way that the hair can be cut such as double crowns, widow's peak, nape whorls, cowlick, etc.

◆ *Product on it* – if products like wax, gel or grooming cream are on the hair you won't be able to cut the hair properly. It will stick together and stop you from being able to cut it correctly; you must wash the hair before you start the cut.

◆ *Any infections or infestations* – if there are any signs of a suspected condition you need to know what it is, so you know whether it is possible to proceed. If you do find something that you are not sure about seek assistance

Check the client's requirements The main aims of hairdressing and barbering are about delivering a continuing, repeated service that satisfies our clients. We can only satisfy the clients if we find out what they want and act upon those instructions. We demonstrate this by getting confirmation of the things we are doing throughout the service. This does a number of things as it:

◆ ensures that we only do things that the clients want

◆ makes them more confident about what we are doing

◆ removes any miscommunication or confusion

◆ gives us more confidence in what we are doing for the client

◆ involves the client and helps to develop a professional relationship.

See Unit G7 Advise and consult with clients, pages 100–136.

TOP TIP

As many men have shorter hair, their nape hair growth patterns will have far more impact on what hairstyle you choose.

BEST PRACTICE

Personal hygiene is especially important to hairdressers. You work in close proximity to the client so make sure that you eliminate body odour, bad breath or dirty hands and nails by taking the appropriate action.

ACTIVITY

Hair growth patterns

Hair growth patterns do have an impact on the way that hair can be styled. For each of the listed growth patterns below, write down in what ways this will influence your cutting options.

Hair growth pattern	Effect on styling
Widow's peak	
Nape whorl	
Double crown	
Cowlick	

Influencing factors affecting style choice

Male pattern baldness Your consultation will cover a wide variety of factors that influence what happens next and male pattern baldness or the early signs of it should be high upon your list of things to look for.

Male pattern baldness (MPB) is a balding or thinning condition the cause of which, regardless of claims, is still eluding the scientists. MPB may be due to high levels of the male hormone testosterone within the body. Many treatments have been developed with little or no long-term remedial effects. Hair transplants have been a possible option in the past, but this type of treatment is expensive and needs a lot of upkeep.

Depending at what stage the MPB is, you need to find out how your client feels about it. If the hair loss is relatively slow, there is no need to rush immediately for the clippers and a grade 2. There could be some considerable time before the condition requires a focused attention and, therefore, you need to provide advice and reassurance with a range of styling alternatives.

If however, the MPB is in a progressed state then it is obviously going to impact on what styles are achievable. For example, if there is a significant general thinning or hair loss on top (MPB type 1) then your styling options are far more limited than if MPB is only apparent in the recession area around the forehead (MPB type 2).

If your client has lost their hair and wears a toupee, you must account for this in your styling. Obviously, there has to be some blending between the natural, remaining hair and the added hair. Be careful not to leave the hair either too long or too short around the blend area. If there is any imbalance in lengths between the two, it is definitely going to show.

If, however, the client wears a full hairpiece then they might just prefer to keep whatever remaining hair very short beneath it. This makes fitting and positioning of the hairpiece easier and will be more comfortable to wear over long periods of time.

Male pattern baldness

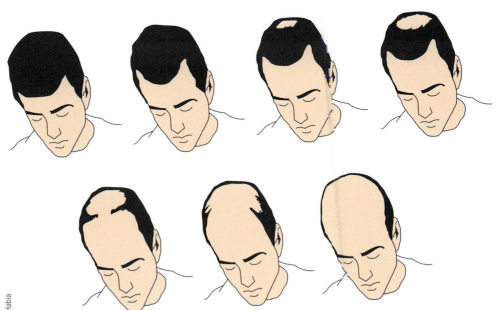

Habia

Facial shapes

Facial shapes	How best to work with it
Square and oblong facial shapes	Square and oblong are typically masculine and provide a perfect base for traditional classic well groomed looks on shorter hair. These facial shapes have less impact on men's longer hairstyles.
Round faces	If shorter, more classic styles are required, the round face is improved by the introduction of angular or linear perimeters. On the other hand, if the hair is to be worn longer the roundness of the face will be reduced, as more will be covered.
Square angular features, jaw, forehead, etc.	Again these are traditionally accepted as a feature of masculinity. They do not really pose any limitations for classic type work. They also work well with longer hair too. Squarer, more angular features are softened with beards and moustaches.
Flatter heads at the back	They are improved by contoured graduation, which creates shaping and tapering that is missing from having a flatter occipital bone. Sometimes the head is both flat and wide and this can make the problem harder to deal with. Wider, flatter heads are made less noticeable by longer hair, if this is not possible then explain what the effect will look like if taken very short.

Examination of hair and scalp While you are looking at the client's hair and scalp, be particularly aware of the texture of the hair. If it is coarse and tightly curled, you will need stronger combs to stretch the hair out from the head before cutting, and firmer movements will need to be applied. The density of the hair is important too: if it is thick, then styles with varied hair lengths are possible.

On the other hand, sparse hair, particularly if it is fine, requires a great deal of attention and expertise If finely textured hair has to cover a sparse area of the head, it will have to be longer than hair of coarser texture. The amount, type and growth patterns of hair are all-important too. Younger men may have distinctly higher forehead hairlines than women of similar age. Thinning crowns and decreasing density of hair marks many male patterns.

Hair grows at a rate of about 1.25cm (12.5mm) each month and this is more noticeable with shorter layered styles. Regular trimming is essential to keep them tidy.

Hair growth patterns Although men can wear longer hair as well as short, a whole range of modern contemporary styling effects has developed since the basic and traditional short back and sides. The application of hair products will often 'dress up' an otherwise professional or classic looking hairstyle, turning it into something with a more distinctive 'fashion look' for social and special occasions.

For more information on hair growth patterns see Unit G7 page 126.

BEST PRACTICE

Always look for contra-indications for cutting and shaping; these could relate to infections, infestations, poor hair/skin condition, difficult hair growth patterns, face shape and physical features.

Now and again a men's named style becomes fashionable. Some of these names, such as a 'Grade 1 all over', a 'David Beckham', an 'EMO', a 'Wigo', a 'Mullet', the Wedge or a Mohawk, have passed at some time or another into the general vocabulary. Always make sure that you know what your client means if he uses a name to describe a style; remember, it may be completely different from your idea of that style.

TOP TIP

How often do you find people using the wrong expression or term to explain what they want? Always make a point of correcting misused terms; it will show that you:

◆ listen to the client and you are hearing what he says

◆ have a professional knowledge of your craft and its skills and techniques

◆ have pride and professional interest in your work.

BEST PRACTICE

Look out for:	Why is it a concern?
Hair density	Scalps with densely populated hair can always be reduced, thinned or controlled in some way, whereas thinner hair or male pattern baldness create a range of limitations that you will need to both express and contend with.
Hair tendency	Curly hair has more styling limitations than straighter hair. Wavy hair is always easier to direct or position than straight hair. Point these factors out before you start.
Hair texture	Fine hair is always difficult to handle, whereas coarser hair when straight will often appear spiky or blunt. Conversely, coarse, wavy hair can often appear dry regardless of natural condition. Each hair texture type creates a different problem.

ACTIVITY

Knowing how to remove, replace and maintain the clipper blades is an essential part of hairdressing. With the electric clippers removed from the power supply or rechargeable clippers 'run down', get your supervisor to show you how the lower blade-retaining screws are undone and removed. This will give you access to both cutting blades and the area below the armature (the vibrating arm that works them) for cleaning purposes.

When you have dismantled the blades get used to checking for signs of corrosion. If a rusted area exists it will look like blackened areas around the blade edges. If blades have been allowed to get to this stage they should be replaced by new ones as their ability to cut cleanly without friction has been greatly reduced.

With the blades stripped down, you can now use clipper oil to lubricate the two blades, wiping any excess away. Now you can replace the blades (the right way up) and partially re-tighten the retaining screws. Finally, readjust the alignment of the blades and tighten the screws. Check the alignment once more: the lower stationary cutting blade should extend around 3mm further than the upper cutting blade with the clippers adjusted fully forwards to the shortest cutting length. Hand them back to your supervisor so that your maintenance can be checked.

Diversion

Good care and regular maintenance of your tools is an essential part of hairdressing and barbering.

Cutting tools and equipment

Clippers Clippers are and have been an essential item of equipment for men's styling. They have been invaluable for the popularity of short hairstyles but are equally important for the shaping and trimming of necklines and facial hair shapes.

The electric clippers cut hair by oscillation: the side-to-side movement of an upper metal blade passing over a lower rigid or fixed one. On each pass of the upper blade, the hair caught between the teeth of the lower blade is cut and falls away.

Regular cleaning and lubrication will prolong the blades' useful life and keep the cutting edges sharp. Without this care the constant friction of one blade passing over another will affect their ability to work properly: electric clippers generate quite a lot of heat and, if they have not been maintained, their ability to cut cleanly and efficiently deteriorates over time. New blades are relatively expensive, as they can often cost half the price of a new pair of clippers. If the clipper blades are unable to cut keenly you will not be able to trim, shape and style neck or facial hair shapes accurately.

You should always take care not to drop them, as this can easily cause damage to the cutting teeth or even break them! Any missing areas of teeth along the blades will be extremely dangerous and could easily cut the client if they were used. So when they are not in use, hang them up out of the way or replace them back in the charger unit.

Clipper blades should always be checked for alignment before each time they are used. The fixed lower blade is adjustable and this allows for small adjustments to be made backwards, forwards or even side to side.

Loosening the small retaining screws underneath allows the blades to be adjusted. This also provides access to the upper blade, for removal, cleaning out the fragments of hair and essential oiling/lubrication.

When the blades are replaced the retaining screws must be retightened properly. If this is not done, the vibration will dislodge the alignment and this could easily take a chunk out of your client's hair, or worse, even cut him!

Well-maintained clippers will cut either wet or dry hair with equal ease, although many stylists prefer to cut the hair first, and then wash the hair after to remove any small fragments and make any final checks.

HEALTH & SAFETY

Always take care when using any sharp items of equipment. Your safety and the safety of the client are in your hands; take care not to be distracted while you are working.

> For more information on looking after these items see Chapter 10.

> See also Unit GH12 Cut hair using basic techniques, pages 266–299, which covers:
> - scissors
> - thinning scissors
> - combs, neck brushes and sectioning clips.

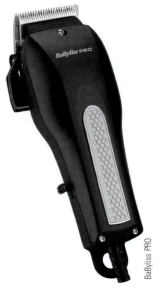

BaByliss PRO

Razor

Standard clipper grades/attachments

Clipper attachment size	Length of cut hair
No attachment/grade fitted	
Grade 1 = 3mm ($\frac{1}{8}$ inch)	Very close to skin, almost as close as shaving. Very short, on darker hair it will only leave a stubbly shadowing effect
Grade 2 = 6mm ($\frac{1}{4}$ inch)	Close cut, will see some skin on finer hair types but short enough for the hair to appear straight even if it is naturally curly
Grade 3 = 9mm ($\frac{3}{8}$ inch)	Popular length grade for short groomed effects. Typically cuts to that of short scissor over comb lengths
Grade 4 = 13mm ($\frac{1}{2}$ inch)	Popular length which has a similar effect to longer scissor over comb type effects
Grades 6–8 = 16mm-25mm ($\frac{1}{2}$–1 inch)	Popular longer lengths used for beard shaping

Note: There are no set standard sizes for clipper attachment combs/grades; you will need to adapt the hair length required by your client in light of the make and model clippers that you have/or your salon provides.

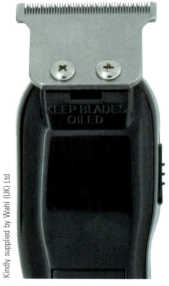

Kindly supplied by Wahl (UK) Ltd

Clipper blade

Razors The open or 'cut-throat' style razor used in shaving is made out of a single steel blade which is hinged and closed into a protective handle. The modern counterpart for this has disposable blades which can be removed and disposed of safely after use. (Note: As a matter of good practice and hygiene – razors with disposable blades are always disposed of after each client in a sharps box, this avoids any risk of cross-infection. A fixed blade 'cut-throat' must be sterilized between use on different clients.)

The razor used for hair styling is called a **shaper**; it too has disposable blades which are fitted into a hinged sheath that provides a handy, safe styling tool. Razor cutting is *always* carried out on wet hair and with sharp blades. This is because of the way in which razors are used, and the angle at which they cut through the hair. Razoring should never be done on dry hair as this will be painful for the client, and pull and tear the hair, possibly causing it to split, even if the blades are new.

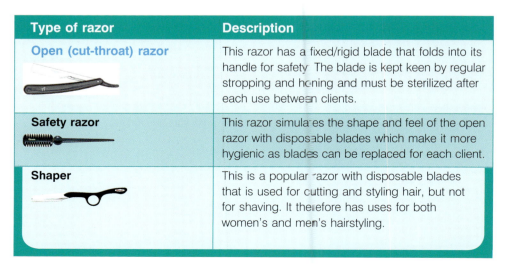

Type of razor	Description
Open (cut-throat) razor	This razor has a fixed/rigid blade that folds into its handle for safety. The blade is kept keen by regular stropping and honing and must be sterilized after each use between clients.
Safety razor	This razor simulates the shape and feel of the open razor with disposable blades which make it more hygienic as blades can be replaced for each client.
Shaper	This is a popular razor with disposable blades that is used for cutting and styling hair, but not for shaving. It therefore has uses for both women's and men's hairstyling.

ACTIVITY

Choosing a hairstyle

The hairstyle that you choose for your client is influenced by a number of different factors. We have listed the main considerations in the table below. What impacts do these features have upon your decisions?

Aspect to consider	Effect/impacts on styling
Head and facial shape	
Body physical features	
Reason and purpose for the style	
Quality, quantity and distribution of the hair	
Hair positioning, type, growth and tendency	
Style suitability	
Age and ability	
Lifestyle	

Cutting techniques

Cutting tools	Techniques that can be achieved	Explanation of technique
Scissors (straight or flat parallel blades)	Club cutting (blunt cutting) Freehand cutting	The most basic and most popular way of cutting sections of hair straight across, parallel to the index and middle finger. The blunt, straight sections of cut hair that it produces are ideal for precise lines. The different angles that the hair can be held will produce either square, graduating or reverse graduating layer patterns.
Thinning scissors	Thinning/texturizing	Thinning scissors will remove uniform bulk from any point between the root area and ends. However, they have more creative uses when they are used to 'feather' the perimeter edges of hairstyles (which is often more difficult with straight bladed scissors).

Cutting tools	Techniques that can be achieved	Explanation of technique
Electric clippers	Clippering with grade attachments	Clipper grades (the attachments that provide uniform cutting lengths) are made in a range of sizes for different purposes, and are numbered accordingly. They will provide closely cut uniform layering or if differing grades are used, they can provide graduation on hair that is too short to hold between the fingers.
Kindly supplied by Wahl (UK) Ltd	Fading Clipper over comb and scissor over comb	A way of blending short hair at the nape or edges of a hairstyle down or 'out' to the skin. It is achieved by using the clippers with the blade 'backed off' creating a very short, tapered effect with a smooth blended effect without any lines. Both techniques are a popular way of layering or fading very short hair into styles that can't be held between the fingers. The hair is held and supported by a comb and the free edges protruding through are removed.

Cutting hair to achieve a variety of looks

Cutting rules

There isn't any mystery about cutting, it's like most other things: if you follow the procedural steps and do each thing at the right time, you will get the right results. These rules maintain a consistent approach to the way that you tackle any hairstyle and the consistency bit ensures that you achieve the correct quality levels during the execution of the work.

These rules are set out below:

Cut hair with natural fall Being aware of and cutting with natural fall is extremely important. Looking for the directions of growth within the hair is an essential part of consultation as it is within the execution of the haircut. If you work with the natural fall in terms of partings, nape hair growth, double crowns, etc., you will be compensating for these anomalies and be able to produce an easier to manage result. Ignore these factors and you will be giving both you and the client a hard job in styling it.

As previously covered in preparation, always try to shampoo the hair, even if you are only doing a dry haircut. This way when you dry the hair off, you will be able to see the natural fall far easier and be able to work with it.

Accurate sectioning   Having made the previous considerations of safety, care and the hair design aspects, you are almost ready to start cutting. The only other thing that you need to consider is how you tackle all that hair, when parts of it can easily get in the way whilst you work. Very short hair doesn't really pose any problem but sectioning isn't just for those with very long hair.

In order for you to be able to manage sizeable amounts of hair at any one time, you must organize and plan the haircut. The planning bit becomes automatic; it's the few moments that you spend thinking:

◆ How do I go about this?

◆ Where do I start?

◆ What is the finish going to be like?

So, if the planning is automatic it's the organization bit that you have to address. Quite simply, being organized is about working in a methodical way. It is the way in which you routinely start at one point, divide and secure all the rest of the hair out of the way, finish that bit, and then take down the next part to work on, and so on.

Each part or section that you work on should be small enough for you to cope with, without losing your way and continuing on blindly! It seems a strange term to use, but 'blindly' is exactly the right word. If the sections are too deep or too wide you will not be able to see the cutting guideline that you need to work to. Accurate sectioning guarantees that every cut is addressed to the same length every time.

Controlling the shape   There are three aspects of cutting that you must get right on every haircut:

◆ *The holding angle* – the angle at which the hair is held out from the head

◆ *The cutting angle* – the angle at which the scissors, razor, etc. cuts the hair

◆ *The holding tension* – the even pressure applied to sections of hair when it is held ready for cutting.

That doesn't seem much to guarantee success, but it does take a lot of practise and concentration. Even if you start well in the haircut you cannot afford to 'lose it' in the closing stages.

Cutting lines, or perimeter lines are the outline shape created when layered hair is held directly out with tension, i.e. perpendicular and without twisting or sagging, from the head. The curves and the angle in relation to the head, determine the shape of the cut style. The main ones are:

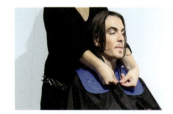

cross checking

◆ the contour of the shape from top to bottom

◆ the contour of the shape around the head, side to side.

When cutting the lines and angles, comb the hair and hold the sections with an even tension. The tension ensures that accuracy is maintained throughout the cut and the position in which you hold and cut the hair determines the position the cut sections take when combed back on the head. The angles and lines of cutting depend on the different lengths required by the style. The first cutting line – the outer perimeter line – may be related to the nape (when starting at the back). The second cutting line – the inner perimeter line – depends on the different lengths required throughout the style.

Creating guidelines The guideline is the initial cutting line that is created as a sort of template for all the subsequent sections that are taken.

As a general rule the simpler or more basic the hairstyle the fewer the guidelines there will be. Conversely, the more complex the hairstyle the more guidelines will be involved.

So at Level 2 the styles that need to be done involve fewer guidelines:

◆ a uniform layered haircut has one

◆ a basic graduation has two.

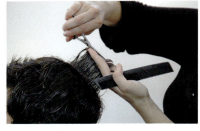

correct tension

A uniform layered haircut has layers of equal length all around the head, so the first cutting guideline dictates the overall length for the rest of the haircut.

For easier control, haircuts are always started at the back; this way the bulk of the hair is tackled and checked before moving onto the sides and top. So after dividing the hair vertically and evenly down the back, take a horizontal section at both sides about 2cm above the hairline and secure with sectioning clips out of the way. Cut this baseline to the length that you need to and after checking, take down the next section 2cm above and secure the remainder.

Cutting guidelines

Uniform layers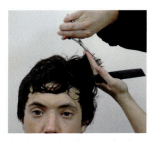

Graduation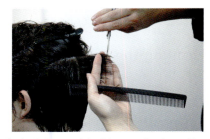

At the point beneath the vertical division in the hair, take and hold a vertical section as shown above, without twisting and with an even tension. Cut this perpendicularly (at a vertical angle) to the head. (The client's head should be horizontal and not chin down, or head back.)

With the guideline cut, you take the next section, parallel to the guideline, with the same even tension, so that you can see the lengths of the previously cut guideline through the held mesh. Cut this to the same length as the guideline. Continue this throughout each section until the complete horizontal area has been cut. Then take down another 2cm on either side and repeat the process, slowly working up the back to the crown.

With the back done, you take a horizontal section above the ears through to the front, cut your perimeter baseline and follow the guideline through from behind the ear working towards the front hairline. Repeat up to the top and cut the other side in the same way.

Finish the haircut over the top working forwards from the known guidelines at the top. Finally, trim the front hairline perimeter shape to complete the hairline profile shape and **cross-check** to see that the sides, back and top are all in balance.

The graduated haircut uses a similar guideline process to that of uniform layering; the only difference is that the hair is held out at an angle from the head as opposed to perpendicular. The steeper the angle is held away from the head, the lower the bulk line will be and the greater the weight distribution for the overlying lengths. Conversely, the shallower the angle of the cut; the higher the bulk line will be and the less weight distribution for the overlying lengths.

(For more information on cutting guidelines on uniform layers or graduation see the step by steps later in this chapter).

Cross-checking the cut

Possibly at different points during the cut, but certainly after the cut, you will need to re-check what you have already done. This is done by taking and holding sections at an angle which is at right angles (90°) to the original cut sections. (In other words, if you originally cut the hair in vertical meshes, your cross-check will be done with horizontal meshes.)

Cross-checking provides a final technique for checking the continuity and accuracy of the haircut. Where you find an imbalance in weight, or extra length that still needs to be removed, it provides you with the opportunity to create the perfect finish.

Neck outlines/shapes

Many short, layered cuts are graduated at the sides and into the nape sometimes by clipper over comb or, when left slightly longer, by scissor over comb techniques. On shorter hairstyles the neck- and hairlines become the main focal perimeters of the hairstyle and, in emphasizing these, you will need to give them careful attention as it is very easy to infringe into the hairline and remove hair that is needed for the outline shape.

Where possible always use the natural hairlines as the limit for the hairstyle. This produces a smoother effect on the eye and produces styles that look balanced and right. If you ignore the natural hairlines and cut above them, you will find that the hair below will grow back very quickly and produce a stubbly effect within a few days. Or, if done on dark hair, it will produce a 'shadowed' effect within 24 hours.

However, natural necklines often lack consistency; the growth is often uneven, intermittent or sparse. Therefore the outline shapes for these men wearing shorter hair need to be defined. The more natural the nape line, the softer and less severe will be the look.

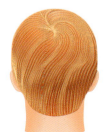
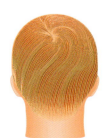
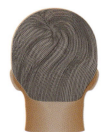

TOP TIP

Hairlines

The higher the cuts made into the hairline the harsher and starker the look becomes.

ACTIVITY

Planning your work

Any service that you provide to the client needs to be thought about before you start. This planning is essential for achieving a successful result, so in this activity, complete the table below to create a checklist of things that you should consider before carrying out the service.

Checklist for cutting

1.

2.

3.

4.

5.

6.

The shaping of front hair into a fringe can produce a variety of facial frames and the focal point it creates changes the overall effect dramatically. In many men the front hairline recedes and this is often a sign of male pattern baldness. This influences the choice and positioning of perimeter fringe shapes. Always give this some thought before cutting the hair.

In men, the side hairlines, **sideburns** or sideboards bridge the hairstyle and beard shape. These need to fit, and care must be taken in shaping them. Lining the hair above the ears and along the sides of the nape is usually carried out with the scissor points or carefully angled inverted clippers.

Common cutting problems

Necklines All of the classic perimeter neckline shapes above can easily be ruined if a lack of care and attention occurs. The detail of the outline of very short hair can easily be spoiled by careless layering or clippering. Every millimetre counts. You need to make sure that your outlining with the clippers is even and smooth throughout. If you do make a mistake and find that you have encroached on the outline shape you would be better off re-cutting the outline slightly shorter to eliminate the fault.

BEST PRACTICE

Always check the clipper blade alignment before using them for each client.

Blending from clipper lengths to scissor length Another common problem on short hair is found at the **blend area** between different clippered grades, or between the clippered and hand-held cut lengths. If a careful blending hasn't been made cutting marks will show at the point where the two areas combine.

There are two ways of tackling this problem:

1 If the hair is still too long on the hand-cut/held side, you can re-fade the two zones together by scissor over comb methods. Be careful not to undercut the longer lengths as this will mean that you will have to re-cut all the clippered area.

2 If the lengths of hair between the two areas are slightly uneven it will definitely show unless you correct it. In any area where clippers fade out to club cut lengths you can

resurface the hair by using thinning scissors over comb just on the very tips of the hair. A light blending of thinned hair produces an optical illusion that cheats the eye by softening the two hard cut edges and the final effect appears correct.

Ears Nature does not guarantee symmetry, and this is particularly true with faces. One side of the face is not exactly the same as the other and this applies to ears too. One may be larger than the other; they may be irregular in shape or at different heights; you need to make sure that you have considered this before you start. Unevenness on long hair doesn't matter, but when it's on short hair the imperfections will be made clear.

You need to find out how your client feels about his facial features. Sometimes these natural imperfections are not a concern; they are merely a characteristic of the client's personality. Don't forget to check on whether your client wears glasses or a hearing aid; take all of these factors into your assessment.

Finally you and your client will be able to agree exactly what look is required, and you will then have a basis on which to decide how the work is to be carried out.

Hair type If your client's hair is very curly, do remember that it will coil back after stretching and cutting. Similarly, wavy hair, when cut too close to the wave crest, can be awkward to style as it tends to spring out from the head. Very fine straight hair will easily show cutting marks or can disclose unwanted lines from clippering if you take too large sections. Make sure that the sections you take are accurately divided and sectioned.

Final points to remember

1 If the hair is dirty, then for hygienic reasons it must be washed before you cut it. Wet hair is a necessity for blow-drying and finishing, but not necessarily a convenient arrangement for a quick trim before work or during lunch.

2 Clean, dry hair should not be cut with a razor because of the discomfort to your client caused by the tearing and dragging action of the razor on the hair.

3 Accurate sectioning and graduation produces fine layering. This is partly determined by how much hair there is to cut. Longer lengths can be sectioned with the comb and taken between the fingers, while short lengths are best tackled either by clipper over comb or scissor over comb techniques. A section (that cannot be held between the fingers) is lifted with the comb and a guideline is created by cutting straight across. Subsequent lifting with the comb to the guideline length produces the next section to be cut.

4 Clippers must be used to tidy the necklines on short styles, graduating from the natural line out from the head. How far up the head and how short the cut needs to be is determined by the style and shape agreed with your client. If longer lengths are required higher in the back hair, then the clippers need to graduate away from the head sharply.

5 Cross-checking is an essential part of cutting. It's your way of including a quality control. As you progress through the cut, you obviously need to change your stance, holding position and holding angle. These factors can lead you to go wrong. Typical problems might be that the back section doesn't integrate with the sides properly or the top doesn't blend with the sides, or the fringe doesn't fit with the top. Whatever the potential problem the easiest way to compensate for this is to cross-check to make sure that the cut works well in different planes.

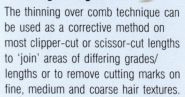

TOP TIP

Removing cutting marks
The thinning over comb technique can be used as a corrective method on most clipper-cut or scissor-cut lengths to 'join' areas of differing grades/lengths or to remove cutting marks on fine, medium and coarse hair textures.

TOP TIP

Men's short hairstyles often benefit from washing again after cutting. This removes all the shorter clippings and makes them more comfortable.

Tapering and thinning encourage the hair to curl at the ends, while club cutting increases density and reduces that tendency.

Feathering and texturizing can produce extra lift and bounce.

If your client has a build-up of wax, gel or moulding crème on their hair you must insist that the hair is washed to get it out or off the hair before you attempt the haircut.

STEP-BY-STEP: CLIPPER GRADUATION

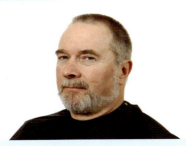

1 This sequence shows a typical men's graduated clipper cut. However there is another sequence that focuses upon the beard shaping, see page 339.

CHECK THE BLADE ALIGNMENT FIRST!

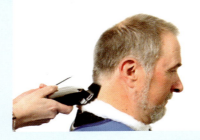

2 When hair is too short to section, you need to start at the bottom with the longest grade attachment first.

This enables you to work up the head cutting the longest hair first and then working down to the shortest required grade and fading through from the shortest to the longest.

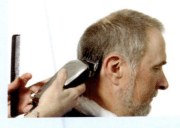

3 Cut all the back hair in direct vertical movements first.

Make sure at this stage that you don't go around the occipital bone as this can often need blending into the top with scissors. (Not in this case)

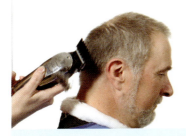

4 After cutting vertically, you can sweep across at an angle to ensure that the clippers have picked up all the hair that needs to be cut.

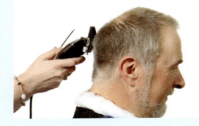

5 Here we see the exit point at the occipital and the hand position which enables the clippers to leave the cutting line at the back of the head, in one complete movement.

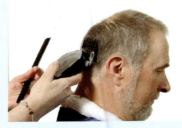

6 Change down to a shorter length grade and re-cut the back, fading out into the longer length grade below the occipital.

Continue with shorter grades depending on the client's wishes. Remember to fade the short grade into the longer grade above at a lower point each time.

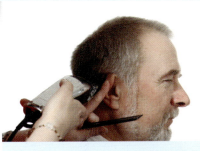

7 When working on the sides, make sure that you hold the ear out of the way.

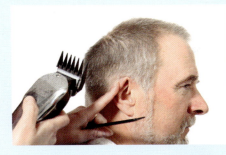

8 Cut upwards, away from the ears.

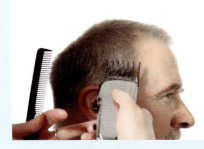

9 Continue around the sides to the frontal area, blending the shorter grades into the longer one at the top.

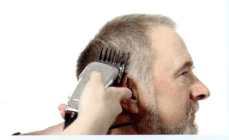

10 Fade out to the longer grade above.

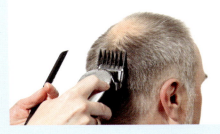

11 Finish blending the clippered area with either:

1   A longer length grade for the top, as shown in step 13 or,

2   The hair can be cut scissor over comb.

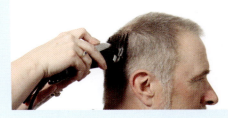

12 Continue this around the back and sides.

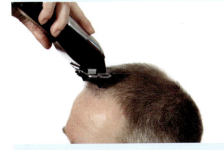

13 With back and side done, work through the top area to the crown (depending on whether the client wants scissor-cut length or clippers).

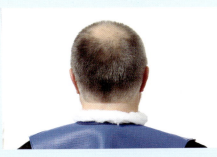

14 Finally, remove the attachments and re-check the blade alignment. You can now profile the back hair by turning the clippers over and cutting 'edge' onwards to create the U, V or square outline required.

STEP-BY-STEP: UNIFORM LAYERING

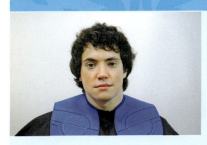

1 Put on a clean gown or cutting square and place a cutting collar around the shoulders.

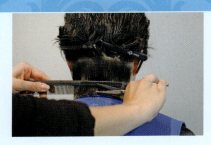

2 Section off the hair at the back so you can cut the lower perimeter length first.

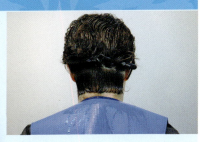

3 With the base line cut, you can tidy the neck hair now or leave it to the end.

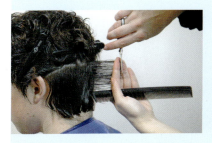

4 Start your guide line at the centre of the back with a vertically held mesh. Now cut all the other sections around the lower nape to the same length.

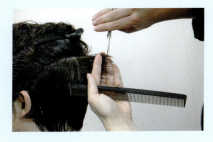

5 Continue up the back by taking a centrally held section directly above your first guide line.

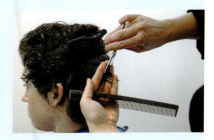

6 Cut the other sections around the back to the same length.

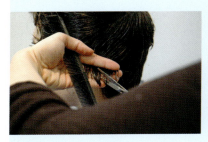

7 Adjust your holding position to suit your stance and comfort.

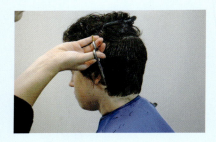

8 Cut the outline shape by safely cutting away from the ears.

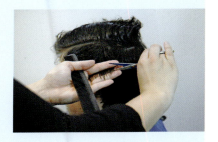

9 Cross-check your layering to maintain the accuracy.

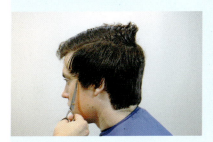

10 Carefully outline the shape to create the profile.

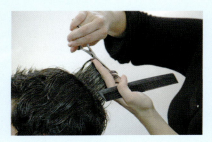

11 Continue into the top by taking your guideline over the crown.

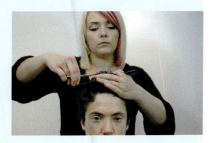

12 Work towards the front by club cutting.

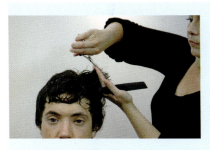

13 Blend in the top to the previously cut sides.

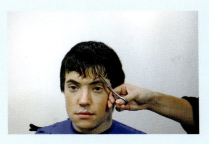

14 Finish off the front by point cutting the fringe to reduce unwanted weight.

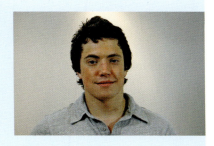

15 Final effect.

CourseMate video: Gents Uniform Layer

Provide aftercare advice

Product knowledge

More information on products can be found elsewhere in this book.

These provide a useful reference and range of products that would be suitable for recommending to men to help them manage their hair between visits.

Please see the styling products table in Unit GB5 Dry and finish men's hair pages 194–197.

Home- and aftercare checklist

✓ Talk through the style as you work; that way the client sees how you handle different aspects of the look.

✓ Show and recommend the products/equipment that you use so that the client gets the right things to enable them to get the same effects.

✓ Tell the client how long they can expect the style to last and when they need to return for re-shaping.

✓ Demonstrate the techniques that you use so they can achieve that salon hair look too.

✓ Tell the client what you are doing, keep them informed

In Unit GH12 we looked at aftercare that you should give the clients. We should follow that procedure for male clients in the barber shop, read pages 296–297 and remind yourself of the procedure.

For further information on how to give advice to clients see Units G7 Advise and consult with clients and G18 Promote additional products and services to clients.

SUMMARY

Remember to:

- ✓ prepare clients correctly for the services you are going to carry out

- ✓ put on the protective wear available for styling and dressing hair

- ✓ listen to the client's requirements and discuss suitable courses of action

- ✓ adhere to the safety factors when working on clients' hair

- ✓ keep the work areas clean, hygienic and free from hazards

- ✓ promote the range of services, products and treatments within the salon

- ✓ clean and sterilize the tools and equipment before they are used

- ✓ work carefully and methodically through the processes of cutting hair, whether wet or dry

- ✓ place, position and direct the hair appropriately to achieve the desired effect

- ✓ communicate what you are doing with the client as well as your fellow staff members.

Knowledge Check

For this project you will need to select two of your clients:

Client 1 should have short clippered hair.

Client 2 should have longer uniform layers.

For each of these clients:

1   Describe what your client's hair was like before you started.

2   Explain how you decided upon the style that was done.

3   Describe what methods, techniques and tools were used to complete the look.

4   Take a photograph (perhaps with your mobile) of the finished effect.

ASSESSMENT OF KNOWLEDGE AND UNDERSTANDING

A selection of different types of questions to check your cutting knowledge, these should also refresh your knowledge gained from Chapter 12.

Q1   Accuracy is achieved by ___ and cutting the hair at the correct angle.   Fill in the blank

Q2   Scissors should be sterilized in Barbicide™.   True or false

Q3   Select from the following list those that are *not* texturizing techniques: Multi selection

Club cutting	☐ 1
Graduation	☐ 2
Slice cutting	☐ 3
Layering	☐ 4
Point cutting	☐ 5
Chipping	☐ 6

Q4   Symmetrical shapes produce equally balanced hairstyles.   True or false

Q5   Which of the following is not a cutting term?   Multi choice

Cross-checking   O a

Thinning   O b

Freehand   O c

Freestyle   O d

Q6   Accurate clipper cutting is dependent upon the angle at which they are   True or false
held in relation to the head.

Q7   Which of the following hair growth patterns will affect the natural fall   Multi selection
and way that a fringe lies after it is cut?

Nape whorl   ☐ 1

Double crown   ☐ 2

Widow's peak   ☐ 3

Low hairline   ☐ 4

Cow lick   ☐ 5

High hairline   ☐ 6

Q8   A ___ is the perimeter shape produced by cutting.   Fill in the blank

Q9   Which of the following cuts would easily describe a disconnection?   Multi choice

Graduation in a long hairstyle   O a

Reverse graduation in a long hairstyle   O b

A fringe in a shoulder-length bob style   O c

Texturizing in a short cropped style   O d

Q10   Clubbing is a technique of cutting that maximizse the hair density.   True or false

14 Trimming beards, moustaches and sideburns

LEARNING OBJECTIVES

◆ Be able to maintain effective and safe methods of working

◆ Be able to cut beards and moustaches to maintain their shape

◆ Be able to provide aftercare advice

◆ Know how to work safely, effectively and hygienically when cutting

◆ Know how to use cutting tools and equipment

◆ Understand the cutting techniques used for trimming and shaping facial hair

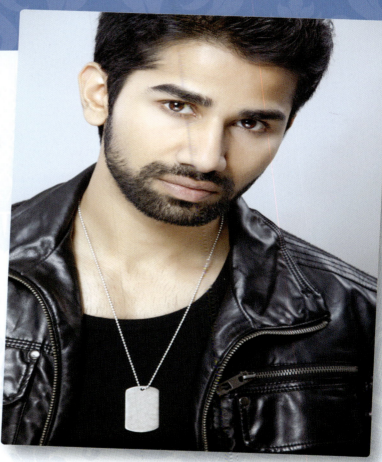

scissor over comb

KEY TERMS

barbering comb

clipper over comb

clipper-grade attachments

cross-checking

exfoliation

freehand cutting

Unit title

GB4 Cut facial hair to shape using basic techniques

Information covered in this chapter

◆ The tools and equipment used during trimming and shaping

◆ The preparations that you should make prior to cutting facial hair

◆ The factors that influence facial hair cutting decisions

◆ Cutting/trimming facial hair techniques

◆ The aftercare advice that you should give clients

INTRODUCTION

This unit looks at the basic skills of trimming and shaping men's beards and moustaches. The techniques involved are quite different to those used in other hair services although you will find that the same equipment keeps cropping up but it is now used in different ways.

These rudimentary practices have always been a feature of men's barbering and this chapter explores the different aspects that you should consider before tackling the skills of this essential barbering service.

Facial hair trimming

If you have already covered the men's cutting unit GB3 you will be familiar with the techniques of freehand, scissor over comb and clipper over comb techniques. These techniques and the other things that you will need to cover are set out within this chapter under the following topics:

- preparation and maintenance
- client consultation
- identifying the influencing factors that affect style choice
- cutting techniques and accuracy
- good customer care.

Be able to maintain effective and safe methods of working when cutting facial hair

Preparing the client

Your duty and responsibilities towards health and safety are reinforced throughout all hair-related services and each service has specific procedures that you should follow. This outcome addresses all of the health and safety issues that you need to consider when styling facial hair.

Gowning the client Always use freshly clean, laundered protective equipment:

- Fasten a gown at the back, or secure the cutting square with a clip ensuring that the covering is close-fitting around the neck and protects the client from any clippings or spillages.
- Place a towel around the front of the client so that the free edges are fastened at the back.
- Tuck a strip of neck wool (or neck tissue) into the top edge of the towel to stop hair fragments from falling inside the client's clothes.

After consultation and just prior to starting, cover the client's eyes with a cotton wool pad to prevent snippings and clippings from entering their eyes.

Positioning the client Facial hair cutting requires the client to tilt their head back so that you can work at an angle that enables you to work safely and carefully. The barbering chair is designed for this with its inbuilt head rest and reclining ability. (If you need to recline the chair do it before the client is seated.)

If you need to make any adjustments to working height or angle you can do this now.

Your working position and posture

Barbering, as you already know, involves a lot of standing and because of this you need to be comfortable in your work. You should always adopt a comfortable but safe work position, but sometimes comfortable and safe are not necessarily the same thing.

Cutting involves a lot of arm and hand movements and you need to be able to get close enough so that your hands and fingers are in a position where you can cut the hair unencumbered, without bad posture.

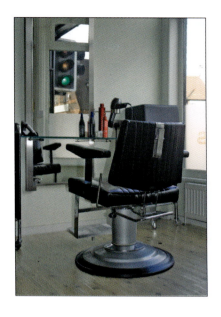

1 You should adjust the seated client's chair height to a position where you can work upright without having to over reach on the top sections of their head.

2 You should clear trolleys or equipment out of the way so that you get good all-round access (300°) around the client.

3 Your equipment should be close enough at hand for you to reach it safely without putting you or the client at risk; the items should be clean, sterile and ready for use.

Your personal hygiene

Personal hygiene can't be stressed enough; it is vitally important for anyone working in personal services. Your personal hygiene, or lack of it, will be immediately noticeable to everyone you come into contact with. You may have overslept, but if you haven't showered it will be very uncomfortable for you, your colleagues and the clients as BO is unpleasant in any situation. Other strong smells are offensive too; the smells of nicotine or smoking are very off-putting to the client, particularly if they are a non-smoker.

Working efficiently, safely and effectively

Working efficiently and maximizing your time is essential, so making the most of the resources available should occur naturally. Always treat the salon's materials in the same way that you would look after your own equipment; always try to minimize waste, being careful with how much product you use.

Make full use of your time: don't leave things to the last minute as this will encroach into the appointment time: Prepare your tools and equipment so that they are cleaned and sterilized.

You need to work in an orderly environment; you must have the materials that you need at hand and the equipment that you want to use in position and ready for action. This is a good exercise in self-organization and shows others that you are a true professional.

Keep an eye on the clock; you must remember that you need to be working to time and that means providing the styling service in a commercially acceptable time. Don't forget your client is expecting to go home at some point too.

BEST PRACTICE

It is important to keep your breath fresh when conversing with clients. Bad breath (halitosis) is the result of leaving particles to decay within the spaces between the teeth. You need to brush your teeth after every meal. Bad breath can also result from digestive troubles, stomach upsets, smoking and eating strong foods such as onions, garlic and some cheeses.

Prevent infection

Infection and disease occur by two obvious methods within the salon/barber shop environment. They are:

- either brought in by a 'carrier' visiting the salon who then cross-infects other people within the salon
- or the result of poor hygiene and cleanliness within the salon.

Most of the preparatory aspects covered in this chapter aim to keep the standards of hygiene within your working environment very high.

But there would be little point in maintaining the healthy environment unless you checked your clients for signs of infections or infestations during your consultation, as a warm, humid salon can offer a perfect home for disease-carrying bacteria. If they can find food in the form of dust and dirt, they may reproduce rapidly.

Good ventilation, however, provides a circulating air current that will help to prevent their growth. This is why it is important to keep the salon clean, dry and well aired at all times. This includes clothing, work areas, tools and all equipment. Sterilization provides the most effective way of providing hygienically safe work implements in salons. Sterilization means the complete eradication of living organisms.

Different types of equipment use different sterilization methods, which may be based on the use of heat, radiation or chemicals.

ACTIVITY

Disposal of sharps

What is your salon's policy for the disposal of sharps?

Contact your local council offices' environmental health department for more information.

For more information see pages 11–12 in the health and safety chapter.

Disposal of waste and sharps

HEALTH & SAFETY

Disposal of sharp items

Used razor blades and similar items should be placed into a safe container ('sharps box'). When the container is full it can be discarded. This type of salon waste should be kept away from general salon waste as special disposal arrangements may be provided by your local authority.

Prepare the client's facial hair

Many men with longer beards never comb them out because they don't want to lose the shape they naturally take on, or they simply don't see the benefits of doing so. Obviously this is a mistake, as regular grooming keeps them free from debris and reduces the chance of infections or ingrowing hair. You should always make a point of giving the clients advice on this or at least tell them how they can manage their own facial hair between visits.

Moustaches and beards get matted as they get longer because the bristles tend to get curlier and lock together. These tangles have to be removed so that the longer hair is revealed, and this allows you to style *all* of the hair and not just part of it.

Cleansing is important too; a beard with debris or grease cannot be styled until it has been cleaned. If you are shampooing the hair as part of another service, then the beard can be done at the same time, or alternatively, you can ask the client to wash their face and beard in the front wash basin or cleanse with facial wipes.

Consultation

Check the client's requirements The main aims of hairdressing and barbering are about delivering a continuing, repeated service that satisfies our clients. We can only satisfy the clients if we find out what they want and act upon those instructions. We demonstrate this by getting confirmation of the things we are doing throughout the service. This does a number of things:

◆ It ensures that we only do things that the clients want.

◆ It makes them more confident about what we are doing.

◆ It removes any misunderstanding or confusion.

◆ It gives us more confidence in what we are doing for the client.

◆ It involves the client and helps to develop a professional relationship.

You need to understand your client fully and be able to negotiate and seek agreement with him throughout the service.

Identify factors that influence the service Be sure to listen to your client's requests. Many mistakes can be avoided if you achieve a clear understanding of what the client is asking for.

The facial style that you choose with your client should take into account each of the following points about the client's:

◆ face and head shape/size

◆ facial physical features (including any scars or blemishes that need disguising)

◆ hair quality, abundance, growth and distribution

◆ age, lifestyle and suitability.

For more information see Unit G7 Advise and consult with clients—Using visual aids in consultation, pages 105–106.

Facial features

Facial features	How best to work with it
Square and oblong facial shapes	Square and oblong are typically masculine and provide a perfect base for traditional classic well-groomed looks. The angular features of the face can be augmented with closer, shorter beards or moustaches and would probably benefit from fewer curves and more angular, linear effects.
Round faces	The effect of a round face can be lessened or increased: it depends what the client wants. If the plan is to reduce the effects, then choose beard designs that lengthen the jawline and incorporate lines and angles rather than curves. If the round features suit the personality and image of the client then work with it by cutting uniform length shapes.
Square angular features, jaw, forehead, etc.	Again these are traditionally accepted as a feature of masculinity. These can be handled in a similar way to that of the squarer features above. Squarer, more angular features can also be easily softened with beards and moustaches.
Small faces	Smaller faces should be balanced with facial hair designs that don't overpower the overall effect. Keep your designs close cut and uniform in length.

Facial features	How best to work with it
Wider heads	These wide features will be increased with full, long beards. Create beard designs that are closer cut at the sides and extend to more length at the chin.
Scars, marks and blemishes	If the client has any scars or blemishes this may be the reason for growing a beard or moustache in the first place. You need to ask if there are any features that the client wants to disguise. *Always make a point of looking for these during your consultation*.
Facial piercing	Facial piercings around the mouth and ears do need to be considered during your consultation as well. It is unlikely that the client will want to remove them/it so you have to be very careful in combing, detangling and cutting anywhere near to the area(s) of the piercing(s).

You need to find out how your client feels about his facial features. Sometimes these natural imperfections are not a concern; they are merely a characteristic of the client's personality. Don't forget to check on whether your client wears glasses or a hearing aid; take all of these factors into account.

Finally you and your client will be able to agree exactly what look is required, and you will then have a basis on which to decide how the work is to be carried out.

Aspects to consider

Some men have a heavy, daily growth of facial hair and they find that they need to shave every day. This heavy growth can be obvious for a range of reasons.

1. The growth appears heavy because of the contrast against the skin due to natural colour.

2. The hair seems to grow particularly fast.

3. The density of hair distributed on the face is particularly thick.

4. Combinations of these factors put together.

So, bearing these aspects in mind – initially, the males that are most likely to choose to grow beards and/or moustaches will have ticked two or more of the above. But they are not the only ones who choose to do this, as many others with a poorer growth or definition will grow facial hair for other reasons.

Mouth and width of upper lip to base of nose The size and width of the mouth forms the basis for any moustache. The distance between the upper lip and the base of the nose creates a sort of canvas for the moustache. If the distance between the two areas is quite deep, it will provide more outline shape options for the wearer than if it were narrow.

Similarly, the width of the face at the cheeks will also determine the best-suited effect. Someone with a wide face will be able to wear a fuller moustache, whereas someone with a narrow face could be *swamped* by this much hair.

HEALTH & SAFETY

Always make sure that the clippers are cleaned before they are used. Any hair caught between the blades will limit their ability to work, and is unhygienic for the client.

Bone structure and facial contours You should take particular care for clients who have a well-defined bone structure, i.e. cheekbones, jaws and facial contour. If they have a particularly linear aspect to their facial features then it would be wiser to retain that similar effect with the overall shapes and outlines. (That's unless they want to disguise themselves or have physical features they want to cover up.)

On the other hand, the man who has a rounder, fuller face can benefit from a shape that defines the face with a more structured effect. Remember that these people can wear beards with fuller effects than those men with narrower facial features.

Width of chin and depth of jawline Facial hair growth forms a frame for the physical features of the face and it is the width of the chin and the depth down to the bottom of the jaw that become the focal point of any facial hair shaping. The outlines of the shapes created here are more noticeable than any others. Historically, beards were left relatively full; this meant that there was very little upkeep for the wearer, apart from keeping the beard from getting too bushy. Latterly, the fashion for wearing more chiselled effects has meant that not only thickness but an outline shape must be maintained.

Tools and equipment

Scissors Scissors are and will always be the most important piece of hairdressing equipment that you will ever own. If you look after them you will be surprised how long a single pair will last. Scissors can be used on either wet or dry hair and vary greatly in their design, size and price. There isn't any single way of choosing the correct pair for you; however, there are a number of aspects that you should consider.

Thinning scissors Thinning scissors can be used on facial hair but have a limited practical use. They have blades with serrated teeth. These cutting surfaces will remove bulk or density from hair but can leave a beard a little endy.

Cutting combs Get into the habit of only using good-quality cutting combs. You will find that by spending only a little more you will get so much more out of them. The design of a cutting comb for hairdressing is quite different to that of barbering.

The hairdressing cutting comb is parallel and rigid throughout its length whereas the **barbering comb** is tapered and more flexible. For trimming and styling beards or moustaches you will probably find that the rigid, hairdressing comb is more useful. It will be easier to comb out tangled facial hair and it also provides a better cutting guide for scissor and clipper over comb work.

There are also two sorts of cutting comb. The first and by far the most popular has two sets of differently spaced teeth: at one end they are finer and set closer together while the other half are wider and further apart. This provides more control with finer sections on fine hair and wider sections on the coarser, more bristly hair. The second type of cutting comb has uniformly spaced teeth throughout the length of the comb.

The length of cutting combs varies greatly. Again, what's best for you depends on the size of your hands and what you can manage and manipulate quite easily. The normal length of a cutting comb is around 15cm but long ones are now very popular and provide a better guide when cutting freehand baselines.

The quality of combs and the materials they are made from varies greatly. The best-quality combs are made from plastics that have the following properties:

◆ They are very strong but flexible; the teeth do not chip or break in regular use.

◆ They remain straight in regular use and do not end up looking like a banana after a couple of weeks!

◆ They are constructed by injection moulding and do not have sharp or poorly formed edges (as opposed to combs that are made from pressings and have flawed seams which tend to scratch the client's ears and scalp).

◆ They are resistant to chemicals, making them ideal for cleaning, sterilization and colouring (as they will not stain).

ACTIVITY

Disorders and diseases

This task will help you to revise your knowledge of hair and scalp disorders and conditions.

Fill in the table below. We have completed the first one for you.

Name	Description	Cause	Treatment
Dandruff	Small, itchy, dry scales of shedding epidermal skin	Overactive cell production	Dandruff scalp treatments and shampoo designed to control the problem
Alopecia areata			
Psoriasis			
Seborrhoea			
Male pattern baldness			
Fragilitis crinium			
Damaged cuticle			
Trichorrhexis nodosa			
Monilethrix			
Barber's itch			

Clippers Clippers are and have been an essential item of equipment for men's styling. They have been invaluable for the popularity of short hairstyles but are equally important for the shaping and trimming of necklines and facial hair shapes.

Maintaining the tools

	Tools	Method of cleaning/sterilizing
	Neck brush	Wash in hot soapy water and place in ultraviolet cabinet for ten minutes
	Sectioning clips	Wash in hot soapy water and immerse in Barbicide™ jar for 30 minutes
	Cutting comb	Wash in hot soapy water and immerse in Barbicide™ jar for 30 minutes
	Scissors	Brush away hair fragments from pivot area and blades with a colouring brush. Carefully wipe the blades with sterile wipes and then place with open blades in the ultraviolet cabinet for 15 minutes each side
	Thinning scissors	Brush away hair fragments from pivot area and blades with a colouring brush. Carefully wipe the blades with sterile wipes and then place with open blades in the ultraviolet cabinet for 15 minutes each side

See pages 312–318 for more information on this topic

Cut beards and moustaches to maintain their shape

Facial hair cutting techniques

Many of the techniques used to cut men's facial hair are common to barbering practices: see Unit GB3 and Unit GH12 for more information on:

- scissor cutting
- **freehand cutting**
- **scissor over comb**
- **clipper over comb**
- controlling the cut
- **cross-checking** the cut.

Every client is different; they all have differing needs, features and requirements. Therefore, they should always be handled with individual care and attention. Your consultation and analysis will need to reflect this and you will have to adapt to their requests. Normally, the process of trimming and shaping beards or moustaches will be the same in any event, that being:

- you remove the bulk from the interior of the feature first, then
- you tidy and shape the outline to finish the exterior effect.

Always work to and with the natural facial hairlines; it's CK to leave length longer than this but encroaching over this natural division will cause you and the client a lot of problems. If you take your outlines shorter then:

- the results will look strange, unnatural and out of balance
- the bristles will show and would need razoring to remove
- it will be difficult for the client to maintain the style, as he would need to change his shaving technique to keep the lines clean.

Work with the natural growth patterns too; you can't change the direction of the bristles as they grow out from the face. You have to accommodate them within the shaping and trimming. No two heads of hair are the same and this goes for the positioning and natural shapes of beards and moustaches on faces too.

Make allowances for any particular anomalies such as:

- strong directional movements, say to one side – this will limit the wearer to a particular length before it is very noticeable
- whorls or circulatory growth patterns – the effects of these are lessened by more length
- missing or thinning areas – again the effects of the affected areas are lessened by extra length or made more obvious if cut short.

Facial hair is bristle; it is stiffer than hair on the head and this is partly due to the frequency with which it is cut in relation to hairstyles. This creates its own problems, as it is more difficult to cut by the scissor over comb method. This leads stylists and barbers

HEALTH & SAFETY

Always take care when using any sharp items of equipment. Your safety and the safety of the client are in your hands; take care not to be distracted while you are working.

HEALTH & SAFETY

Maintain your scissors

Carefully wipe over the blades at the end of the working day to remove any fragments of hair and then apply a little clipper oil to the pivot point to prevent any corrosion around the fastening screw. This will prolong their life and stop them from binding or getting stiffer to use.

HEALTH & SAFETY

Always look for any contra-indications before you start any facial hair shaping. Look carefully for any suspected infestations or viral or bacterial infections.

to choose clipper over comb, as the mechanical advantage makes the job far easier. But as you need to use one hand to steady and position the comb, you can only use one to hold the relatively heavy clippers. This technique is more complex than using clippers held with two hands and **clipper-grade attachments**.

ACTIVITY

Service timings

Complete the table below to answer the following:

1. How much time is allocated for each of the following services in your place of work?

2. What are the correct tools to use for each?

Service	Timing	Tools/equipment
Dry cut		
Wet cut		
Beard trimming		
Cut and finish		

Clipper over comb

The clipper over comb technique should start by combing and lifting away the ends, then skimming over these to remove wispier bits first. The benefit of this will be to allow you to:

◆ see if any areas show less density in growth than others

◆ make sure that you don't reduce these areas, resulting in skin showing through in a patchy effect.

Bristles are strong and when they are cut into smaller fragments they can fly all over you and the client. This can be dangerous as bristles can stick in any areas of unprotected skin! Or worse, they can enter into the eye. To prevent this happening to the client, it is safer to get him to close his eyes while you trim or, alternatively, place damp cotton wool pads over his eyes to protect them from the fragments.

When the interior of the facial hair shape has been cut, you can then concentrate on defining the shape by creating the outside perimeter line. Hair growth can often be uneven across the head, let alone the face. Even if the client is a regular visitor to the salon you will need to check for balance throughout the shaping, to make sure that the growth doesn't occur thicker and deeper on one side than the other.

Although comfort is always a major concern, for beard trimming it may be easier to start your outlining with the clippers, centrally up the neck, to the point below the chin to start the profile shape. By doing this, you can define the exact position where you stop and you will find that you can then work on either side of the client to create an even symmetrical finish. After this you can complete the shape behind or over the jaw, and finally from the cheek area down to the desired top profile of the beard.

HEALTH & SAFETY

Remember to check the clipper blade alignment before trimming the outline shape of beards and moustaches.

On the other hand, most moustaches are trimmed at or above the upper lip using scissors, which are easier to handle and stops the vibration of the clippers tickling the client and causing him to pull back. The upper perimeter line can then be augmented by the clippers to give a clean, finished profile shape.

HEALTH & SAFETY

Safety

Always take care when using sharp implements on the client's skin. Concentrate on the job in hand and ignore other distractions.

If you do cut the client:

1. Put on a pair of disposable non-latex gloves.
2. Use a medical sterilized wipe to clean the area and remove any hair or bristle.
3. Apply pressure to the cut to stem the flow of blood.
4. When the wound has stopped bleeding finish the service and give the client a clean, dry tissue for any minor seepage.

BEST PRACTICE

Always make the skin taut when you are working with clippers around the outlines or removing hair outside of the desired design line. This provides a closer cut finish and acts as a safety feature for the client if he has 'rugged' or heavily lined features.

Removing unwanted hair outside the desired style line

Finishing and tidying is the last part of the service; you need to clean up any hair or stubble that lies outside the desired style line. After you have agreed with the client that the overall shape and design is OK, you take the electric clippers and turn them so that the fixed blade works away from the design line. You may find that you need to stretch the skin around the neck and face to get a cleaner, straighter, cut close to the skin. Then, working back from the design line, draw the clippers away over the neck/cheek or jaw to create a clean finish. Take a neck brush and carefully brush away any fragments. Then finally re-cut any areas still with signs of uncut bristle. A final brush and the cutting part is over.

Examples of beard shapes

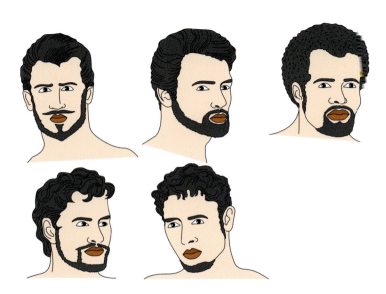

STEP-BY-STEP: BASIC BEARD TRIMMING

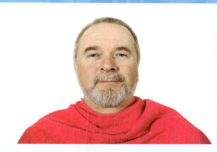

1 Prepare the client by placing neck wool around the cutting collar and then cover this with a clean fresh towel.

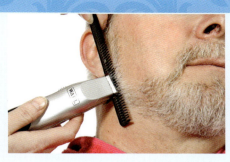

2 With lighter facial growth, a normal set of clippers may be too aggressive, so a cordless profiler/trimmer may be better.

Use your cutting comb to detangle the facial hair and cut a guideline length for the shaping.

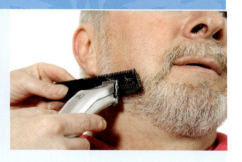

3 With the guideline cut you can cut clipper over comb up that guide.

Keep your comb (and subsequently the trimmers) angled away from the face.

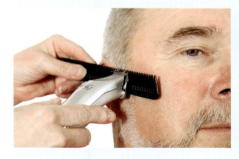

4 Check around the face on both sides to ensure evenness.

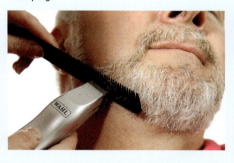

5 Work underneath the neck, ensuring that all the loose hair is removed by combing away or brushing.

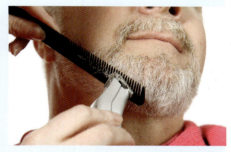

6 Work forwards, up and around the chin to trim and shape the front beard shape to the required length.

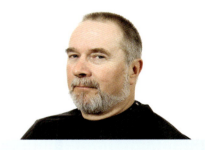

7 Hair and beard final effect.

STEP-BY-STEP: BASIC MOUSTACHE SHAPING

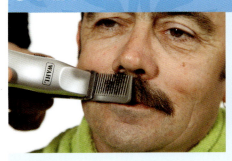

1 Some men prefer a moustache that has longer top length without any layering, these moustaches only require lip lining as in step 4/5.

For shaped moustaches, remove any tangles by light combing, then using cordless trimmers over comb, remove the longer bristles.

CHECK THE BLADE ALIGNMENT FIRST

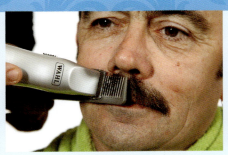

2 Take care around the nose as the edges of the clippers are still very sharp. Also ask the client if they want to wear eye protection to avoid hair fragments entering the eyes.

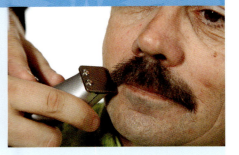

3 With the length of the moustache cut to the required length, you can now start at the outer edges to trim the lower profile shape.

Do not cut above the natural hairlines as this will make it very difficult for the client to maintain, and it will look very odd.

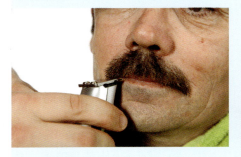

4 Continue the lip lining on both sides.

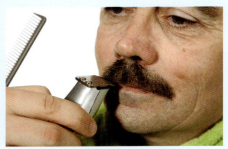

5 Working from the outer edges towards the centre.

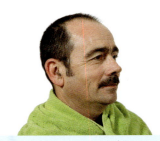

6 Remove any loose hairs and brush the client's face. (They may want to use a towel.)

STEP-BY-STEP: BASIC SIDEBURNS TRIMMING

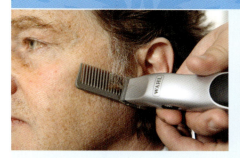

1 Sideburns can be cut scissor over comb, but it is far easier cutting bristly, coarse hairs with electric trimmers, but remember to check the blade alignment before you start. If the client has longer hair, clip it out of the way, as electric clippers will quickly take it away! Comb through to detangle.

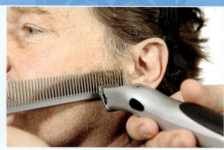

2 Lift the sideburns to trim the length within the sideburn before any shaping or profiling.

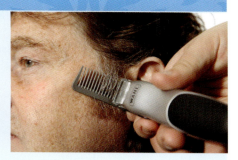

3 Work through the areas from the lower part, up to the upper parts.

Remember, the growth may be uneven, and you will need to check this before you start. Here we see some white hair in and amongst the darker growth. This is often different in texture and will need to be taken into consideration.

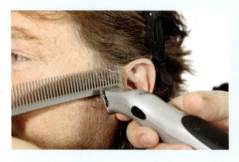

4 As you work through you may find that because of thickness, the effect and balance in the mirror is disproportionate for the client and you may have to take the complete sideburn even closer and shorter.

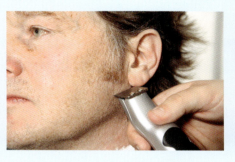

5 When you are satisfied with the length, you can then tidy the outline shape.

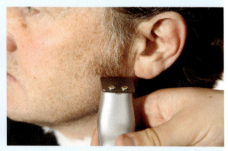

6 For lining and profiling, you will need to turn the trimmer over to create a neater edge.

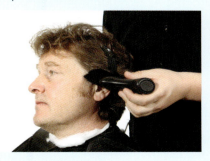

7 Finally, when you have done both sides, brush away any loose hair and check the final shape with the client in the mirror.

HEALTH & SAFETY

Don't forget to use damp cotton wool pads to protect the client's eyes from hair clippings if necessary.

ACTIVITY

Home care advice

Good home-aftercare advice is about giving the client the correct advice on looking after their hair and skin at home.

This will include advice on:

◆ products
◆ tools and equipment
◆ future salon services.

1. What advice should you give regarding products?

2. What advice do you need to provide regarding tools and equipment?

3. What advice could you provide regarding future salon services/treatments?

Providing aftercare advice

See Unit GH12 on pages 296–297 for more information on this topic.

Much of the homecare advice relating to products, maintenance and handling is covered elsewhere.

No service is complete unless the client leaves in the knowledge that he can achieve the same result as that done in the salon. If he can't achieve a similar effect he is unlikely to return. You can make sure that he does, and the real sign of client satisfaction is the booking of his next visit before he leaves the salon.

You can help to achieve this by making sure you tell him

◆ how long the effect will last and when he needs to come back

◆ which products and equipment you have used and how they might benefit the client at home

◆ how to maintain the effect himself.

How long will it last?

Facial hair grows at an average 1.25cm per month, so a shorter, closer styled beard or moustache will have grown out within a month, whereas longer facial designs will last longer. (Or, more to the point, the growth won't be quite as noticeable and therefore the client will tend to go longer in between visits.) Remember, if the effect incorporates a moustache, then it will need trimming anyway, as it will over fall the upper lip fairly quickly.

Whatever the length or effect created, you need to tell your client from the outset how long they can expect it to last, so that they don't have any unrealistic expectations.

Products and skin care

Explain to the client how they can manage the effect themselves. You need to provide advice on cleansing – what to use, in relation to their hair and skin types, how often to use it and what products wouldn't suit them and therefore should be avoided and your reasons why.

Skin care for men is now a very popular and growing business area. It is as important to men as it is for women; the only difference is the range of products that is available. Men who shave regularly will already know that blunt razors and shaving creams are contributing factors for minor skin infections or blocking pores and follicles and starting inward-growing hairs. When this occurs, a spot forms on the surface of the skin and the bacteria will have started a small infection. This, like ingrowing hairs, is uncomfortable and itchy and can easily be avoided if you give the client the correct advice.

Exfoliation is beneficial to the client as it removes dead skin cells from the epidermis and stimulates blood circulation, which will generally improve the skin's condition. There are many different products now available for men and these can be bought as grains that are mixed with water and applied as a paste or, alternatively, a wide range of ready-to-use products with a variety of bases such as fruit acids or herbals with essential oils.

Home maintenance

Finally, no complete service can end without the professional advice on how a look or effect can be maintained between visits. You need to give your client the tips and advice on how he can keep the beard and moustache tidy. The hair will continue to grow between visits and the first thing that the client will be aware of is longer perimeter hair over falling an upper lip or a beard that is getting rather bushy.

We don't expect the client to try and maintain the denser, inner parts of facial hair shapes, but he will want to tidy edges if they become an irritation or look wild!

A few suggestions on what tools he can use (such as trimmer edges on electric shavers, nail scissors for slight trimming) and some advice on how to use them will suffice; you can sort the rest of it out when they return.

SUMMARY

Remember to:

- ✓ prepare clients correctly for the services you are going to carry out
- ✓ put on the protective wear available for styling and dressing hair
- ✓ listen to the client's requirements and discuss suitable courses of action
- ✓ adhere to the safety factors when working on clients' facial hair
- ✓ keep the work areas clean, hygienic and free from hazards
- ✓ promote the range of services, products and treatments within the salon
- ✓ clean and sterilize the tools and equipment before they are used
- ✓ work carefully and methodically through the processes of cutting hair whether wet or dry
- ✓ place, position and direct the tools and facial hair appropriately to achieve the desired effect
- ✓ communicate what you are doing with the client as well as your fellow staff members.

Knowledge Check

For this project you will need to collect historical examples of different beard and moustache shapes.

Use the Internet to find your examples, giving:

A. a brief description for each of the styles, and

B. the following details for each look:

1 the source for the style/shape,

2 its historical time point in history and

3 either an image or sketch of the selected looks.

ASSESSMENT OF KNOWLEDGE AND UNDERSTANDING

A selection of different types of questions to check your knowledge of cutting facial hair.

Q1 Closer cutting is achieved by using the clippers without the _____ attached.　　Fill in the blank

Q2 Razors should be sterilized in Barbicide™.　　True or false

Q3 Select from the following those tools that need sterilizing in a UV cabinet:　　Multi selection

Cutting collar	☐ 1
Cutting square	☐ 2
Scissors	☐ 3
Clippers	☐ 4
Thinning scissors	☐ 5
Clipper grades	☐ 6

Q4 Outline shapes for beards are best cut with clippers.　　True or false

Q5 Which of the following is not a cutting term?　　Multi choice

Cross-checking	O a
Fading	O b
Freehand	O c
Freestyle	O d

Q6 Close accurate cutting is dependent upon cutting angles and tensioning on the skin.　　True or false

Q7 Which of the following is not a facial hair term?　　Multi selection

Goatee	☐ 1
Side burns	☐ 2
Handlebar moustache	☐ 3
Mohawk	☐ 4
Full beard	☐ 5
Mullet	☐ 6

Q8   The pre-application of hot ___ will soften facial hair making it easier to cut.   Fill in the blank

Q9   Which of the following should not be used for trimming facial hair?   Multi choice

Clippers   O a

Shaper   O b

Scissors   O c

Razor   O d

Q10   Thinning is a technique of cutting that maximizes the hair density.   True or false

15 Basic hair patterns and designs

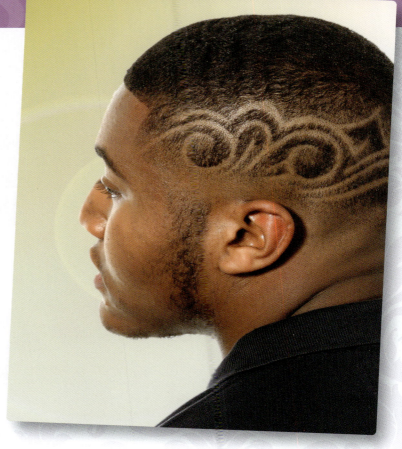

LEARNING OBJECTIVES

◆ Be able to maintain effective and safe methods of working

◆ Be able to plan and agree hair patterns for your client

◆ Be able to create patterns in your client's hair

◆ Know how to work safely, effectively and hygienically

◆ Understand how you can create designs in hair

◆ Know about preparation, the cutting techniques, and how to resolve simple problems

◆ Know how to provide maintenance information and advice to your clients

KEY TERMS

avant-garde

contra-indications

cowlicks

double crowns

eczema

hair whorls

mini clippers

pre-cutting

sharps box

storyboard

T liner/outliner

tramliner

visual aids

widow's peaks

AH21 Create basic patterns in hair

Information covered in this chapter

◆ The tools and equipment used for cutting patterns in hair

◆ The preparations that you should make prior to cutting

◆ The factors that influence cutting decisions

◆ Creating a design and a cutting plan

◆ The aftercare advice that you should give clients

INTRODUCTION

Intricate hair designs and scalp tattoos have tribal and ethnic origins, and now play a big part in helping to produce individuality and unique effects for the wearer. At a senior level, we are amazed at how art and design can be introduced to hair in new and exciting ways. But even at a basic level, the effects created enable the wearer to stand out in a crowd, and for the stylist, hair art is only a few steps away.

Maintain effective and safe methods of working when cutting patterns in hair

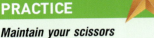

For specific information on the following topics, review the pages specified.

Much of the preparation of materials, tools and clients needed for this service are similar to that elsewhere in this book. If you are not familiar with this aspect of the service then see Units GH12, GB3 and GB4 to cover this work.

- Tools and client preparation – see Unit GB4 Cut facial hair to shape using basic techniques pages 326–345 and Unit GB3 Cut hair using basic barbering techniques pages 300–325.
- Hygiene and sterilization – see Unit GB4 Cut facial hair to shape using basic techniques pages 326–345 and Unit GB3 Cut hair using basic barbering techniques pages 300–325.
- Cutting techniques – see Unit GH12 Cut hair using basic techniques pages 266–299 and Unit GB3 Cut hair using basic barbering techniques pages 300–325.
- Working position, comfort and safety – see Unit GB4 Cut facial hair to shape using basic techniques pages 326–345.

BEST PRACTICE

Maintain your scissors

Carefully wipe over the blades at the end of the working day to remove any fragments of hair and then apply a little clipper oil to the pivot point to prevent any corrosion around the fastening screw. This will prolong the scissors' life and stop them from binding or getting stiffer to use

HEALTH & SAFETY

Disposal of sharp items

Used razor blades and similar items should be placed into a safe container ('**sharps box**'). When the container is full it can be disposed of. This type of salon waste should be kept away from general salon waste as special disposal arrangements may be provided by your local authority.

Cutting tools and equipment

Clippers Clippers are and have been an essential item of equipment for men's styling. They have been invaluable for the popularity of short hairstyles but are equally important for the shaping and trimming of necklines, facial hair shapes and design patterns in hair.

You will find specific information about scissors, clippers, thinning scissors and combs, etc. in Chapters 12 and 13 pages 266–299 and 300–325.

ACTIVITY

Hair design consultation

A. List five main factors you should consider when carrying out a consultation for hair design/patterning work.

1. _____
2. _____
3. _____
4. _____
5. _____

B. Give a brief explanation for each of the points listed stating why you think these are important and how they will affect the techniques and methods you use.

HEALTH & SAFETY

Always look for any contra-indications before you start any hair patterning. Look carefully for any suspected infestations or viral or bacterial infections.

Clipper type	Blade profile	Uses
Standard clipper	WAHL *Kindly supplied by Wahl (UK) Ltd*	Standard width clippers are a general 'catch-all' piece of equipment. Available in mains or rechargeable power options; they will comfortably manage the cutting of large amounts of hair very quickly. They can be fitted with a variety of grade attachments and are essential to men's barbering.
T liner/outliner	FORFEX® BaByliss PRO FX702 *BaByliss PRO*	**'T' liners/outliners** are a more specialized clipper that have a T-shaped blade. The fixed blade extends beyond the width of the clipper body enabling them to be used around the ears or facial hair shapes; providing a closer (yet safe) cut finish than that of standard clippers.
Tramliner	FORFEX® BaByliss PRO *BaByliss PRO*	A **tramliner** is a specialist narrow blade clipper, designed for intricate lining and detailing of hair. This type of clipper enables you to cut free-form designs without inverse etching techniques that you would need to use with the other types of clipper.
Mini clipper	FORFEX® BaByliss PRO *BaByliss PRO*	**Mini clippers** are usually battery powered or have a rechargeable power supply. They have a narrower cutting width than standard clippers and are particularly useful for hair detailing or precision designs. They produce less vibration than standard clippers and are therefore more comfortable for the client when working across the scalp.

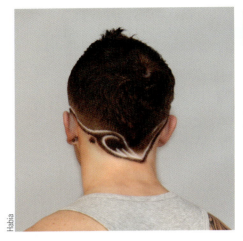

Habia

Plan and agree hair patterns in hair

Creating a portfolio of work and examples

Imagine that you were going to have a tattoo and you didn't have a visual idea that you could convey to the tattooist. How would they know what you wanted? Well fortunately, they have a backup; because they keep photographs of the work they have done, and many more illustrations of designs for you to choose from. Collectively, these **visual aids** form the basis for their portfolio.

In building your own portfolio you could collect sources from all sorts of things. Remember: patterns and textures can occur in anything and you can start a comprehensive portfolio from very small beginnings. At a basic level you would do well to start with the patterns or textures that appear in nature. Everything from snowflakes to snail shells, or ripples on water to cloud formations, have been catalysts which have eventually become the basis of good design.

In hair dressings the basic shapes, patterns and designs have clear roots in tribal, ethnic and historical cultures. In the past (and still in the present day) hair dressings and adornment are associated with social grouping and within those groupings, the different levels of status by those wearing the different effects. You can look into the historical origins yourself as there is plenty of research material available on the Internet.

From a design point of view there are three distinct modal themes, and knowing which one to use with a client will depend upon personal image, preference and motivation. You must get a clear indication of what is suitable for your client during your consultation.

Be warned, you need to create a range of designs, to suit all sorts of clients. This type of work is not a *personal crusade*; it is about providing a public service to those people who are willing to pay for your advice and expertise.

The three different mode lines are:

◆ classic or traditional

◆ current fashion

◆ futuristic or **avant-garde**.

Classic or traditional work could be defined as timeless. That is to say the effects are neither in nor out of fashion. Classic themes were created at a time when the basic design rules were first established. Classic work tends to be quite different from the other two groups of styles as it has the following distinct qualities:

◆ the effects tend to be quite simple in their design construction

◆ simple designs have greater impact because they are clearer; they have a less 'busy', 'uncluttered' appearance that creates better visual contrasts

◆ the effects are durable and last well.

Current fashion trends are changing with the seasons. These fashions are different to classic styling in that they are of the moment. They often start on the catwalks of fashion shows of London, Paris and New York, or on stages in arenas around the world, worn by music artists. Current fashion and the drivers that support it can easily be researched and found, as they appear on TV and fill printed media (and waste bins) every day.

Future (avant-garde) fashions try to push the boundaries of what is acceptable and what can be worn. The clients that warm to these emerging fashions are going to be confident at the very least, but more likely outrageously extrovert in their individual appearances. These people want exclusivity; they don't want to share their look with others; they are more than happy to carve out their own individual look.

Try to show breadth and depth in your portfolio of work; try to cover aspects that address all sorts of design modes, as this will indicate to others that you have the ability to adapt to/in any situation.

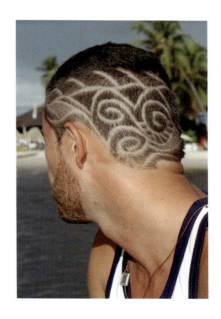

Working with designs
In looking for material to add to your portfolio, you are more likely to find aspects or elements of images that you want to use within larger designs or images. It is unlikely that you will find complete, finished compositions of work to show clients and without these finished effects, you can't expect a warm, enthusiastic response from clients.

Very few people have the artistic ability to visualize a photograph of a finished look, let alone an element of a design or a pattern upon them. You need to find ways of:

◆ making the design or pattern larger

◆ incorporating the design into a finished effect.

Developing a portfolio of ideas
When you find a pattern or a design that you want to add to your portfolio, you need to keep the original image or source and create your artwork from it as the design that you will use as a visual aid with clients. This will become both the source for themes and ideas for the client as well a tool to prompt discussion about the work.

You should have two physical components to the work:

1 The first is the original research or source item – this could be in the form of a photograph, magazine cuttings, Internet downloads or sketches. These original compositions could be on paper, textiles and packaging or on digital media. How you keep them for your portfolio is up to you, but you will need to show your themes to assessors as part of a 'storyboard' of ideas. (A **storyboard** is a creative narrative that is composed of ideas leading to a finished, physical result.)

2 The second is the composition of finished effects – for usefulness, it is more likely that you will want to use this within a working environment and therefore the research material is superfluous in a portfolio that you want to share with clients. The journey that you take in finding sources of design material and turning them into finished works is a personal, learning activity. It is unlikely that the design roughs will be of much interest to the client, other than the fact that they might be a topic for discussion – e.g. 'So where did you get the idea for this design?' 'Well, actually it was a photograph of an airbrushed design on the fuel tank of a Harley Davidson motorbike I saw on holiday.' The collections of finished works will probably be in an album: a visual aid that you can show and share with the client, compiled with individual pages and themes.

This is only an idea and depends on the extent of presentation media you have in the shop. For example, a tattooist will cover their walls with themes and examples of their work. A swish, up-to-the-minute, computer-minded barber's may use projected slideshows or compositions burned to DVD and run as a visual presentation as part of the in-shop entertainment. The way that you put your ideas together, work and develop them and finally present them, is up to you.

TOP TIP
Keep all the source material in your originating portfolio so that you can provide your assessor with a 'storyboard' of the elements that create your final designs.

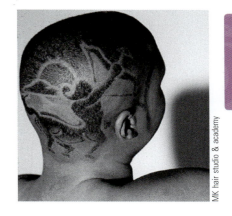

MK hair studio & academy

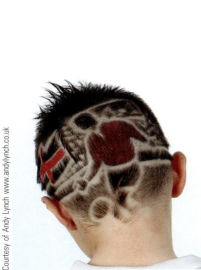

Courtesy of Andy Lynch www.andylynch.co.uk

Style aspects

Head and facial shape The proportions balance and distribution of weight in the design will be a frame for the head and face. Therefore you need to examine the head and face carefully: if you look at the outline of your client's face, you will see that it's round, oval, square, heart-shaped, oblong or triangular. Imagine what the head will look like with less hair; will it expose features that enhance the design plan, or will the factors work against your preliminary ideas?

Would the design benefit from more hair? Is the client's hair long enough to produce the 2D effect? These are the sorts of questions that you need to answer before embarking on some 'flashy' self-advertisement campaign.

Do the client's physical features present some form of styling limitations? These are is-sues that are critical to the achievement of a satisfactory result.

Hair design considerations The perimeters and design outlines formed by the hair in relation to the shape of the face is the first thing people will see. It is this effect that people make decisions upon and comments about, for example: 'That's a great effect'. 'I think that really suits you'. The complete hair design is based upon suitability matched to personality or image aspects. How you fill in' the detail – the movement, direction, colour and patterning – is down to your interpretation and understanding of the client and what is suitable for them. Don't expect them to be the best at self-visuali-zation. If they produce ideas that seem off beat or random, ask them if there is any par-ticular reason why they would want to take that line.

Hair positioning, type, growth and tendency Hair growth direction and distribution should be a major consideration for what is achievable within a hairstyle. You need to make allowances for strong movement, high or low hairlines, natural part-ings, **hair whorls**, **cowlicks**, **widow's peaks** and **double crowns**. Look for these be-fore shampooing. The client cannot compensate for these themselves, so when the hair is in need of washing, they will be plain to see. After the hair is washed the degree and strength of the feature can be seen and then you can reconsider how you will tackle it.

Hair pattern suitability Pattern suitability refers to the effect of the hair design in relation to the face and on the features of the head and body. From an aesthetic point of view, a hair design is suitable when it 'looks right'. But this is a difficult or certainly a sub-jective thing to quantify.

Aesthetically and artistically speaking, the client's hair will 'look right' when the design does one of two things:

- ◆ it harmonizes, i.e. fits and works with the shape of the face and head – and therefore provides an enhancement to an overall image; or

- ◆ it contrasts, i.e. it accentuates features of the face and head – by creating a prominent, strong or stark overall image.

For example, when working with harmonizing aspects, the features and lines of the face and its underlying bone structure are accentuated when the linear (straight) lines and patterns within the hair design are continuous with them.

Hair designs which contrast are not continuous and cross at right angles to the lines and features of the face.

Courtesy of Andy Lynch www.andylynch.co.uk

Similarly, a softening effect is created when curves move away from the hairlines producing harmonizing effects.

As a general rule linear, straight-lined effects and box-like shapes are visually harder and can appear more threatening or brutal than those designs incorporating curves, circles and ellipses.

Basic principles of design

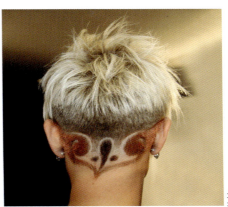

Habia

Balance Balance is the effect produced by the proportions and distribution of detail throughout the style. The opposite, i.e. imbalance, is lack of those proportions. Symmetry or symmetrical even balance occurs when the effects are distributed equally as in a mirrored image through a vertical or horizontal plane. Asymmetry or asymmetric effects occur when the overall shape does not have the same distribution on either side.

However, both symmetrical and asymmetrical shapes can be balanced. Here the aspect of perspective is brought into play where a visually larger component is counterbalanced by a smaller one further away.

Style line Style lines are the directions in which the hair design is positioned or appears to flow. When a break occurs within this flow the eye is immediately drawn to it. A break can only happen for two reasons: either it's a style feature and accentuates what the observer is meant to see, or it's a mistake made by the inexperienced.

Partings and divisions Partings or divisions in hair have a strong impact. Lines created upon the head will draw the attention of the eye and can be used to create flow and movement away from the face to the detail that lies beyond.

Movement Movement refers to the variance of line direction within a hair design. The more variety in direction the more movement there will be. Sometimes this movement is because of natural tendency – to accommodate curls or waves – sometimes it is deliberately created by design shaping and placement.

Hard and soft effects Hard and soft effects result from the balance or imbalance within a hair design or from the movement or lack of movement within it. Subtle lining will convey softer harmonizing effects, whereas stronger lines produce contrasting effects, which work better in achieving more dramatic results.

The combinations of the above and the way in which these style variables are used will give you the basic rules for which you can create your own original effects. Creating completely new styles requires a great deal of thought and work, and your clients will want to benefit from your creative abilities.

Finalizing the portfolio

With a collection of work done, your basic portfolio is complete. You now have designs covering a range of themes and along with this, you may want to give a small description or brief on how you found the sources for your artworks.

You may be very pleased with the results that you have achieved, but don't spoil things by not presenting the information properly. You need to compile your designs in a way that protects them from handling and keeps them all safely together. You also need to choose how you are going to present the collection to clients; would they be better bound in an album or would transparent pockets in a ring binder be better? The choice of presentation is up to you, but whatever medium you choose make sure that the portfolio shows:

◆ professionalism in the way in which it is compiled

◆ a variety in its themes

◆ quality in its reproduction, and

◆ that it portrays realistic options for the clients that *you* can do.

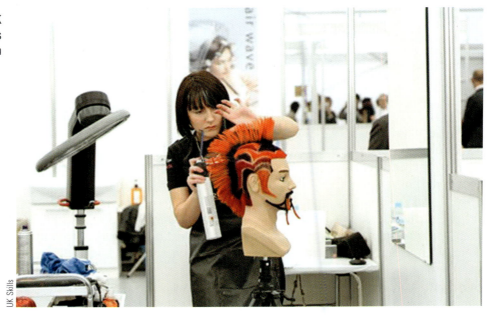

Donna Leach representing the UK in WorldSkills 2007 Team UK Medals Shizuoka, Japan

Consultation

With most of the planning and preparations done, your main concern is establishing with the client exactly what is going to happen and gaining from them the confirmation that what you have selected as a design is both appropriate and satisfactory. If there is any hesitation or uncertainty, you need to either provide more information about what you intend to do, or look again at the visuals from your portfolio to explore other options.

The other aspects for consideration in general consultation relating to adverse or influencing factors are covered elsewhere in this book.

Review Chapter 6 Unit G7 Advise and consult with clients for more information see pages 100–136.

Contra-indications to hair design work The request for a hair design or close-cut patterning may be wanted by the client, but not every client will be able to have the service. Always look closely for signs to see if the service *can* be provided and *ask* the client if they have any reasons that they know of that would *not permit* the service to be conducted.

Do not provide this service when:

◆ there are signs of cuts or abrasions on the scalp

◆ there are signs of reddening from conditions like **eczema** or skin sensitivity or skin allergies

◆ there are any other adverse symptoms such as infections or infestations

◆ the skin surface is too uneven to produce a successful, finished result.

If you have any doubts about symptoms and contra-indications, always ask a senior member of staff for their assistance. You may be putting the salon at risk from legal action or claims for compensation if you don't follow this process properly. Make sure that you keep a record of your consultation and the responses made by the client after the service, for future reference.

ACTIVITY

Create a portfolio

This section has explored the aspects of design and looked at the possible sources for gaining and developing a working portfolio that you could use and continue to build upon when you are working with clients in the barber shop.

Use the information covered within this chapter to create your own portfolio of work. How you choose to display this information depends upon your skill and artistic abilities. Whether you want to collect examples of work you find, sketches from ideas or pictures of your own work, it's all up to you.

BEST PRACTICE

If you have any doubts about symptoms and contra-indications; always ask a senior member of staff for their assistance. You may be putting the salon at risk from legal action or claims for compensation if you don't follow this process properly.

Pre-cutting   In order to work with manageable lengths of hair, you need to pre-cut the client's hair to a length that will enable you to transfer your designs to the head allowing for the longest parts of the detailing. Carefully look at the length you are working with and make sure that you don't undercut the hair length that you need to complete the total effect.

Inaccurate detailing   The most common cutting problem is that of inaccurate detailing. It happens when clippers take too much hair away from the area you want to work with.

1   Make sure that you remove all loose clippings as you go along. Any cut hair left on the scalp will lead you into believing that there is still more to work with; keep brushing away the area that you are working with so that you clearly see where you are.

2   If you do take too much hair away in a particular area, you need to stop and see how much impact it will make on the overall design. You can then choose between modifying your patterning to incorporate a different detailing or re-working the design plan to accommodate another theme or effect.

BEST PRACTICE

Don't try to cover up mistakes; be honest and keep the client informed. In nine cases out of ten they won't mind a slight modification to the overall plan.

Create patterns in hair

Clippers

Intricate design requires accurate cutting and having the correct tools to do the job is everything. Normal everyday clippers are fine for removing large amounts of hair very quickly; but when it comes to working the detail of smaller textures and designs, the other varieties of smaller, narrower-bladed clippers are essential.

General purpose, mains-electric clippers have a cutting blade width of approximately 3cm. This is OK for cutting straighter lines (i.e. more linear patterns), but for anything more detailed, you need to use lighter and narrower, rechargeable clippers, that have blade widths down to less than 1cm. These can be easily manipulated without having trailing leads in the way, so that you can create both curves and lines just as easily.

There are two ways of holding clippers for cutting purposes:

1. **Fixed blade down** the normal way for removing hair and for using the different sized clipper grades.

2. **Inverse, i.e. fixed blade up** this provides a lining tool for cutting outline perimeter shapes such as necklines, or as an etching tool for creating detail within a hairstyle

Clippers held for normal and inversed cutting techniques

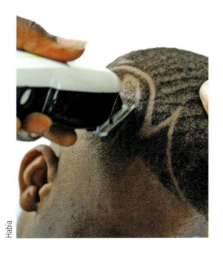

Habia

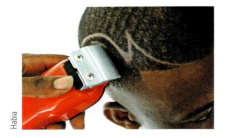

Habia

Different types of clippers

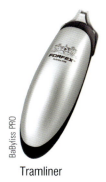

BaByliss PRO

Tramliner

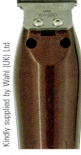

Kindly supplied by Wahl (UK) Ltd

T-liner

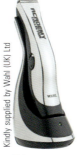

Kindly supplied by Wahl (UK) Ltd

Trimmer

Cutting a 2D pattern

With the outlines and detail drawn on to the pre-cut hair, you can carefully start etching away the unwanted hair; using the correct size clippers in the inverse holding technique. As the clippers remove the hair and create the desired lines, make sure that you brush away the cut hair so that you can clearly see the patterning/lining that you are creating. Any cut hair left in position will mislead you into thinking that the area still needs work. Beware: this is the simplest way for mistakes to be made.

HEALTH & SAFETY

Clippers used in the inverse position are used for lining, neckline shapes and detailing, so more care must be taken as the cutting edges are very close to the skin.

ACTIVITY

Health & Safety

With reference to this particular unit, AH21:

A. What health and safety things do you need to be particularly aware of for this type of work?

B. List your responsibilities under the Health and Safety at Work Act 1974.

HEALTH & SAFETY

Always use the clippers carefully and safely at all times and make sure that you *always* level the clipper blades before using them upon the client.

TOP TIP

Machine clippers cut hair very quickly, so clear away any loose clippings so that you can see exactly where you are within the design.

If you do make a mistake within the design by cutting too much hair away, you will need to adapt your overall design to compensate for the missing hair, possibly by making a design feature of the area.

STEP-BY-STEP: CUTTING A 2D PATTERN

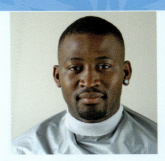

1 Client preparation for creating patterns in hair; ensure a thorough consultation is carried out first.

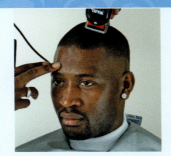

2 Clipper cut hair length to client's requirements.

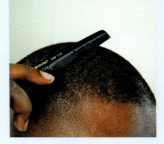

3 Comb against the growth pattern to check evenness of clipper cut and observe for critical influencing factors such as warts, moles or scars, etc.

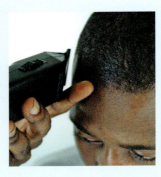

4 For delicate designs, use extended fingers to steady clippers – always be aware that the client may move!

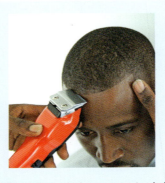

5 For delicate designs, use extended fingers to steady clippers – always be aware that the client may move!

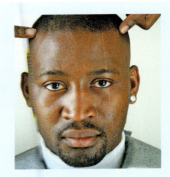

6 Check through mirror for accuracy of hairline width using your fingers as reference points

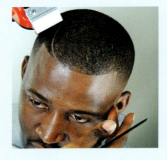

7 Begin the design keeping a sense of proportion. A good tip is to regularly step back to observe all the emerging pattern.

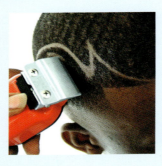

8 Use the corners of the clippers to create curves – a powerful clipper is considered more advantageous than outliners at this stage.

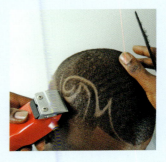

9 If required, hold head still with free hand.

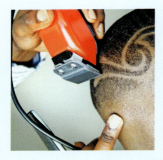

10 Clippers can be held at any angle.

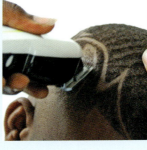

11 Shorten areas within the design to create a three dimensional effect.

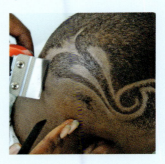

12 Continue technique.

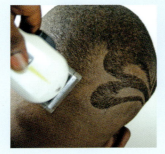

13 Note how the faded area contrasts with the lines and curves – this is sometimes termed creating 'light and shade'.

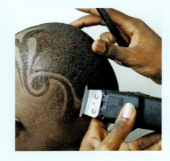

14 Outliners are very useful for pronouncing edges.

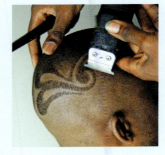

15 Continue technique.

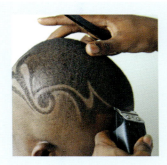

16 Continue technique.

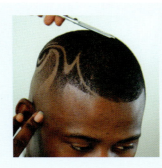

17 Trim off any loose hairs using the scissors freehand.

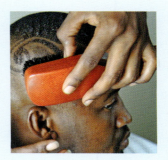

18 Use a soft bristle brush to remove loose clippings and groom the hair.

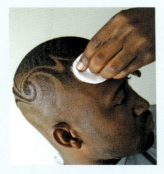

19 Using finishing products of your choice, apply with a pad to produce a gloss finish.

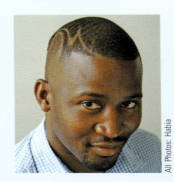

20 Final effect.

All Photos: Habia

Provide aftercare advice

Design work and patterns created on close-cut hair need very little maintenance, the effects are long-lasting (in hairstyle terms) and easy to maintain. They will withstand frequent washing and normally need little more than a rub with a towel.

However, some design work involves colouring too, and if different areas of hair have contrasting colour segments, you may need to provide your client with advice for which type of shampoos will work best by not causing the colours to fade or 'run' together. If the hair has had a permanent colour service then the effects should be less problematic.

Finally, tell your client how long the effects will last: as hair grows longer the impacts of lining lessen. This is particularly true where the lining and detail is created by showing the scalp. The contrasts created by showing skin as opposed to just hair are far more striking, so tell them how long the effect will last before they need to return.

For more information covering general aftercare advice and the following essential knowledge see Unit GH12 Cut hair using basic techniques pages 266–299.

SUMMARY

Remember to:

- ✓ prepare clients correctly for the services you are going to carry out

- ✓ put on the protective wear available for styling and patterning hair

- ✓ listen to the client's requirements and discuss suitable courses of action

- ✓ adhere to the safety factors when working on clients' hair

- ✓ keep the work areas clean, hygienic and free from hazards

- ✓ promote the range of services, products and treatments within the shop

- ✓ clean and sterilize the tools and equipment before they are used

- ✓ work carefully and methodically through the processes of cutting hair

- ✓ place, position and direct the templates or hair appropriately to achieve the desired effect

- ✓ tell the client what you are doing, keep them informed.

Knowledge Check

For this project you will need to gather information from different sources.

Collect photos, digital images or magazine cuttings for different types of hair designs.

Include designs that are motivated by:

A. modern music themes

B. cultural or ethnic themes

C. general artistic designs.

Give a brief description of each and reasons why you included it in your personal collection.

ASSESSMENT OF KNOWLEDGE AND UNDERSTANDING

A selection of different types of questions to check your basic hair patterns and designs knowledge.

Q1 Inverse clippering is a technique used to create ___ neck shapes. Fill in the blank

Q2 Scissors should be sterilized in Barbicide™. True or false

Q3 Select from the following list the items that are a type of machine clipper: Multi selection

Tram liner	☐ 1
Steam liner	☐ 2
Eye liner	☐ 3
T liner	☐ 4
Z liner	☐ 5
White liner	☐ 6

Q4   Linear shapes are curved.   True or false

Q5   Which of the following is not a cutting term?   Multi choice

Graduation   O a

Straightening   O b

Freehand   O c

Fading   O d

Q6   Precision cutting is dependent upon cutting angles and even tension.   True or false

Q7   Which of the following are contra-indications for patterning hair?   Multi selection

Bumps and lumps on the scalp   ☐ 1

Double crown   ☐ 2

Widow's peak   ☐ 3

Alopecia totalis   ☐ 4

Nape whorls   ☐ 5

High hairline   ☐ 6

Q8   A ___ is a type of clipper with a tapered, narrow blade for detailing designs on hair.   Fill in the blank

Q9   Which of the following will affect the natural fall and the way that neck hair lies after it is cut?   Multi choice

Double crown   O a

Cowlick   O b

Nape whorl   O c

Widow's peak   O d

Q10   Clubbing is a technique of cutting that maximizes the hair density.   True or false

16 Colouring hair

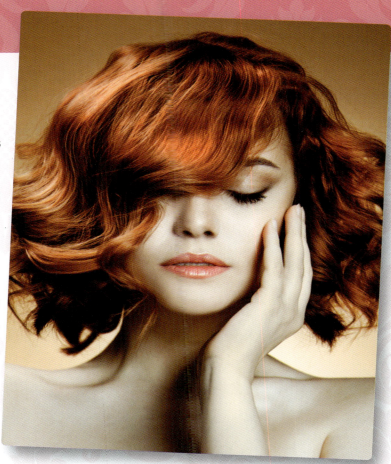

LEARNING OBJECTIVES

◆ Be able to maintain effective and safe methods of working

◆ Be able to prepare for colouring and lightening hair

◆ Be able to colour and lighten hair to create a variety of effects

◆ Understand how to work safely, effectively and hygienically

◆ Know and understand the tests for colouring hair

◆ Understand the basic science of colouring and lightening

◆ Understand colouring products, equipment, and their uses

◆ Know and understand different colouring techniques

◆ Know how to give aftercare advice to clients

KEY TERMS

activator or booster	anti-oxidizing treatment	colour accelerator
activators	boosters	contra-indication
allergic reaction	canites	controllers

depth	over-processing	retouch/regrowth
developer	oxidation	semi-permanent colours
elasticity test	oxymelanin	steamer
eumelanin	para-dyes	temporary colour
full head application	patch test/sensitivity test	tone
incompatibility test	permanent colours	tone on tone colour
incompatible	pheomelanin	toners/toning
incompatible products	porosity test	under-processing
manufacturer's instructions	PPD	virgin hair
melanin	progressive dyes	
oil or gel	quasi-permanent colour	

Unit title

GH9 Change hair colour and GB2 Change men's hair colour

Information covered in this chapter

◆ The preparations that you must make before carrying out any colouring service

◆ The science of hair colouring and colouring products

◆ The tools and equipment used during colouring

◆ The factors that influence successful colouring services

◆ A range of colouring techniques on differing hair lengths and types

◆ The aftercare advice that you should give

INTRODUCTION

Colouring is arguably the most exciting and often the most difficult aspect of hairdressing. The increasing demands and expectations of clients have made colouring, and in particular special colour effects, the 'must have' of hairdressing. Our clients are better informed, have a better understanding, are more aware of what's on offer and are often keen to have a go themselves. This has led to a change in salon colouring. The amount of business done by the home colouring market is huge and this has had a particular impact on salon-based work. It is now more technically demanding than ever before, but this new challenge is not a threat. It now enables all hairdressers to be more professional in their role, explore their creativity and further develop their technical skills.

Colouring for men and women

The hairdressing unit for colouring GH9 and the barbering unit for men's colouring GB2 are very similar. Each one is made up of the same performance criteria and essential knowledge. The only differences that can be found are within their application, i.e. the range statements. Because of these similarities, this book combines the units and only draws attention to specific differences within the colouring processes themselves.

The principles of colour and colouring

Seeing colour When you look at an object, what you are actually seeing is light reflected from it. White light is really a mixture of many colours – that is why sunlight refracted through falling rain can produce a rainbow. This splitting of white light creates what we see as seven different colours: red, orange, yellow, green, blue, indigo and violet. (<u>R</u>ichard <u>O</u>f <u>Y</u>ork <u>G</u>ave <u>B</u>attle <u>I</u>n <u>V</u>ain)

A white object reflects most of the white light that falls upon it; a black object absorbs most of the light falling on it. A red object reflects the red light and absorbs everything else.

Hair colour depends chiefly on the pigments in the hair, which absorb some of the light and reflect the rest. The colour that we see is also affected by the light in which it is seen, and (to a lesser extent) by the colours of clothes worn with it.

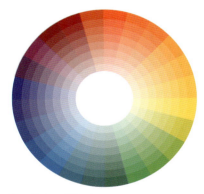

The Colour Wheel

◆ White light from halogen bulbs and full daylight will show the hair's natural colour.

◆ Yellowish light emitted from standard electric light bulbs adds warmth to hair colour, but neutralizes blue ash or ashen effects.

◆ Bluish/green light from fluorescent tubes reduces the warmth of red/gold tones in hair.

Mixing colours The colours of the pigments in paints arise from three primary colours – red, blue and yellow. Pairs of these give the secondary colours – i.e. red and blue mixed together create violet, yellow and blue create green, and yellow and red create orange. White and black can be added to vary the tone of the colour.

The primary colours in light are different – red, green and blue. (These are the three colours used in digital cameras, computer screens and television.) The secondary colours are yellow, cyan and magenta.

The ways in which colour pigments are mixed together in paint to produce other new colours is similar to that used in hairdressing. Like paint, permanent hair colours can be mixed together to create different shades.

Natural hair colour

The natural colour of hair is determined by the colour of pigments within the hair's cortex. These are formed when the hair is in its germinating stage of growth.

Hair colour pigments (known as **melanin**) are deposited into the hair shaft at the region of the papilla and germinal matrix. The smaller pigments responsible for black and brown tones within hair are called **eumelanin** (U-mel-an-in); those responsible for red and yellow tones in hair are larger and are called *pheomelanin* (Fay-oh-mel-an-in). There is another large pigment called Trichosiderin (Try-co-sid-er-in), which is only found in hair derived from Celtic origins.

The hair colour you actually see is affected by the amount and proportion of the pigments present, by the light in which the hair is seen and – to a certain extent – by the colours of the clothes and make-up worn.

With age, or after periods of stress, the production of natural pigments may be reduced. The hairs already on the head will not be affected, but the new ones will. As hairs fall out and are replaced, the proportion that have the original pigmentation diminishes and the hair's overall colour changes. It may become lighter. If no pigment is produced at all, then the new hairs will be white.

The proportion of white hairs among the naturally coloured ones causes the hair to appear grey. Grey hair or greyness (**canites** pronounced 'can-a-sheez') is often referred to as a percentage; for example, '50 per cent grey' means that half of the hairs on the head are white and the rest are pigmented.

It is not uncommon for young people to exhibit some grey hairs – this does not necessarily mean that they will go grey, or completely white, at an early age.

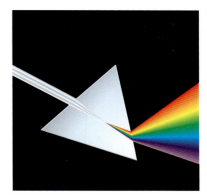

The colour spectrum

Depth and tone

Hair science When we talk about colour we often use the words **depth** and **tone**. Depth is used to describe how light or dark the colour is and tone is used to describe the colour or hue that we see, such as brown, golden red, etc. **Depth = how light or dark it is. Tone = the colour or hue** – ashen, golden, mahogany, etc.

These terms are easier to understand if we tabulate them in the following way.

Depth				
	Very light			
	Light			
	Medium			
	Dark			
	Very dark			
		Gold	Red	Violet
Tone				

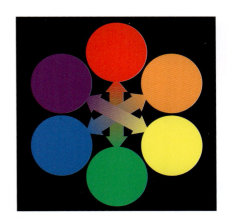

The colour circle

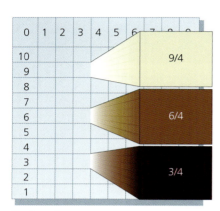

Depth and tones

International Colour Chart system

Taking this principle further, the International Colour Chart (ICC) offers a way of defining hair colours systematically (although charts may vary between manufacturers). Shades of colour are divided and numbered, with black (1) at one end of the scale and lightest blonde (10) at the other.

Tones of other colours (/1 /9 or also stated as .1 .9) are combined with these, producing a huge variety of colours. Charts are usually arranged with shades in rows down the side and tones in columns across the top. To use them, first identify the shade of your client's hair: that row of the chart then shows the colours you could produce with that hair.

For example, if your client has medium blonde hair (depth 7) and you colour with a copper tone (.4), the result should be a rich copper blonde (7.4). The possibilities are almost endless, as these examples indicate:

◆ to produce ash shades, add blue

◆ to produce matt shades, add green

◆ to produce gold shades, add yellow

◆ to produce warm shades, add red

◆ to produce purple or violet shades, add mixtures of red and blue.

ACTIVITY

Depth and tone – warm and cool shades

The natural 'depth' of hair refers to how light or dark it is, whereas 'tone' refers to colouration, e.g. red, blue or green.

Task 1. With your friends and using the salon shade chart, take it in turns to select the nearest natural shade for each of them. Don't make the mistake of looking at the rest of the chart, just keep to the natural bases.

Warm tones are yellow or golden based. Cool tones are bluish or green based.

What tones are produced from red? Well, that depends on whether the red is orange based or pink based.

Task 2. Again in a group work through your salon's shade chart and for each shade note down its shade name, number or code, then decide as a group whether it is a warm tone or a cool tone.

Save the information from both of these tasks in your portfolio for future reference.

How many warm shades were there?

How many cool shades were there?

How many were neither warm nor cool?

Did you find any surprising results?

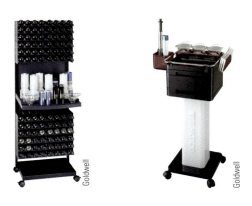

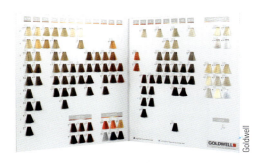

Goldwell   Goldwell   Goldwell

L'Oréal – Majirel

		Ash ,1	Mauve ,2	Gold ,3	Copper ,4	Mahogany ,5	Red ,6	Metallic ,7
10	Lightest Blonde							
9	Very Light Blonde	Very Light Natural Ash Blonde 9,1		Very Light Deep Golden Blonde 9,33	Very Light Natural Copper Blonde 9,04			Very Light Natural Cool Blonde 9,07
8	Light Blonde		Light Iridescent Blonde 8,2	Light Golden Blonde 8,3				
7	Blonde	Ash Blonde 7,1			**Deep Copper Blonde 7,44**		Extra Iridescent Red Blonde 7,62	
6	Dark Blonde		Dark Deep Iridescent Blonde 6,22	Dark Natural Golden Blonde 6,03	**Dark Copper Red Blonde 6,46**	Dark Mahogany Golden Blonde 6,53	Dark Extra Red Blonde 6,66	Dark Natural Cool Blonde 6,07
5	Light Brown	Light Deep Ash Brown 5,11			Light Extra Copper Red Blonde 5,46	Light Mahogany Iridescent Brown 5,52	Light Red Brown 5,6	Light Cool Ash Brown 5,71
4	Brown		Extra Burgundy Brown 4,20	Golden Brown 4,3		Mahogany Ash Brown 4,51		
3	Dark Brown							
1	Black							
	Natural/ Basic, 0	Ash ,1	Mauve ,2	Gold ,3	Copper ,4	Mahogany ,5	Red ,6	Metallic ,7

In the table above we see how the L'Oréal shades are positioned within the colour table. Row 1, containing Black (1), denotes the *darkest* shades, gradually going up in numbers to Row 10, containing 'Lightest Blonde' (10.0). This denotes the lightest shades.

Within the table two shades, 'Dark Copper Red Blonde' (6.46) and 'Deep Copper Blonde' (7.44) are highlighted. These two examples identify additional colour properties. These shades are denoted, as are many others in the table, with having a second number after the decimal point.

Shade	Depth	Primary tone	Secondary tone
Dark Copper Red Blonde	6●	4	6

1 The primary tone denotes the range that the shade is in.

2 Secondary tone indicates the additional pigmentation within the shade. This provides lots of extra colouring permutations.

Sometimes colour manufacturers want to increase a shade's intensity and vibrancy. This is achieved by adding double the tone to the particular shade, doubling the tonal effect.

Shade	Depth	Primary tone	Secondary tone
Deep Copper Blonde	7●	4	4

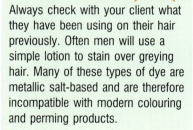

BEST PRACTICE

Always check with your client what they have been using on their hair previously. Often men will use a simple lotion to stain over greying hair. Many of these types of dye are metallic salt-based and are therefore incompatible with modern colouring and perming products.

Types of synthetic hair colour

Temporary colour Temporary colours are available in the form of lotions, creams, mousses, gels, lacquers, sprays, crayons paints and glitter dust. On hair in good condition these do not penetrate the hair cuticle, nor do they directly affect the natural hair colour: they simply remain on the hair until washed off.

Temporary colours are ideal for a client who has not had colour before, as they are readily removed if not liked. They have subtle colouring effects, particularly on white hair. Hair condition, shine and control are enhanced.

If used on badly damaged or very porous hair, the temporary colour may quickly be absorbed into the cortex, producing uneven, patchy results.

Features and benefits

Feature	Benefits
Have large molecules and sit on the surface of the hair	Easy to remove as they are washed away during the next shampoo
Come in a variety of types as mousses, setting lotions, gels, creams, colour sprays and colour shampoos	Easy to apply as they can either be applied during the shampoo process or alternatively as a styling or finishing product
Come in a variety of shades and colours	Can be used as a fashion statement or alternative to enhance natural tones by either adding depth to faded hair or neutralizing unwanted tones from hair

Points to remember

- Temporary colours only last for one wash (unless the hair is porous).

- They are often difficult to remove totally from hair that is extremely porous or lightened.

- You cannot lighten hair with temporary colours.

- You cannot target a shade in the same way as you can with longer-lasting colours.

- They may not give you an even coverage on the hair.

Semi-permanent colour Semi-permanent colours are made in a variety of forms – some ready-mixed for immediate use, others needing to be mixed and prepared before use as necessary. Always check the manufacturer's instructions to ensure that you know which type of colour you are going to use.

Semi-permanent colours contain pigments which are deposited in the hair cuticle and outer cortex. The colour gradually fades each time the hair is shampooed. Some colour will last through six washes, others longer.

Generally, these colours are not intended to cover large percentages of white hair – for instance, black used on white hair would not produce a pleasing result. Choose colours carefully.

Diluting permanent colour

Some permanent colour may be diluted for use as semi-permanents. These products may contain skin sensitizers, however, so skin tests must be performed before use in this way. Check manufacturer instructions for more information.

Features and benefits Semi-permanent colours are ideal for those people who want to try colour but are not ready yet to take a big step forward into the maintenance of permanent colour effects. They last up to six or eight shampoos and do not produce any regrowth; the hair loses the colour on each subsequent shampoo so the effect fades over time. Conditioning agents form part of the colouring package to add shine and improve style manageability while the colour is deposited on to the hair.

Semi-permanents also provide an ideal solution for livening up faded mid-lengths and ends for clients who have permanent colours; this is particularly useful if the hair is not really ready yet for another treatment of peroxide-based colours.

Semi-permanents will colour white/grey hair to some extent, although the penetration doesn't extend beyond the cuticle layer, so colour density is relatively poor. (White hair tends to have a very smooth cuticle so there are fewer spaces for the pigments to bond on to.) The colour range is varied, ranging from fashion effects to many of the shades you would expect to see in a standard shade chart. They are simple to use and require no developer and hence no mixing.

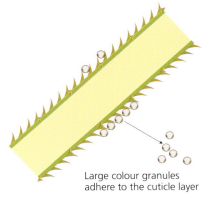

Large colour granules adhere to the cuticle layer

Temporary hair colouring

TOP TIP

Hair products and the under 16s.
All chemicals that are used within hair and beauty products are controlled under European laws (EU Directives). Some chemicals found in permanent and quasi colours, lighteners, permanent waving, relaxers and chemical straighteners, are restricted, and no longer permitted for use on young people under 16 years of age. Any hair preparation that falls within this group is now prohibited and you will find that these products are clearly marked 'This product is not intended for use on persons under the age of 16'

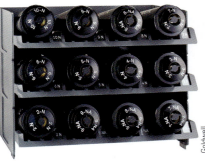

Goldwell

Feature	Benefits
Have large molecules that sit on the surface of the hair whilst other smaller ones penetrate deeper into the hair.	A great way to introduce clients to colour without long-term commitment. Fairly easy to remove as they are washed away in six or eight shampoos.
Come in a variety of types as mousses, liquids, gels, creams. Come in a variety of colours as fashion effects or as standard shade chart references.	Easy to apply, normally requires no mixing, take a short time and leave no regrowth. Can be used as a fashion statement or alternatively as a trial for a permanent colour effect.
(* At Level 3) Can be used in colour correction work. Add tone to white/grey hair.	A simple and quick pre-filler and pre-pigmentation shade. Provide some masking/coverage for unwanted greys.
Provide an alternative to permanent colour.	Note* may need a patch/skin test beforehand. See tests page 387.

Points to remember

◆ Semi-permanent colours only last for up to six or eight washes.

◆ They are often difficult to remove totally from hair that is extremely porous or lightened.

◆ You cannot lighten hair with semi-permanent colour.

◆ They will not colour white/grey hair with 100 per cent coverage.

◆ They cover with far better results than temporary colours.

Now that 'frequent use' shampoos have become popular, semi-permanent colours fade quickly. Therefore a new generation of longer-lasting, quasi-permanent colours have been introduced which are more practical and economical. These colours allow for a greater coverage of white hair and last for up to 12 washes.

Quasi-permanent colour
Quasi-permanent colours (also called tone on tone colours) are nearly permanent – they last for a longer period of time than semi-permanent colour but not as long as the true permanent colour. When using them, follow the manufacturer's instructions carefully.

Features and benefits
Quasi-colours are used a lot in the home-retail sector. They are not true permanent colours but do require the mixing of colour with a low-strength developer. They last for at least 12 washes and anything up to 24 and, regardless of advertisers' claims, *they do leave a regrowth*. These types of colours do have a better ability to cover white/grey hair and this is the main reason why they are so popular as home colours.

Quasi-colour should be treated like a permanent colour or lightener; they do require a skin test 24–48 hours beforehand.

Feature	Benefits
Are processed with a developer and have similar molecules that penetrate deeper into the hair.	Easy solution for all-over colouring; last a long time, generally up to 12–24 shampoos.
Come as gels or creams.	Require mixing with developer and have been made easy to apply for home use. Leave a regrowth.
Come in a variety of colours as fashion effects or as standard shade chart references.	Can be used as a fashion statement or as an alternative to more permanent-based colour.
(* At Level 3) Can be used in colour correction work. Add depth and tone to white/grey hair.	Are an alternative longer-lasting pre-pigmentation shade. Provide up to 50 per cent coverage for unwanted greys.
Provide a different alternative to perma-nent para-dyes.	Tend to be used regularly and more often than salon-provided treatments.
Good conditioning properties, add shine and improve manageability.	Leave hair in good condition, manageable and with added shine.

Points to remember

- Quasi-permanent colours always require a skin test.

- They last for 12–24 washes, leaving a regrowth.

- They can only be removed by colour reduction (not by colour or lightener).

- They often provide the basis for colour correction work if wrongly used at home.

- They offer good coverage; colour white/grey with better saturation than semis.

- They have similar effects to permanent colours.

Permanent colour
Permanent colours are made in a wide variety of shades and tones. They can cover white and natural-coloured hair to produce a range of natural, fashion and fantasy shades.

Hydrogen peroxide is mixed with permanent colour. This oxidizes the hair's natural pigments and joins the small, synthetic pigments together with the natural ones in a process called *polymerization*. The hair will then retain the colour permanently in the cortex. Hair in poor condition, however, will not hold the colour and colouring could result in patchy areas and colour fading.

The use of modern permanent colour can lighten or darken the natural hair colour, or both together in one process. This is achieved by varying the percentage strength of hydrogen peroxide.

Main points to remember
True permanent para-dyes are the only colours that cover white/grey hair with 100 per cent saturation/coverage. The colours tend to come in easy-to-dispense tubes as creams or gels which are then mixed with hydrogen

Tiny colour granules are mixed with hydrogen peroxide – they pass through the cuticle layer into the cortex

peroxide, as the developer, to create lasting effects that grow out. Even if the colour used is darker than the natural depth and deposits only, the colour effect will remain until it is either cut or grows out.

The para-dyes contain **PPD** (*para-phenylenediamine*). This is a known allergen and it is this compound that necessitates the need for conducting skin or sensitivity tests before any colouring service is carried out. There are other chemicals within para-dyes and they all do different things:

◆ Ammonia/resorcinol is alkaline and when it comes into contact with the hair it swells the hair shaft in preparation for the pigmentation. It also acts as an **activator or booster** for the hydrogen peroxide by releasing oxygen and starting the **oxidation** process.

◆ Conditioning agents improve the hair during the colouring process, enabling it to be smoother and shinier as a result.

◆ During the process hydrogen peroxide oxidzes the natural pigments of the hair and this enables the synthetic pigments to bond with them, creating a permanent change within the hair's cortex.

Vegetable-based colour
As well as being a popular source for conditioning agents, plant extracts have been used as dyeing compounds for thousands of years. These were the only sources of colour until chemists developed synthetic alternatives. Natural henna (Lawsonia) is still used widely today in many countries and it is used for dyeing skin as well as the hair. Natural plant-based dyes do not present any problems for hairdressing treatments; however, these ingredients are sometimes added to other elements to form compounds, mixtures of vegetable extracts and mineral substances. One that is still available is compound henna – vegetable henna mixed with metallic salts. This penetrating dye is incompatible with professional products used in hairdressing salons and will react with professional salon colours and perming products.

Metallic dyes – incompatibles
Metallic dyes (**progressive dyes**) are surface-coating colour. They are variously known as reduction, metallic, sulphide and progressive dyes. These types of dye are also **incompatible** with chemical hairdressing services and are still found in men's colour restorers; such as 'Just for Men' and 'Grecian Formula 2000'.

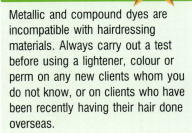

Artificial depth and tone are added. Lightening of the natural pigments can occur with some shades.

The granules swell and join together becoming permently trapped.

ACTIVITY

Solve the following problems and record your answers in your portfolio.

What could be the reasons for:

1. permanent colour fading on the ends of long hair?

2. permanent colour not taking properly on the roots?

3. grey/white hair resisting semi-permanent colour?

4. permanent copper red colour not taking on mid-brown hair?

5. blonde hair looking ashen or green?

The effects of hydrogen peroxide on hair

Hydrogen peroxide strength	Effect upon the hair
5 vol (1.5%)	◆ Assists the deposit of quasi-permanent colour and some toners into very sensitized hair, adding depth, making it darker.
10 vol (3%)	◆ Assists the deposit of quasi-permanent and some* permanent colours into natural/virgin or sensitized hair, adding depth, making it darker.
20 vol (or 6%)	◆ Assists the deposit of colour into the hair, adding depth, making it darker. ◆ Enables coverage of white/grey hair. ◆ Will lighten two levels above base 6 (on fine hair). ◆ Will lighten one level below base 4.
30 vol (or 9%)	◆ Will lighten hair three levels above base 6. ◆ Will lighten hair two levels below base 4.
40 vol (or 12%)	◆ Will lighten hair four levels above base 6 (with high lift colour).

Special note: When hydrogen peroxide lightens hair to any level it will remove the smaller pigments first. The larger, warmer pigments (*pheomelanin*) within the hair are more difficult to remove, so unwanted golden or even orange tones are often left within the hair.

Diluting hydrogen peroxide This illustration shows you how the strengths that you have in stock can be diluted to make lesser-strength hydrogen peroxide.

The first column refers to the strength peroxide that you have, the second refers to the peroxide you want to create. The last three columns show you how many parts of the peroxide you need and how many parts of distilled water you need to add to it.

BEST PRACTICE

Mixing colour
Don't mix permanent colours together until you are ready to use them. Mix the colours carefully, making sure that you measure the amounts accurately. If the proportions are wrong the final effect will be wrong!

Diluting hydrogen peroxide

Strength you have	Strength you want to create	Peroxide	Add	Water
40 vol (i.e. 12%)	30 vol (i.e. 9%)	3	+	1
40 vol	20 vol (i.e. 6%)	1	+	1
40 vol	10 vol (i.e. 3%)	1	+	3
30 vol (i.e. 9%)	20 vol (i.e. 6%)	2	+	1
30 vol	10 vol (i.e. 3%)	1	+	2
20 vol (i.e. 6%)	10 vol (i.e. 3%)	1	+	1

ACTIVITY

Complete the following sentences.

1. a. 6% is <u>2</u> times stronger than 3%.
   b. 9% is __ times stronger than 3%.
   c. 12% is __ times stronger than 3%.
   d. 12% is __ times stronger than 6%.

2. a. 20 vol. is <u>2</u> times stronger than 10 vol.
   b. 30 vol. is __ times stronger than 10 vol.
   c. 40 vol. is __ times stronger than 10 vol.
   d. 40 vol. is __ times stronger than 20 vol.

3. a. 6% is __ times stronger than 10 vol.
   b. 9% is __ times stronger than 10 vol.
   c. 12% is __ times stronger than 10 vol.

Lightening hair

Lighteners have alkaline chemicals within them that achieve lightened effects by dissolving the natural tones (pigments) within hair. Similar to para-dyes, lightening products are mixed with hydrogen peroxide to activate the oxidizing process, and they are used in three main forms:

- *high lift colour* – which is a non-bleach process for lightening hair partially or whole head

- *powder lightener* – which is used for highlighting and partial lightening techniques

- *gel/oil lightener* – which is suitable for whole-head applications including the scalp.

The alkaline compound acts upon the hair by swelling and opening up the cuticle. This enables the peroxide at six per cent or nine per cent to release oxygen and oxidize the natural pigments of melanin from within the cortex. This creates **oxymelanin** and is seen as it reduces the natural colour through the different degrees of lift.

The colour control during lightening is not the same as with colouring though. Often when full-head lightening is done the result is quite yellow (although the control of warm pigments during lightening is better with high lift colour).

Toning colours

Level of depth	Tone required	Tonal quality	Pre-lighten to
10	Silver, platinum, mauve/violet	Cool	Very pale yellow
9	Ashen blondes, light beige blonde	Cool	Pale yellow
8	Beige blonde	Cool	Yellow
8	Sandy blonde	Warm	
7	Golden blonde	Warm	
7	Chestnut, copper gold	Warm	Orange
6	Red copper	Warm	
5	Mahogany	Cool	Red/orange
4	Burgundy, plum	Cool	

Toning is the process of adding colour to previously lightened hair. A variety of pastel shades, such as silver, beige and rose, are used to produce subtle effects. Different types of **toners** are available; read the instructions provided by their manufacturers to find out what is possible.

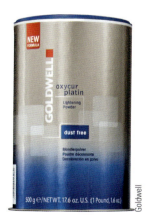

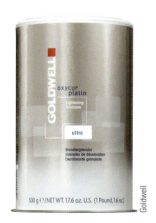

Choice of lightening method

High lift colour All manufacturers produce a special range of colours that are used to lighten hair. As these are mixed with six per cent or nine per cent volume peroxide their ability to achieve very high lift results are limited by the natural depth that you are starting with.

The colour control and condition of the hair is generally better than that produced by using lightener, since the colour can deposit ashen, beige or warm tones as the colour works and the hair lightens. And because you are using a hair colour and not lightener, less moisture is removed from the hair during the process, so a better condition is guaranteed at the end.

High lift colours are similar in composition to normal hair colours with one exception: they use an alkaline component (e.g. resorcinol) which swells the hair shaft enabling a better penetration of the chemicals into the cortex and hence able to lighten as well.

Removing high lift colour

You can remove high lift colour by emulsifying the colour, by adding a little warm water to the colour and gently massaging all over. This mixes the colour with the water and helps to release the products from the hair enabling you to use a lighter action within the shampooing process. The hair can be conditioned as normal at the end or an anti-oxidant can be applied to help close the cuticle and lock in the colour results.

Emulsion lightener Emulsion lighteners are slow acting. They are made up of two compounds that are added together and then mixed with hydrogen peroxide:

- **oil or gel** lightener
- **activators**, **boosters** or **controllers**.

This type of lightener is specially formulated for use directly onto the roots of the hair, and is suitable for contact with the scalp. It is kinder and gentler during the lightening process and is mixed with 20 vol. hydrogen peroxide for root, mid-length and ends application. The lift through the undertone shades is aided and controlled by the addition of activators. These boost the power whilst maintaining relatively low hydrogen peroxide strength.

Emulsion lighteners also contain additives which control the resultant colour as the hair lightens. As mentioned earlier, these tend to make hair yellow, so they have matt emulsifiers which neutralize unwanted yellow tones whilst the lifting process takes place. Heat may be used during the development of the process, but the client must be monitored closely (particularly if a **colour accelerator** or **steamer** is used to aid development) as these types of lightener can often be more viscous and mobile and might drip!

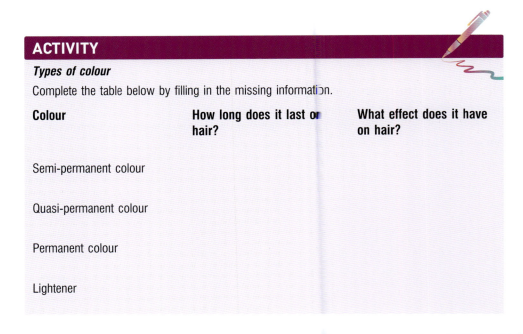

ACTIVITY

Types of colour

Complete the table below by filling in the missing information.

Colour	How long does it last on hair?	What effect does it have on hair?
Semi-permanent colour		
Quasi-permanent colour		
Permanent colour		
Lightener		

Removing emulsion lightener

Make sure that when the lightener is removed you rinse without massaging and with only tepid or warm water. The client's scalp has been subjected to chemicals and could be sensitive; the cooling action of the rinsing will stop the lightening process and make the client more comfortable. After the emulsion has been rinsed away the hair can be shampooed with a mild colour shampoo and conditioned with an **anti-oxidizing treatment**.

Powder lightener Powder lighteners can be mixed with six, nine or twelve per cent hydrogen peroxide, depending upon the level of lift required. Powder lighteners are fast acting and are used for a variety of highlighting techniques. When they are mixed in the bowl the consistency is that of a thick, 'porridge-type' paste. The stiffness of the consistency prevents spillages and enables the lightener to work like a poultice. As the process continues the mixture will expand. This action is speeded up more if accelerated by heat, so a careful eye should be kept on the development timings.

Removing powder lightener

Again, as with emulsion lightener, make sure that when it is removed from the hair you rinse it without massaging, using only tepid or warm water. The removal of powder lightener can be far more problematic than that of emulsion lightener and this has more to do with the colouring technique that has been used. If different coloured highlights have been done with Easi-Meche™, foil, wraps, etc. these need to be removed carefully and individually as one colour may affect another. Although the client's scalp has not been subjected to chemicals, it still might be sensitive from the colouring technique; again, the cooling action of the rinsing will stop the lightening process and make the client more comfortable. Afterwards the hair can be shampooed with a mild colour shampoo and conditioned with an anti-oxidizing treatment.

TOP TIP

The degree of lift required in emulsion lightener is controlled by the number of activators added into the mixing bowl with the oil. It is not boosted by stronger hydrogen peroxide levels. Always follow the manufacturer's instructions when using lightening products.

HEALTH & SAFETY

Avoid inhalation of powder lighteners

Be very careful when you dispense powder lightener into a bowl. The particles are very small and tend to 'dust' into the air very easily. This is a hazardous chemical compound which can cause respiratory conditions. You must avoid contact through inhalation; wherever possible only use 'dust-free' powder lightener.

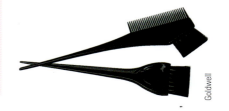

Goldwell

Lightening service required	What you need to check for	Technique/application	Lightener type
Whole head (on virgin hair)	**Test results:** ◆ (Skin tests etc).		
	Natural hair depth: ◆ Lightener will lift five levels quite happily on hair with brown/ash pigments. However, strong red content will be difficult to remove.	Lightener must be applied to mid-lengths and ends first. A plastic cap should envelop the contents and can be developed with gentle heat until ready.	Only emulsion oil-based lighteners or creams are suggested for application to the scalp. These are used with six per cent hydrogen peroxide and sachet controllers to handle levels of lift.

Lightening service required	What you need to check for	Technique/application	Lightener type
	◆ Hair beyond base 5 will not lift safely beyond base 9. Suggest other colouring options.	When the hair has lightened two to three levels of lift, the root application can be applied.	
	Hair length: ◆ Lengths up to 10cm lighten evenly, provided manufacturers' instructions are followed. ◆ Lengths over 15cm are not recommended, as evenness of colour will be difficult to guarantee.	◆ Always follow manufacturers' instructions.	
	Hair texture: ◆ Finer hair needs extra care and lower hydrogen peroxide strengths, i.e. six per cent. ◆ Medium and coarser hair present fewer technical problems.		
	Hair condition: ◆ Only consider hair in good condition for lightening. Lightening removes moisture content during the process, hair that is porous or containing low moisture levels has insufficient durability for lightening.		
Full head (on previously coloured)	◆ Not recommended		
Root application (pre-lightened ends)	**Existing client:** ◆ Yes, check previous records and current hair condition and carry out service. ◆ No, new client: go through all the checks in the **full head application** table and find out the previous treatment history.	Roots only without overlapping previous lightened ends. ◆ Always follow manufacturers' instructions.	Only emulsion oil or cream-based lighteners are suggested for application to the scalp.
Highlights (fine even meshes on natural, i.e. virgin hair)	**Test results:** ◆ (Skin tests etc). **Natural hair depth:** ◆ Lightening products will lift five levels quite happily on hair with brown/ash pigments. However, strong red content will be difficult to remove and require stronger developer and/or additional heat.	◆ Plastic self-grip meshes (e.g. Easi-Meche™ L'Oreal Professionnel). ◆ Foil meshes. ◆ Colour wraps.	High lift powder type with suitable hydrogen peroxide developer at six per cent, nine per cent or for highest lift twelve per cent (providing no product is allowed to make contact with the skin/scalp).

Lightening service required	What you need to check for	Technique/application	Lightener type
	◆ Hair beyond base 5 will not lift safely beyond base 9. Suggest other lightening technique.		
	Hair length: ◆ Hair length will have an impact on evenness of colour. However a small tolerance is acceptable, and 'visually' indistinguishable on longer hair lengths.		
	Hair texture: ◆ Finer hair needs extra care and lower hydrogen peroxide strengths, i.e. six per cent. ◆ Medium and coarser hair present fewer technical problems but generally take longer.		
	Hair condition: ◆ Only consider hair in good condition for lightening. Lightening removes moisture content during the process, hair that is porous or containing low moisture levels has insufficient durability for lightening.		

Cap highlights Highlight caps are a safe, simple and popular choice for cost-effective, single-colour or lightened highlights on short layered hair. Even with the application of a single colour a multi-toned effect can be achieved. The reason for this is more to do with the cut and styling though, rather than the introduction of a solitary tone. Highlight caps can produce basic effects, whilst more complex, technically involved, multicolour effects are achieved through other techniques.

Woven highlights Woven highlights in foil, Easi-Meche™ or wraps are the preferred technique for multi-toning hair. The visual effects are unlimited and new exciting colour combinations and techniques are happening each year. The application of this type of colouring is both creative and artistic, and is only limited by the vision that the stylist has.

TOP TIP

The success of highlights on coloured hair is often poor. This work is often undertaken in salons, but ends seldom lighten effectively, whilst the roots lighten very quickly. In this instance, colour should be removed with a synthetic colour remover-decolour, before highlights are attempted.

ACTIVITY

With your colleagues, each collect from styling magazines a selection of (say six) partial/highlight effects.

Now take it in turns to show the others each of your pictures and then explain how each effect was created, providing the technique, application and colours used. Record these details along with the relevant pictures for use in your portfolio. Check your assessment with your supervisor or a senior member of staff.

Maintain effective and safe methods of working when colouring and lightening hair

Safety and preparation

Although Chapter 1 covers much of the general aspects of heath and safety that you need to know, each technical procedure has specific things that relate to that area of hairdressing alone. Hair colouring is particularly problematic as it involves the application of a variety of potentially harmful chemicals. Therefore the care that you take in handling products and preparing yourself and the client is absolutely critical to safe and successful colouring.

Records

These should be found and put ready at the beginning of the day. The appointment book identifies all the expected clients, so all their treatment history – dates of visits, who provided the services, previous chemical services, records of any tests and any additional comments – can all be collated long before the clients arrive.

Similarly, when clients have been in, any results of tests or notes following treatments must always be updated as soon as practically possible. The records are essential for keeping things going smoothly, by maintaining services even if key staff are away, let alone if things go wrong and they are needed in any pursuance by insurers.

Tests

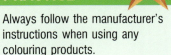

For more information on tests see pages 386–389.

Collect together the results of any tests carried out prior to the appointment. If there have been any adverse reactions or contra-indications no permanent colour service can be carried out. Have you made this clear to the client and made plans for alternative services such as temporary or semi-permanent colouring?

BEST PRACTICE

Always follow the manufacturer's instructions when using any colouring products.

Materials

After the records have been found it is advisable to get all tubes, cans or bottles of colour put aside and ready along with the client's record information. Doing this earlier has several benefits. It can save valuable time later when you need to mix them, particularly if you are running on a tight schedule. But it has useful benefits for the salon's stock control systems too: when products are removed from stock you can see when certain colours are running low. These can be noted and the relevant person made aware.

Gowning

Always make sure that the client and the client's clothes are adequately protected before any process is started. Most salons have special 'colour-proof' gowns for colouring and lightening processes. These gowns are resistant to staining and are made from finely woven synthetic fabrics that will stop colour spillages from getting through onto the client's skin or clothes. When you gown the client, make sure that the free edges are closed and fastened together. On top of this and around the shoulders you can place a colouring towel and over this a plastic cape. This needs to be fastened but loose enough for the client to be comfortable throughout the service. Remember that this may be over an hour or so.

Using barrier cream

Barrier cream can be used as physical barrier to prevent staining around the client's face/hairline. It is also particularly useful if the client has any general sensitivity to chemical-based products. Remember it is not an excuse for poor slapdash application, allowing you to extend the colour application beyond the root area to the skin. But it will help in areas where colour seeps off the hair onto the skin.

Apply barrier cream to the skin with a finger or cotton wool close to the hairline, taking care not to get it onto the hair, as this could stop the colour from taking evenly.

It can be removed later after you have shampooed the colour from the hair and before any other services are conducted.

Seating position

The chair back should be protected with a plastic cover. If this is not available a colouring towel can be folded lengthwise and secured with sectioning clips at either end. The client should be seated comfortably, in an upright position, with their back flat against the cushioned chair pad.

Trolley

You should have your colouring trolley prepared and at hand with the materials you will need. Foils for highlighting should have been previously prepared to the right lengths and combs, brushes, sectioning clips, etc. should be all cleaned, sterilized and ready for use.

Protecting yourself

Your personal hygiene and safety are also important. The care you take in preparing for work should be carried through in everything you do and this is made even more important when you are about to handle hazardous chemicals. Put on a clean colouring apron and fasten the ties in a bow. Then take a pair of disposable vinyl gloves and put them on ready for the application. It is recommended as best practice to wear a glove of 30cm length to offer protection to the wrist area. There should be a variety of sizes for staff to choose from to ensure best fit.

Use your time effectively; each salon allocates different times for different services. A retouch may only take 20 minutes to apply on shorter hair whereas a long hair set of full-head woven highlights could be booked for an hour.

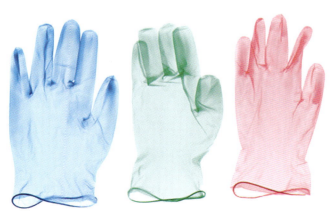

> **BEST PRACTICE**
>
> When mixing colouring products, never add colour or developer together by guesswork. The amounts that have to be added together are critical to a successful outcome. Don't take unnecessary risks!

For more information about working position and efficiency, personal hygiene, avoiding dermatitis, etc., see Unit G20 Make sure your actions reduce the risks to health and safety, pages 2–23.

For more information about using and checking electrical equipment during processing see Unit GH8 Shampoo, condition and treat the hair and scalp, pages 138–163.

ACTIVITY

Make sure that you are up to speed with your colouring

You can always practise your timing for different colouring services by working on a modelling head and applying conditioner instead of colour. This allows you to get the feel of product application without any problems arising from uneven application.

TOP TIP

Always follow the manufacturer's instructions for mixing the correct amounts together. If the proportions are wrong the colour will be wrong.

TOP TIP

Colouring materials are expensive. The profitability of the job you are about to do relates directly to the amount of colour you use. Always mix a small amount up to work with. If you do run out you can always mix up some more.

BEST PRACTICE

Dos and Don'ts

Dos

When a client's hair is developing under a Climazone, Rollerball or any other colour accelerator, do check at intervals during the processing to see that they are comfortable and that the equipment is not too hot.

Do check the equipment controls so that the timing and temperature settings are correct.

Do check the manufacturer's instructions before you mix any products. They will give you the recommended amounts and quantities to mix together.

Always do a skin test on the client before any colouring process.

Do put screw tops and lids back on colouring products immediately. Their effectiveness will be impaired if they are exposed to the air for any longer than needed.

Do make a note of low levels of stock as product is removed from storage.

Do make good use of your time. Always prepare your work area and the materials you will need before the client arrives; this saves valuable time later.

Don'ts

Never handle electrical equipment with wet hands, always dry them first.

Never leave colour spillages until later. Mop them up straight away while you still have your protective gloves on.

Don't mix up too much product at one time, it is wasteful and expensive. If you need more you can always mix up more when you need it.

Never mix products up before they are needed. Colour products have a set development time and oxidization will start if they are exposed or mixed too soon.

Never attempt to do any colouring procedure without wearing the correct PPE.

Don't work in a cluttered environment. Always make sure that the work area is prepared properly and ready for use.

Don't forget to complete the client details/records after doing the service. Make sure that all aspects – dates, times, changes in materials, etc. – are recorded accurately.

ACTIVITY

Hair tests

Complete this activity by filling in the missing information in the spaces provided

Type of test	What is the purpose of the test?	How is the test carried out?
Elasticity		
Porosity		
Incompatibility		
Patch		
Strand		

Prepare for colouring and lightening hair

Colour consultation

Before you start any colouring treatment there are a number of things that you should do.

Choosing colours

First of all	Things to consider
Does the client know of any reasons that would affect your choice of service?	Ask the client about their hair to find out if there are any known reasons why the service can not continue – are there any contra-indications?
What colour would be best to suit their needs?	Should you be using temporary, semi-permanent or permanent colouring?
How can the desired effect be best achieved?	Does the colour need to be applied to the roots first, the mid-lengths and ends, or can it be applied all over? Would the effect benefit more from partial colouring such as highlights or lowlights?
How long will it last?	Will the colour fade off or does it have to grow out?
How much will it cost?	Is this affordable and something that can be kept up in the future?
How will it affect the hair?	Will the long-term effects be what the client expects?
Is the hair suitable for colouring?	Have you tested the hair and skin beforehand to see if there are any contra-indications or hair condition issues that will affect the result?

Now consider

What are the client's expectations?	How will the colour enhance the style and natural colour of the hair? What are the benefits for them?
What are the results of your tests?	Examine the hair: does it present any limitations for what you intend to do?
What is the hair condition like?	Are there any factors that will change the way in which colouring will work on the hair? What previous information is available?
What do the client's records say?	Does this information influence the choice and colour process?
How will you show the effect to the client?	Have you got any illustrations of the finished effect? Does the colour chart give a clearer picture of the shade the hair will go?
How long will the process take?	Is there enough time to complete the effect? Has anything changed as a result of the consultation? Would this service now need to be re-booked or do you have the time to complete it still?

What contra-indications should I be looking for?

Contra-indications are	How could you find out?	How else would you know?
Skin sensitivity	Ask the client if they have ever had a reaction to hair or skin products in the past.	Patch test/sensitivity test.
Allergic reaction	Ask the client if they have ever had a reaction to hair or skin products in the past.	Patch test/sensitivity test.
Skin disorder	Ask the client if they know about any current skin disorders.	Examine the scalp to see if there are any physical signs of skin abrasions, discolouration, swellings, infestation or infections.
Incompatible products	If you see the results of any previous colour ask what type it was, how was it done?	Look for discolouration or unnatural colour effects on the hair. Test for incompatibles.
Medical reasons	Ask the client if there are any current medical reasons why colouring can not be performed.	Examine the hair; look for signs of healthy active growth. If there are signs of weakened, damaged, broken or missing hair, ask for more information. Test for elasticity and porosity.
Damaged hair	Ask the client if there are any current known reasons why the hair is in its current state/condition.	Examine the hair; look for signs of healthy active growth. If there are signs of weakened, damaged, broken or missing hair, ask for more information. Test for elasticity and porosity.

What sort of colour should I use?

Type, PPE and timings	Preparation	Suitability	Effects
Temporary colour. PPE – wear gloves and apron. Whole head application done at workstation takes five minutes.	No mixing required, colour applied straight from the can, bottle etc. as coloured mousses, setting lotions, hair mascara.	No skin test required. Most hair types (including coloured and permed) although it can be more difficult to remove from lightened hair. Colour control – poor, shade guide targeting can only be used as an approximation.	The colour only lasts until the next wash. Subtle toning on grey hair. Hair condition may be improved. Surface colour without chemical penetration. Does not lift natural colour, only deposits.

Type, PPE and timings	Preparation	Suitability	Effects
Semi-permanent colour. PPE – wear gloves and apron. Whole head application done at workstation or at basin takes five minutes. Left on up to 15 minutes.	No mixing required, although transference to an applicator may be necessary.	Skin test may be required. Most hair types (including coloured and permed) often used as a colour refresher between permanent colour treatments. Can cover small amounts of greying hair. Colour control – poor, shade guide targeting can only be used as an approximation.	Lasts up to six shampoos. Colour fades/diffuses after each wash. Does not lift natural colour, only deposits. No regrowth, natural colour unaffected.
Quasi-permanent (tone on tone colour). PPE – wear gloves and apron. Whole head brush application done at workstation, takes up to 25 minutes. Alternatively, using an applicator bottle can save time and takes up to 15 minutes. Left on up to 40 minutes.	Mixed with developer or activators. These can be in liquid or crystal form. Measurement and mixing must be accurate.	Skin test required. Most hair types (including coloured and permed) often used as a colour refresher between permanent colour treatments. Will cover up to 30 per cent grey hair. Colour control – good, will achieve shade guide targeting.	Lasts up to 12 shampoos. Colour fades a small amount after subsequent shampoos. Does affect natural colour, bonds with natural pigments. Can produce a regrowth.
Permanent colour (para-dye) PPE – wear gloves and apron. Regrowth brush application done at workstation, takes up to 25 minutes. Left on up to 40 minutes. Whole head colouring will depend on length and order of application.	Mixed with hydrogen peroxide at 10, 20, 30 or 40 volumes (3 per cent, 6 per cent, 9 per cent or 12 per cent). Measurement and mixing must be accurate.	Skin test required. All natural hair types and most coloured and permed hair (providing hair not too porous or damaged). Will cover all grey. Can lift up to two shades – high lift colour will lift three or four shades.	Permanent colour or para-dyes are made in a wide variety of shades and tone. Long lasting and grows out. Will change natural hair pigments.

Note: All timings are approximated. Partial colouring techniques – highlights, slices, dip ends, etc. – may take longer depending on operator experience, the amount of colour applied and the technique used.

Measuring flasks and mixing bowls

Measurement of hydrogen peroxide at any strength must be accurate; the amount used in relation to colour is a critical factor to a successful outcome. Different types of colour are formulated to be used with particular developers. For example, L'Oréal's Dia-Richesse™ should be mixed with DiaActivator™ developer. If you use a different developer the consistency will be wrong and this will make the application difficult. All gel and cream colours, when mixed, will be stiff enough not to run or drip when either on the brush or on the hair. Using unmatched, alternative developers will do the opposite and could be a potential hazard for the client.

When you measure developer into a measuring flask you must make sure that your eye line is at the same level as the liquid in the flask so that the measurement is accurate.

When you mix **developer** with colour from tubes, you will notice that all tubes have markings on the side showing the quarter, half and three-quarter points. These enable you to squeeze from the bottom of the tube up to these points, knowing that your measurement will be accurate.

If you are mixing two or more shades of colour together, always mix these well in the bowl first before adding any developer. This allows the different pigments to be evenly distributed throughout the colour and also throughout the hair when it is applied!

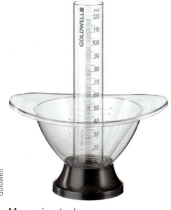

Goldwell

Measuring tools

Skin and hair tests

Skin or sensitivity test The sensitivity test is used to assess the reaction of the skin to chemicals or chemical products. In the salon it is mainly used before colouring. Some people are allergic to external contact with chemicals such as PPD (found in permanent colour). This can cause dermatitis or, in even more severe cases, permanent scarring of skin tissue and hair loss. Some have an allergy to irritants to which they react internally.

To find out whether a client's skin reacts to chemicals in permanent colours, carry out the following test 24 to 48 hours prior to the chemical process.

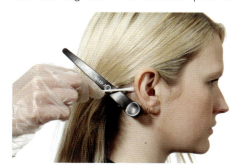

Carrying out a skin test

1 Use a small amount of dark, natural, colour shade for your test (darker, natural shades 1, 3, 3.0., etc. contain higher concentrations of PPD).

2 Clean an area of skin about 5mm square, behind the ear with warm water.

3 Apply a little amount of the colour to skin.

4 Don't cover the area, but ask your client to report any discomfort or irritation that occurs over the next 24 hours. Arrange to see your client at the end of this time so that you can check for signs of reaction.

5 If there is a positive response – a **contra-indication**, a skin reaction such as inflammation, soreness, swelling, irritation or discomfort – do not carry out the intended service. *Never* ignore the result of a skin test. If a skin test shows a reaction and you carry on anyway, there may be a more serious reaction that could affect the whole body!

6 If there is a negative response – no reaction to the chemicals – then carry out the treatment as proposed.

7 Record the details of any tests on the client's treatment and service history.

BEST PRACTICE

Always ask your client if they have had a (black) henna tattoo. These may contain PPD and will increase the chance of your client having a skin sensitivity to hair colouring.

Hair tests

Incompatibility test	When is it done	How is it done
This will show if there are any chemicals present, i.e. metallic salts or other mineral compounds, within the hair that will react against any new proposed services.	Prior to colouring, highlighting and perming treatments.	Place a small sample of hair in a mixture of 20 parts hydrogen peroxide (six per cent) and one part ammonium-based compound from perm solution. If the mixture bubbles, heats up or discolours do not carry out the service.

Incompatibility test

Elasticity test	When is it done	How is it done
This determines the condition of the hair by seeing how much the hair will stretch and return to its original length. Overstretched hair will not return to the same length and indicates weakness and damage.	Prior to chemical treatments and services. (Ideal for hair that has impaired elasticity, e.g. from lightening or colouring.)	Take a single strand of hair between your fingers, holding it at the root and the end. Gently pull the hair between the two points to see if the hair will stretch and return to its original length. (If the hair breaks easily it may indicate that the cortex is damaged and will be unable to sustain any further chemical treatment.) 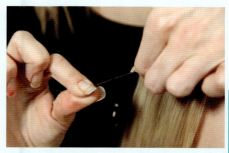 Elasticity test

Porosity test	When is it done	How is it done
This test also indicates the hair's current condition by assessing the hair's ability to absorb or resist moisture from liquids. (Hair in good condition has a tightly packed cuticle layer which will resist the ingress of products.) Hair that is very porous holds on to moisture; this is particularly evident when you try to blow-dry it. The hair takes a long time to dry.	Before chemical services. If the cuticle is torn or damaged, the absorption of moisture and therefore hydrogen peroxide is quicker, so the processing time will be shorter. Over-porous hair will quickly take in colour but will not necessarily be able to hold colour as the cuticle is damaged and allows the newly introduced pigments to wash away.	Take a single hair and hold it out, then with your other hand, run your finger and thumb, back along the hair towards the scalp (against the natural lie of the cuticle layers) If it feels roughened or *bumpy*, as opposed to just thicker, it is likely that the hair is porous. 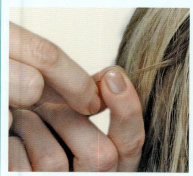 Porosity test

Strand test	When is it done	How is it done
Most colouring products just require the full development time recommended by the manufacturer – check their instructions. However, some hair conditions take on the colour faster than others. A strand test will check the colour development and see if it needs to come off earlier.	A strand test or hair strand colour test is used to assess the resultant colour on a strand or section of hair after colour has been processed and developed. A strand test is also useful prior to lightening natural pigments from hair or prior to removing synthetic pigments (i.e. decolour or colour reducer) to see how the hair will respond.	1 Rub a strand of hair lightly with the back of a comb to remove the surplus colour. 2 Check whether the colour remaining is evenly distributed throughout the hair's length. If it is even, remove the rest of the colour. If it is uneven, allow processing to continue, if necessary applying more colour. If any of the hair on the head is not being treated, you can compare the evenness of colour in the coloured hair with that in the uncoloured hair. 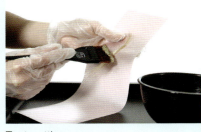 Test cutting

Strand test done as a 'test cutting' (more suitable for helping with colour selection. The test helps to see the colour result on a client's hair. Don't forget to label the hair so that you don't get it mixed up with other test cuttings)

Recording the results Make sure that you record the details of all tests that you conduct. Update the client's record card in full and immediately after you have done the test. Don't leave it until later, you might forget! These records are essential information that will be needed again and help to show that a competent service has been provided at that time.

This would be vitally important if there was a problem at some later stage, particularly if it involved any legal action taken against the salon.

BEST PRACTICE
If you are not sure about the results of any tests that you perform, ask a senior member of staff for their second opinion.

BEST PRACTICE
Record the results
After any treatment or tests have been carried out always update the client's records immediately. These tests and the findings are critical to the client's well-being and the salon's good name. You should record the:

◆ date
◆ the test carried out
◆ development times
◆ results
◆ recommended home-care or follow-up advice given.

BEST PRACTICE
Record the client's responses to your questions and the comments about how the results of any tests affected their hair and skin.

Colour and lighten hair and Colour and lighten (men's) hair

Colour selection

Colour selection, i.e. the process you go through in choosing the right target shade for your client's hair and the correct mixture of products to achieve that target shade, is based upon:

◆ customer choice (initially)

◆ current state of your client's hair (i.e. if it has already undergone processes such as highlights)

◆ existing condition of your client's hair.

1 If the hair has been regularly coloured before and there is a clear regrowth, with ends that have faded, you may only need to do a straightforward regrowth application with the same colour. Then, later in the development process, the residual colour can be diluted and taken through to the rest to refresh the total effect. So in this instance a regrowth that takes 20 minutes to apply can be left for 30 minutes' development (depending on manufacturer/colour type). Then, in the last 15 minutes, it can be taken through to the ends, until it is ready to be removed.

   However, if your client's hair has been coloured before, you also need to remember that it will not be possible to make the hair lighter by colouring. Permanent colour does not reduce permanent (synthetic) pigments in the hair. (If this is required you will have to use a colour remover first.)

2 If you need or want to counteract and neutralize unwanted tones in the hair, you will need to apply the principles of the colour wheel. If the client wants to reduce or 'calm down' unwanted red tones then you will be choosing a colour slightly darker in depth but which has the matt tones capable of neutralizing that effect. Conversely, if your aim is to eliminate ashen matt tones (e.g. the colour often seen on fairer hair colours that are regularly subjected to chlorinated swimming pools) then you will be introducing warmer tones to the hair. So in this situation a 'greeny'-looking base 6 blonde will be improved by a shade depth 6 but with a tone warmth .03.

   If you had to reduce a tonal effect that was too yellow, say on a head that had been lightened, then (although the principle of toning lightened hair is slightly different) you would still be applying the principles of the colour wheel. Therefore a violet-based ash colour should be used to neutralize the unwanted tones.

Correcting unwanted tones/effects

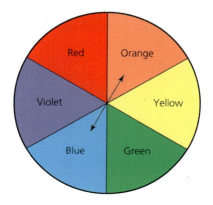

The colour wheel is set out with the three primary colours: red, yellow and blue. In between these three are the secondary colours: orange, green, and violet. These are a direct result of mixing the two adjacent primary colours.

Red + Yellow = Orange

Yellow + Blue = Green

Blue + Red = Violet

However, a colour's tonal effects can be neutralized if it is mixed with a colour directly opposite in the circle.

Hence unwanted:

Red tones are lessened or neutralized by *green*.

Orange tones are lessened or neutralized by *blue*.

Yellow tones are lessened or neutralized by *violet*.

3 If your client has never had any colour on their hair before (**virgin hair**) then colour targeting is easy. Your client will be able to choose practically any shade on the permanent shade chart, providing it is at the same depth or darker. (It is possible to lighten a shade or two with colour in certain situations.)

4 If your client has grey or greying (i.e. white) hair then you will have to decide and agree on what reduction of grey is necessary. If the client wants to cover all the grey, then this is only achievable by using or adding base shades to the target colour, i.e. a natural shade or a natural shade plus the target shade.

The amount of base added to the target shade is directly proportional to the amount of grey. Grey hair is referred to as a percentage of the whole head; therefore a client who has about a quarter of their hair that is grey is referred to as 25 per cent grey. Similarly, a client one tenth of whose hair is grey is 10 per cent grey.

So, the formula for mixing base shades works out like this:

◆ If a client has 25 per cent grey/white then you need ¼ of the base shade added to three-quarters of the target shade.

◆ If a client has 50 per cent grey/white then you need half of the base shade added to half of the target shade.

◆ If a client has 75 per cent grey/white then you need three-quarters of the base shade added to one quarter of the target shade.

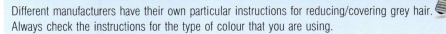

TOP TIP

Different manufacturers have their own particular instructions for reducing/covering grey hair. Always check the instructions for the type of colour that you are using.

Existing hair condition The hair's existing condition is a major contributing factor in the way in which it will respond when it is coloured. Hair that is too porous will absorb the colour differently. The porosity of hair is never even along the hair length, let alone across the hairs throughout the head. This is because the porosity of the hair is directly related to areas of damaged cuticle. Areas of high porosity occur at sites along the hair shaft where cuticle is torn or missing. At these points, moisture or chemicals can easily enter the inner hair without cuticle layer resistance.

This changes the rate of absorption, which ultimately affects the final evenness of the colour and the hair's ability to retain colour in subsequent washing etc. pH balancing conditioners help to even out the hair's porosity and return chemically-treated hair back to a natural pH 5.5.

During processing the only other factors that affect the achievement of an even and expected final colour result (providing your selection is correct) are:

◆ timing

◆ temperature.

Timing the colour development

The level of colour saturation is proportional to the length of time that the hair is exposed to colour. Under-processed hair will not achieve the same saturation as hair that has had full development. The longer that colour is left on, the more density the colour will have.

This can be explained in another way. Imagine that you wanted to redecorate a plain, smooth, white wall. First of all, you choose the colour and shade of paint that you want it to be. Then, after some preparation, you take a brush and start by applying the first coat. When this is dry you look at the colour, only to find that the effect is uneven and patchy. You can see that the tone you wanted is there but it is often thin and almost transparent in places. So you repaint the wall. When this extra layer of paint dries, the saturation of colour is better and more even, but still a little patchy in places. Finally you apply a third coat to the areas that are still patchy and when it dries the colour has an even density throughout. This effect is called *saturation*; it is achieved by the evenness of the density of the colour throughout the hair.

How temperature affects colouring

Temperature is also a contributing factor to colour development. The warmer the salon environment the quicker the colour processing will be. We know that when colour is introduced to heat it takes even more quickly; this can be localized to the client or relate to the whole salon. For instance, the salon temperature may be cool but the colour can be accelerated by putting the client under a *Climazon* or *Rollerball*.

But, remember, the human body produces heat too. In fact up to 30 per cent of body heat is emitted through the top of your head! (This is why wearing a hat in winter keeps you warm.) This heating effect has a dramatic impact on the development of colour and is even more critical when lightening!

So with this extra heat around the scalp area, you can see there are potential problems in controlling the colour and aspects of the client's safety. To help control this process you must make sure that, when the colour is applied to the root area, the hair is lifted away from the scalp so that the air is able to circulate and ventilate the scalp evenly. This ensures that there are no 'hot spots' anywhere that might take more quickly or become a safety hazard to the client.

TOP TIP

If you are in doubt about the timing of colouring always follow the manufacturer's instructions.

For more information on faults and correction see the table later in this chapter.

HEALTH & SAFETY

Always make sure that you remove all colouring products from the hair. This not only stops the action from developing further, but more importantly, it ensures that the client will not get any irritation or discomfort from chemicals deposited on the skin.

HEALTH & SAFETY

When the scalp becomes warm during the processing of colour the skin attempts to regulate the overheating by producing sweat. At this point when the skin is moistened by sweat the colouring products become more viscous and spread more easily onto and even into the skin! This is extremely dangerous and will cause scalp burns as chemicals enter the skin through the hair follicles!

Initially, the client will not be able to distinguish between the heat from the processing and the burning sensation from the chemicals. By the time that they do, the longer-term damage is done. Chemical burns continue to act upon the skin long after the colour has been removed. You *must* avoid this happening.

If this does occur, the client must seek medical attention immediately at hospital.

Colour selection checklist

- ✓   What is the client's target shade?
- ✓   What is the percentage of white/grey hair?
- ✓   What is the difference in depth between the natural hair and the target colour?
- ✓   If the target shade is lighter than the natural shade, is it achievable by colouring alone?
- ✓   What colouring products would be needed to achieve the effect?
- ✓   What developer will be needed to achieve the effect?
- ✓   If the hair appears porous or porous in areas, do you need to do a test cutting first?
- ✓   If the hair has a small percentage of white/grey, what amount of base shade will you need to add to the target shade to stabilize the effect?

ACTIVITY

You have a client who has recently been on holiday in a hot country. The hair colour that you applied to her hair beforehand has now faded off. On questioning her, you find out that she has been swimming in the pool every day. You observe that her hair colour has taken on a greenish tone.

1.   Why has the hair colour changed?

2.   What is your recommended course of action to rectify this problem?

Record this **case study** and your response in your portfolio.

TOP TIP

If the hair is very porous the colour produced by temporary colours may be uneven or difficult to remove.

TOP TIP

The higher the strength of the hydrogen peroxide, the more free oxygen is available and the more oxygen is released into the hair, the higher degree of lift that is achieved. When colour deposit only is required then a lower-strength hydrogen peroxide will suffice.

BEST PRACTICE

Only work on manageable amounts of hair at any one time. Always secure the hair that you aren't working on out of the way with sectioning clips.

Refreshing the colour of the lengths and ends

When you are re-colouring the roots on longer hair you will often find that the ends of the colour need refreshing too. This doesn't mean that a full head colour is necessary: the refreshing can be done during the application

Appearance	1st step	2nd step	3rd step	4th step
When the colour looks the same at the ends as the target shade	Apply to regrowth	Allow to develop and then 15 minutes before full development time	Add 15–20cc of tepid water to the mixture in the bowl, then apply this to the lengths and ends	Leave for a further five-to-ten minutes, to complete the development process
When the tonal quality has faded but the colour is still the same depth	Apply to regrowth	Allow to develop, then 25 minutes before full development time	Add 15–20cc of tepid water to the mixture in the bowl, then apply this to the lengths and ends	Leave for a further 15–20 minutes, to complete the development process
When both the tonal quality and depth has faded on the ends	Apply to regrowth	Add 15–20cc of tepid water to the mixture in the bowl, then apply this to the lengths and ends immediately	Leave all the colour on for full development for 35–40 minutes	

Regrowth/retouch application: quick checklist

Consultation	◆ Find out what needs to be done. ◆ Are there any modifications needed to do the regrowth?
Prepare the client	◆ Make the usual protective preparations. ◆ Brush the hair through to remove the tangles. ◆ Apply a barrier cream to the hairlines (if necessary).
Prepare the materials	◆ Make sure that you have everything you need at hand. ◆ Put on your disposable gloves and apron. ◆ Mix the products correctly.
Method/technique	◆ Divide the hair into four equal quadrants. ◆ Start the application with a brush to the roots at the top of the head, working down and along each quadrant. ◆ Pick up a horizontal section of hair within a back quadrant and with the tail of the brush. ◆ Apply the colour/lightener to the regrowth evenly. ◆ Repeat down the back of the head and through the sides.
Development	◆ Monitor the colour development throughout the processing. ◆ Apply heat if needed to speed up the development process. ◆ Check with the client throughout to ensure their comfort.
Removal	◆ When processing is complete, take the client to the basin and rinse the hair with tepid/warm water, gently massage to emulsify the colour. ◆ Rinse thoroughly until the colour is removed. ◆ Shampoo and condition with an anti-oxidizing agent.

TOP TIP

If you used dry heat to accelerate the development of permanent colours, don't let the heat dry out the products as this will stop the colour from developing further.

STEP-BY-STEP: REGROWTH APPLICATION

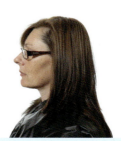

1 Before
Prepare the client by protecting them with a clean gown, towel and cape.
Put on your apron and gloves.

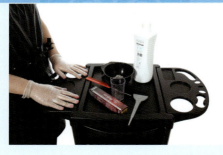

2 Prepare your trolley with the materials you need.
Mix the colour according to manufacturer's instructions.

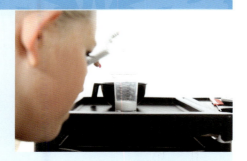

3 When measuring hydrogen peroxide you should always get down to eye level, this ensures accurate measurement.

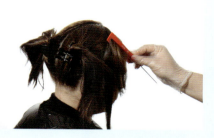

4 Prepare the client's hair by brushing through to remove any tangles.

Then divide the hair into four quadrants ('hot cross bun') and section each one out of the way.

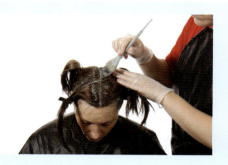

5 Start applying the colour directly to the regrowth.

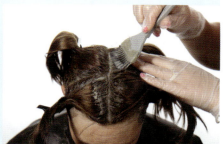

6 Continue without overlapping onto the previously coloured hair.

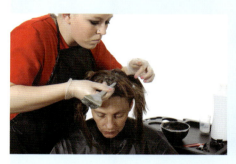

7 After applying the colour to the 'hot cross bun' area you can start to take sections within the quarters, horizontally.

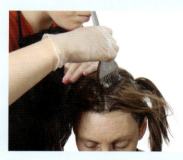

8 Work down through each section.

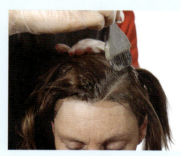

9 Move the hair that has been coloured over, and out of the way.

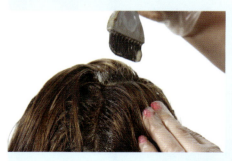

10 Work down through each section and move the hair that has been coloured over, and out of the way.

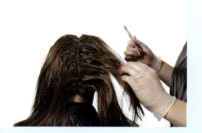

11 With all of the sections completed, just quickly check where you have applied and the hairlines to make sure that everywhere has been covered.

Then allow to develop for the recommended time.

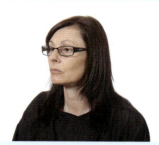

12 Final effect.

Full head: quick checklist

Consultation	◆ Find out what needs to be done. Are any modifications needed to the application, colour(s) or lightener?
Prepare the client	◆ Make the usual protective preparations. ◆ Brush the hair through to remove the tangles. ◆ Apply a barrier cream to the hairlines.
Prepare the materials	◆ Make sure that you have everything you need to hand. ◆ Put on your disposable gloves and apron. ◆ Mix the products correctly.
Method/technique	◆ Divide the hair into four equal sections. ◆ Start the application with a brush to the mid-lengths and ends at the top of the head, working down and along each quadrant. ◆ Pick up a thin 5mm horizontal section of hair within a back quadrant and with the tail of the brush. ◆ Apply the colour/lightener to the mid-length and ends evenly. ◆ Repeat down the back of the head and through the sides.
1st part of development	◆ Allow the mid-length and ends to develop sufficiently first. ◆ Monitor the colour development throughout the processing. ◆ Apply heat if needed to speed up the development process. ◆ Check with the client throughout to ensure their comfort.
2nd part of development	◆ Pick up each of the horizontal sections of hair with the tail of the brush. ◆ Apply the colour/lightener to the root area evenly. ◆ Repeat down the back of the head and through the sides. ◆ Monitor the colour development throughout the processing. ◆ Apply heat if needed to speed up the development process. ◆ Check with the client throughout to ensure their comfort.
Removal	◆ When processing is complete, take the client to the basin and rinse the hair with tepid/warm water, then apply gentle massage to emulsify the colour. ◆ Rinse thoroughly until the colour is removed. ◆ Shampoo and condition with an anti-oxidizing agent.

STEP-BY-STEP: FULL HEAD APPLICATION

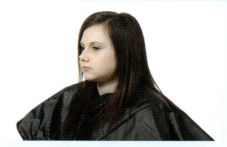

1 Before

Prepare the client by protecting them with a clean gown, towel and cape.

Put on your apron and gloves.

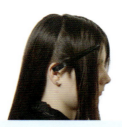

2 Prepare the client's hair by brushing through to remove any tangles.

Then divide the hair into four quadrants ('hot cross bun') and section each one out of the way.

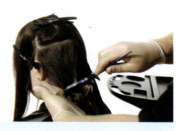

3 A full head colour on longer hair must be applied to the mid-lengths and ends first because these areas will need longer time to develop

Mix your colour according to the manufacturer's instructions, then, starting with one of the lower, back sections, apply your colour to the mid-lengths and draw down to the ends.

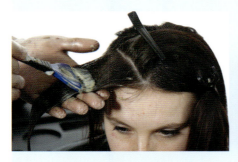

4 The sections for full head application to mid-lengths and ends are three or four times the thickness of that applied to the roots.

With all the back sections done, you can start to work on the sides in a similar way.

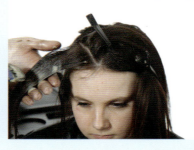

5 Again, draw the colour through the lengths, to cover all the ends.

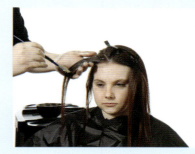

6 Continue technique.

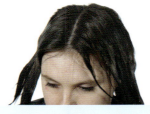

7 When the mid-lengths and ends are complete, you can leave the colour to develop for the recommended timings.

You can use an accelerator to speed up the process.

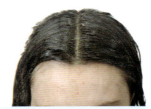

8 After the mid-lengths and ends have developed, you can apply the root application.

See regrowth colour steps for more details.

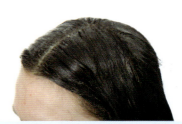

9 Develop all of the colour until processing is complete.

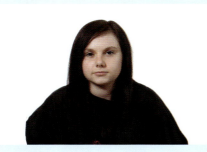

10 Final effect.

Cap highlights: quick checklist

Consultation	◆ Find out what effect your client is trying to achieve. ◆ How much lightened or coloured hair in relation to natural colour is expected – 5 per cent, 10 per cent, 25 per cent? ◆ How will you explain the effect to the client? ◆ Do you have any visual aids to help? ◆ Explain everything that you are going to do.
Prepare the client	◆ Make the usual protective preparations. ◆ Brush the hair to examine the growth patterns and to remove any tangles. Look for areas where highlights would be conspicuous or unsightly. ◆ Look for natural part/parting areas; confirm how the hair is to be worn. ◆ If the hair has slightly longer layers or tends to tangle apply some talcum powder to the hair and work through with your hands. This will help the hair to come through the holes, reducing any discomfort from tugging and picking the sections.
Prepare the materials	◆ Check the quality of the highlight cap. When a cap has previously been used for colouring it starts to wear. ◆ Look for enlarged holes or splits where colour/lightener can seep through on to the hair. ◆ Make sure that you have everything you need at hand. ◆ Put on your disposable gloves and apron. ◆ Mix the products correctly. ◆ Ask the client to take hold of the front of the cap, ensuring it is centrally positioned at the forehead. ◆ Pull the cap down smoothly, ensuring that the fit hugs the contour of the head correctly.
Pull the highlights through	◆ Start at the nape area. ◆ Pull the highlights through by taking enough hair to complete each one in a single movement. Always pull through at an acute (narrow angle) to the cap. ◆ Complete the pattern of repeated highlights, i.e. the percentage required, all over the head.

Apply the lightener or colour	◆ Carefully apply the mixture to all of the highlights evenly. ◆ Lift the pasted hair slightly with the tail of a comb for even ventilation, so that no hair is trapped and can overheat or overdevelop.
Development	◆ Carefully place a clear, polyethylene cap on and around the highlights, to stop any spillages and to aid an even development. ◆ Monitor the colour development throughout the processing. ◆ Apply heat if needed to speed up the development process. ◆ Check with the client throughout to ensure their comfort.
Removal	◆ When processing is complete, rinse thoroughly until all the product is removed (a slight shampoo may be needed). ◆ Lift the flanges of the cap into the basin area and remove in one smooth and even pull. ◆ Shampoo and condition with an anti-oxidizing agent.

STEP-BY-STEP: CAP HIGHLIGHTS

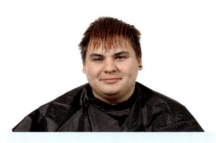

1 Before
Prepare the client by protecting them with a clean gown, towel and cape.
Put on your apron and gloves.

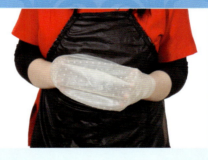

2 Wash, dry and then talc the cap – then check the highlight cap for splits, holes and tears.

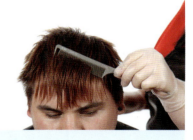

3 Brush/comb through the hair to remove any tangles before placing the cap on the client's head.

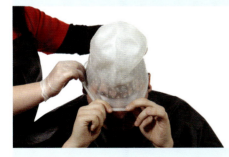

4 Check where the front of the cap is and ask the client to take hold of the cap at the centre of the forehead. Pull down at the back being careful around the ears.
Make sure that the cap fits closely down to the scalp area.

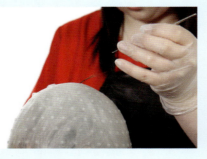

5 Start at the top and lift through a small section of hair with the crochet hook.

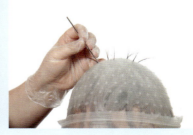

6 Carry on taking sections through in an evenly balanced pattern, all over the cap, i.e. every hole, every other hole or every third hole.

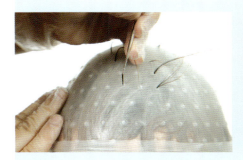

7 Be careful not to pull as this can be extremely painful for the client.

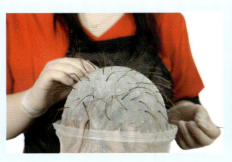

8 When you have finished, check that you have an evenly balanced highlighting pattern.

Fold back the rim so that the fold will collect any runny product or drips.

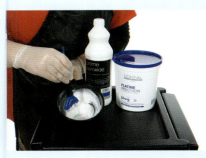

9 Never mix up your product until you are ready to use it.

Always follow the manufacturer's instructions when mixing.

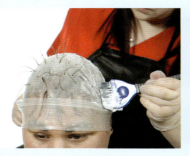

10 After mixing the required products, i.e. colour or lightener.

start to apply evenly from the brush without 'blobbing' or dripping.

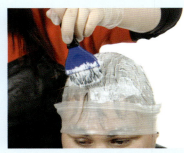

11 Continue all over the cap's surface.

Allow the colour/lightener to develop under an accelerator or steamer for the correct length of time.

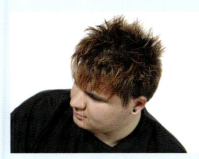

12 Final effect.

STEP-BY-STEP: SHOE SHINE COLOUR

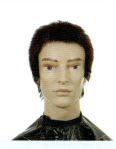

1 Prepare your work area and materials.

Wash and cut the hair so that it is lifted away from the head.

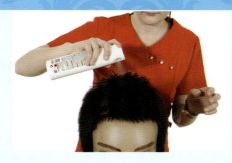

2 Apply spray to help it stand up.

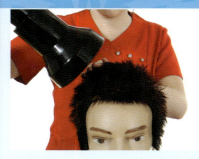

3 Make sure that the hair is totally dry and standing in 'peaks'.

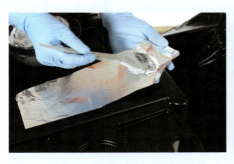

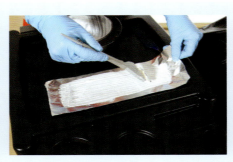

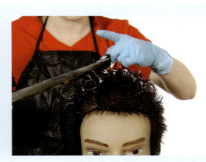

4 Depending on whether you are 'shoe shining' with colour or lightener, prepare a section of foil by applying the pre-mixed product to the central part.

Make sure that the product is 'stiff' enough to work with.

5 Make sure that the colour or lightener is applied to the foil, in a smooth, consistent way. Any excess product, could drop off the foil, and on to the client's hair if you don't!

6 Now turn the foil upside down and sweep it across the points of the hair very lightly so that only the last cm or so gets coloured.

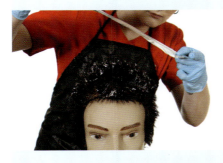

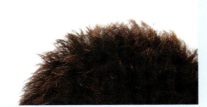

7 'Polish' the surface of the hair in the areas requiring colour.

Develop for the recommended time.

8 Finished effect.

STEP-BY-STEP: COLOUR SLICES

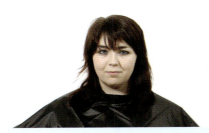

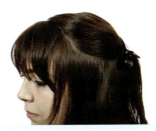

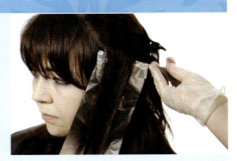

1 Colour slices are a way of introducing colour to emphasize the hairstyle in some way.

Prepare the client by protecting them with a clean gown, towel and cape.

Put on your apron and gloves and prepare your trolley with the mixed colour, your foils, bowl, brush, etc.

2 Section off the area and secure any hair not being coloured out of the way.

3 Hold the area for intended colouring to see where it appears in the mirror.

Then take a slice of hair and place it in a long enough foil.

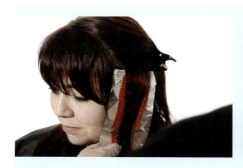

4 Apply the colour to the hair.

Note* unless the slice is to be worn on the surface hair, you don't need to go right to the root, it will never be seen.

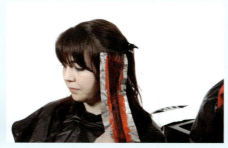

5 Don't allow the colour to seep near the edges.

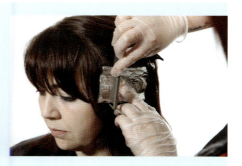

6 Fold your foil to encapsulate the hair and the colour.

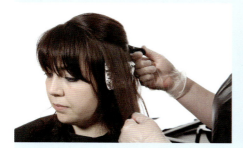

7 Repeat the slices wherever they are required.

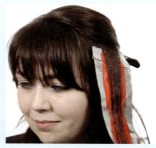

8 Apply and secure the foil.

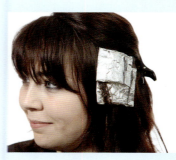

9 Continue technique.

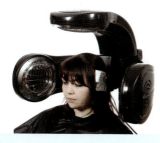

10 Allow to develop for recommended time. If you use an accelerator it will help to speed up the process.

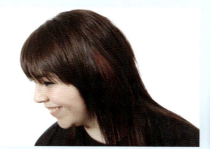

11 Final effect

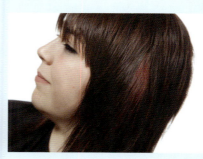

STEP-BY-STEP: HIGHLIGHT T SECTION

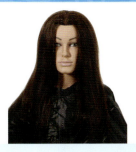

1 A T-Section of highlights follows the parting through the top and extends down the sides to colour the front hairline.

Prepare a trolley with foils, colouring bowl, brush, sectioning clips, tail comb.

Brush through the hair to remove any tangles.

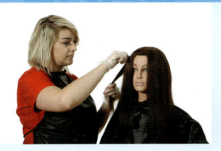

2 Check where the width of your foils will impact on the width and proportions of the head.

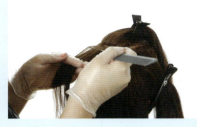

3 Section off any hair that you are not working with and create a section no wider than the foil you are putting in.

Then, holding your first section, weave off a uniform amount of hair that will become highlights.

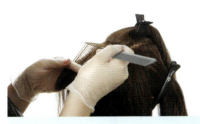

4 Lift them off the held section, and hold them with your finger and thumb.

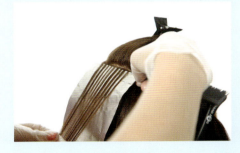

5 Neatly place a foil beneath the highlights and pull the highlights onto the foil, to trap it in place.

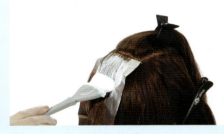

6 With your other hand, apply colour/lightener to the section, starting near the root…

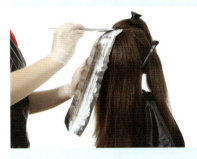

7 And extending down to colour all of the hair.

Fold the foil up in half, making sure that no product seeps out at the sides.

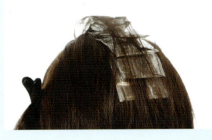

8 You can fold the sides of the foils up to make parcels that encapsulate all of the product.

Carry on working upwards, and through the top to the front hairline.

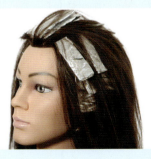

9 Start at the bottom of the sides and repeat the process as you work up to the parting area.

Woven highlights: quick checklist

Consultation	◆ Find out what effect your client is trying to achieve. ◆ How much lightened and/or coloured hair in relation to natural colour is expected? What percentage of each is needed – 5 per cent, 10 per cent, 25 per cent? ◆ How will you explain the effect to the client? ◆ Do you have any visual aids to help? ◆ Explain everything that you are going to do.
Prepare the client	◆ Make the usual protective preparations. ◆ Brush the hair to examine the growth patterns and to remove any tangles, look for areas where highlights would be conspicuous or unsightly. ◆ Look for natural part/parting areas; confirm how the hair is to be worn.
Prepare the materials	◆ Make sure that you have everything you need at hand including foils cut to the required length. ◆ Put on your disposable gloves and apron. ◆ Mix the products correctly.
Method/ technique	◆ Divide the hair into four equal sections. ◆ Start at the back of the head at the nape. ◆ Divide the remaining hair and section and secure it out of the way. ◆ Pick up a horizontal section of hair and, with your pin-tail comb, weave out of the section a mesh of fine amounts of hair. ◆ Place underneath the mesh a foil long enough to protrude beyond the hair length. ◆ Apply the colour/lightener to the mesh evenly. ◆ Fold in half and half again (fold the edges too, if required). ◆ Continue on to next section with the alternating colour(s) or lightener. ◆ Repeat up the back of the head and through the sides.
Development	◆ Monitor the colour development throughout the processing. ◆ Apply heat if needed to speed up the development process. ◆ Check with the client throughout to ensure their comfort.
Removal	◆ When processing is complete each foil must be removed individually by rinsing thoroughly until all the product is removed (this ensures that the colours do not run and bleed together). ◆ Shampoo and condition with an anti-oxidizing agent.

STEP-BY-STEP: WOVEN HIGHLIGHTS

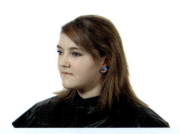

1 A full head of highlights provides tonal colour effects to all of the hair. Sometimes done with colour to form lowlights but more often done with lightener or lightener and colour to create multi-tonal effects.

Prepare a trolley with foils, colouring bowl, brush, sectioning clips, tail comb.

Brush through the hair to remove any tangles.

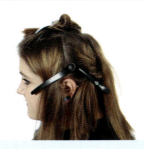

2 Section off the hair first to gauge the width of your foils and the effect over the head.

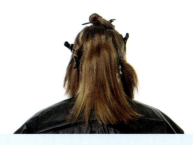

3 Section off any hair that you are not working with and create a section no wider than the foil you are putting in.

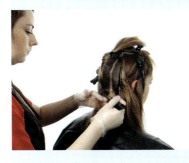

4 Then, holding your first section, weave off a uniform amount of hair that will become highlights.

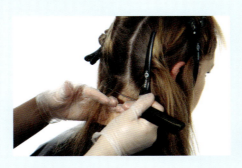

5 Continue technique.

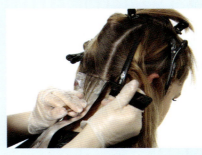

6 Lift them off the held section and hold them with your finger and thumb.

Neatly place a foil beneath the highlights and pull the highlights onto the foil, to trap it in place.

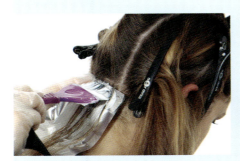

7 With your other hand, apply colour/lightener to the section, starting near the root.

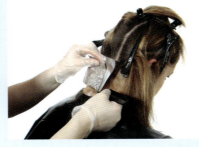

8 You can fold the foil in half and then the sides of the foils, to make parcels that stop the colour product seeping out.

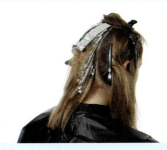

9 Carry on working upwards, repeating the process in a uniform way.

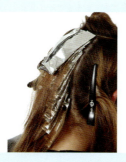

10 Carry on working upwards, repeating the process in a uniform way.

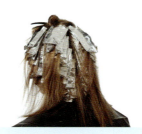

11 Full head of woven highlights

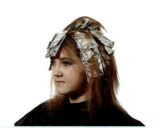

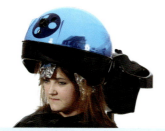

12 Use a steamer (or accelerator) for the recommended development time.

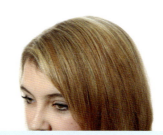

13 Final effect.

Colouring problems and corrective measures

Problem or fault	Possible reasons why	Corrective actions
Colour patchy or uneven	Insufficient coverage by colour Poor application Poor mixing of chemicals Sectioning too large Overlapping, causing colour build-up **Under-processing** (colour was not given full development)	Spot colour the patchy areas
Colour too light	Incorrect colour selection Peroxide strength too high causing lightening Peroxide strength too low Under-processed Hair in poor condition	Choose a darker shade Check strengths and re-colour Check strengths Re-colour Apply restructurants
Colour fades quickly	Effects of sun or swimming Harsh treatment: over-drying, ceramic straighteners, etc. Hair in poor condition Under-processing	Recondition before next application

Problem or fault	Possible reasons why	Corrective actions
Colour too dark	Incorrect colour selection **Over-processing** Hair in poor condition Metallic salts present	Process correctly Senior assistance required
Colour too red	Peroxide strength too high revealing undertone colour Hair not lightened enough Under-processing	Apply matt/green tones
Discolouration	Hair in poor condition Undiluted colour repeatedly combed through Incompatibles present	Use colour wheel to correct unwanted tones Senior assistance required
White hair not covered	Resistance to peroxide/colour Lack of base shade within the mixed colours	Pre-soften Re-colour with correct amount of base and tones
Hair resistant to colouring	Cuticle too tightly packed Under-processed Incorrect colour selection Poor mixing/application	Pre-soften Re-colour Senior assistance required Senior assistance required
Scalp irritation or skin reaction	Chemicals not removed from hair properly after processing Peroxide strength too high Poor quality materials, causing abrasions to the scalp Client allergic to chemicals	Wash hair again and condition with anti-oxidants Senior assistance required Refer to doctor/hospital
Breakage	Lightening/highlighting hair that has previously had lightener on it before	Use restructurant on remaining hair to strengthen the weakened hair

Providing aftercare advice

Clients need your help to look after their hair at home, you need to give them the right advice so that they can make the most of their new colour and style between visits.

You should tell them what sorts of products they could use that would make their colour last and reduce the risk of fading. Also make a point of telling them what they should avoid, as some products will reduce the effects of your colouring, causing it to fade prematurely or lose its intensity or vibrancy.

Explain the benefits of maintaining their hair in good condition, as hair in good condition is easier to manage, it looks better and is noticeable to everyone else as well.

If you would like to see more information on aftercare advice, see Units GH8 Shampoo, condition and treat the hair and scalp pages 138–163 and GH12 Cut hair using basic techniques pages 266–299.

SUMMARY

Remember to:

- ✓ prepare clients correctly for the services you are going to carry out
- ✓ check the results of any tests that have been undertaken
- ✓ put on the protective wear available for colouring and lightening
- ✓ listen to the client's requirements and discuss suitable courses of action
- ✓ adhere to the safety factors when working on clients' hair
- ✓ keep the work areas clean, hygienic and free from hazards
- ✓ promote the range of services, products and treatments within the salon
- ✓ clean and sterilize the tools and equipment before they are used
- ✓ apply the science aspects you have learnt relating to colouring and lightening
- ✓ work carefully and methodically through the chemical processes
- ✓ time the development of any chemical processes carefully
- ✓ communicate what you are doing with the client as well as your fellow staff members
- ✓ record the processes in the client's treatment history.

Knowledge Check

Project 1

For this project you will need to collect and test a range of hair samples. You will need to create three sets of sample batches of:

- ◆ grey/white hair
- ◆ coloured hair (with high lift colour)
- ◆ lightened hair
- ◆ coloured hair (base 6)
- ◆ natural virgin hair (base 6).

Each of the different types listed above will be coloured with:

- ◆ a base shade 8
- ◆ a copper shade 8
- ◆ an ash/beige shade

Mark each hair sample so that you know which one is which. Now mix up your three selected shades with 6 per cent (20 vol) hydrogen peroxide, then apply a little of each colour to each of the three collected sample batches. Allow time for the full development, then rinse each one and dry it off.

Record the changes for each sample:

- ◆ Which ones reached target shade?
- ◆ Which ones had no effect?
- ◆ Which ones have little or no coverage?
- ◆ Which ones have discoloured?

Write up the findings of your project in your portfolio. (If you have enough of each sample repeat the exercise again but now with 3 per cent (10 vol) hydrogen peroxide for a differing set of results.)

Case study

Your salon is recommended to a client who has moved to the area. She walks into the salon with lightened hair and requests a root retouch. The hair is coarse, dry and below the shoulders.

She says that her work had tended to move her around and previous attempts by other salons have resulted in inconsistent colouring.

How would you deal with this?

List the process of events that should take place in your portfolio. Include in your responses:

◆ consultation aspects, questions, examination and tests

◆ selection of suitable products and equipment

◆ the precautions you would take

◆ the advice and conclusion you would provide.

Project 2

For this project you will need to collect and test a range of hair samples.

You will need to create sample batches of:

◆ grey/white hair

◆ coloured hair (base 6)

◆ natural virgin hair (base 7)

◆ natural virgin hair (base 6)

◆ natural virgin hair (base 5).

Each of the different types listed above will be lightened to test the effects upon each prior to highlighting.

Mark each hair sample so that you know which one is which. Now mix up your lightener with 9 per cent (30 vol) hydrogen peroxide, and then apply a little lightener to each of the sample batches.

Allow time for the full development, then rinse each one and dry it off.

Record the changes for each sample:

◆ Which ones reached a suitable shade for highlights?

◆ Which ones were unsuitable for highlights?

◆ Which ones had no effect?

Write up the findings of your project in your portfolio.

Case study

Your client recently had her hair highlighted at another salon whilst on holiday. The client did not think that the result was at all satisfactory. The resultant highlight effect was uneven, and also patchy in places that were too gold.

How would you deal with this situation?

Make notes of what you would say and do. List the questions you would ask, and the order in which you would ask them. Retain notes for your portfolio.

Here are some things you should consider:

◆ Find out why the hair was not successfully treated at the other salon.

◆ Find out whether the client returned there to complain and what the outcome was.

◆ Record what you think might have caused the unsatisfactory results.

◆ Record what you think would have been a successful course of action.

◆ Find out whether the hair is in a fit state for further treatment.

ASSESSMENT OF KNOWLEDGE AND UNDERSTANDING

A selection of different types of questions to check your colouring knowledge.

Q1 A ____ test will identify a client's sensitivity to colour products.   Fill in the blank

Q2 A quasi-permanent colour lasts longer than semi-permanent colour.   True or false

Q3   Which of the following products are likely to be an incompatible?   Multi selection

Permanent colour containing PPD   ☐ 1

Retail permanent colour containing PPD   ☐ 2

Vegetable henna   ☐ 3

Compound henna   ☐ 4

Single step applications for covering grey, i.e. 'Just for men' ?   ☐ 5

Single step toners for application to lightened hair   ☐ 6

Q4   Lighteners and high lift colours are the same.   True or false

Q5   Which of the following tests do not apply to colouring services?   Multi choice

Skin test   ○ a

Incompatibility test   ○ b

Porosity test   ○ c

Development test curl   ○ d

Q6   Permanent colours alter the pigmentation of hair within the cuticle.   True or false

Q7   Which of the following colour products do not require the addition of hydrogen peroxide as a developer?   Multi selection

Powder lightener   ☐ 1

Semi-permanent colour   ☐ 2

Quasi-permanent colour   ☐ 3

Temporary colour   ☐ 4

Vegetable henna   ☐ 5

High lift colour   ☐ 6

Q8   Green tones within hair are neutralized by adding ____ tones.   Fill in the blank

Q9   Hair lightened from natural base 7 should be capable of maximum lift to: Multi choice

Red   ○ a

Pale yellow   ○ b

Yellow   ○ c

Yellow/orange   ○ d

Q10   Lightened hair that appears too yellow can be neutralized by adding mauve.   True or false

17 Perming and neutralizing hair

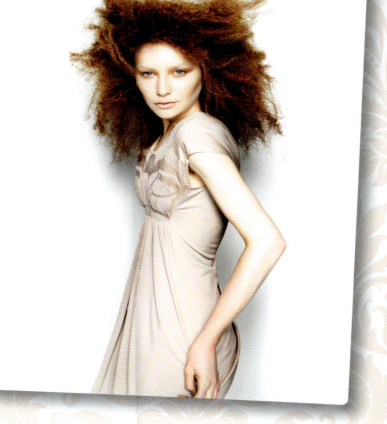

LEARNING OBJECTIVES

◆ Be able to maintain effective and safe methods of working

◆ Be able to prepare for perming and neutralizing

◆ Be able to perm and neutralize hair

◆ Understand how to work safely when perming and neutralizing hair

◆ Know about the tests for perming and neutralizing

◆ Understand the basic science for perming and neutralizing

◆ Know the products, equipment and their uses

◆ Understand perming and neutralizing techniques and problems

◆ Know how to provide aftercare advice to clients

KEY TERMS

acid wave solutions

allergic reaction

ammonium thioglycolate

COSHH

development test curl

disulphide bonds

elasticity test

incompatible chemicals

metallic salts

personal protective equipment

polypeptide chains

porosity test

pre-camping

pre-perming treatments

reduction

Unit title

GH14 Perm and neutralize hair

Information covered in this chapter

◆ The preparations that you must make before carrying out any perming and neutralizing service

◆ The tools and equipment used during perming and neutralizing, their maintenance and the preparations that you should make

◆ The factors that influence successful results in perming and neutralizing services

◆ A range of perming techniques to be used on different hair lengths

◆ The aftercare advice that you should give to clients

INTRODUCTION

Ask a hundred clients with fine hair what they really want and you will get a unanimous response: lasting volume. Only one service in hairdressing or barbering can deliver this and that is the permanent wave.

Perming is a complex technical operation that involves the careful and accurate application of potentially damaging chemicals to the client's hair. If you get it right then quite possibly, no-one will ever know that the hair has been permed (except the client that is).

Successful perming relies heavily upon having a sound knowledge and the experience in knowing how different hair textures, types and densities will react when the movement is added. Without this knowledge, the only thing that can be guaranteed is failure. But like many things in life it is easy when you know how. This chapter provides you with all the essential information you need in the future to get it right every time.

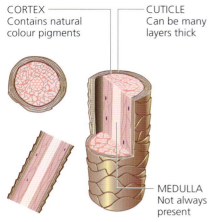

CORTEX
Contains natural
colour pigments

CUTICLE
Can be many
layers thick

MEDULLA
Not always
present

Cross-section of hair

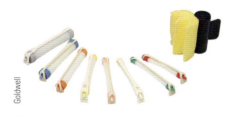

Changing the keratin

Before going ahead with this section, refer to 'the physical properties of hair' in Unit G7 (Chapter 6, page 109).

How perms work

The chemical changes that take place within the hair

'Perming' is the term given to the physical and chemical processing of hair, changing it into waves or curls. Unlike the movement and curl or smoothness produced by blow-drying or setting, the adding of movement to hair produced by perming is permanent: the hair does not return to its previous state when it is dampened. However, hair continues to grow and the new hair retains its natural shape. So, the waves and curls produced by perming gradually get further and further away from the scalp as the hair grows. To keep the same style the hair will, at some point, need to be permed again.

Because perming really does make a permanent change to the hair, you cannot easily correct mistakes (as you can with blow-styling, for example). The process also involves a variety of chemicals. It is therefore important that you make sure you understand what you are doing.

Changing the keratin

Of the cross-links between the **polypeptide chains** of hair keratin, the **disulphide bonds** or bridges give hair its shape. Each disulphide bridge is a chemical bond linking two sulphur atoms between two polypeptide chains lying alongside each other. During perming some of these links or bridges are chemically broken, making the hair softer and more pliable, allowing it to be moved into a new position of wave or curl. Only 10–30 per cent (depending on lotion strength) of the disulphide bridges are broken during the action of perming. If too many are broken, the hair will be damaged beyond repair. You need to keep a check on the progress of the perm to ensure that:

◆ perm movement is optimized

◆ the chemical action is stopped at the right time.

You do this by rinsing away the perm lotion and neutralizing the hair. During neutralizing, pairs of broken links are joined up again at different sites along the hair. The newly formed cross-links hold the permed hair firmly into its new shape.

Changing the bonds

The hair is first wound with tension on to some kind of former, such as a perm curler or *bendy waver*. This is the *moulding* stage. Then you apply perm lotion to the hair, which makes it swell. The lotion flows under the cuticle and into the cortex. Here it reacts with the keratin, breaking some of the disulphide bonds between the polypeptide chains. This *softening* stage allows the tensioned hair to take up the shape of the former: you then rinse away the perm lotion and neutralize the hair. This fixing stage permanently rearranges the disulphide bonds into the new shape.

This process can also be described in chemical terms. The softening part that breaks some of the cross-links is a process of **reduction**. The disulphide bridges are split by the addition of hydrogen from the perm lotion. (The chemical in the perm lotion that supplies the hydrogen is called a 'reducing agent'.)

The final neutralizing stage re-creates or fixes the bonds at different positions between polypeptide chains. It occurs by an oxidation reaction. New disulphide bridges form and the hydrogen that was previously introduced as hydrogen peroxide is chemically changed. The hydrogen reacts with the oxygen in the neutralizer, forming water. (The chemical in the neutralizer that supplies the oxygen is called an 'oxidizing agent' or 'oxidizer'.)

BEST PRACTICE

Always bear in mind how your perm will affect the client's hair structure.

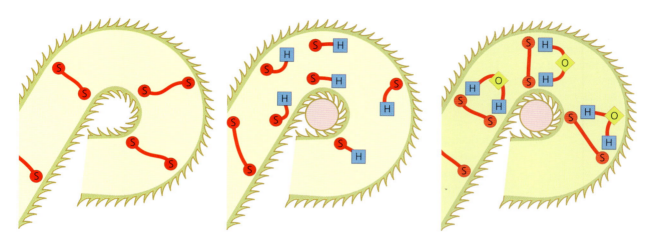

Disulphide bridges   Reduction: Breaking disulphide bridges   Oxidation: Forming new disulphide bridges

Maintaining effective and safe methods of working when perming hair

Protect the client

Gown, towel and cape – the client's PPE Perming lotions are alkaline chemical compounds that are applied by the post-damping method, i.e. after the curlers have been wound in. So potentially they could become a hazard if they were to drip or soak into the gown or client's clothes, unless adequate protection was provided. This is potentially very dangerous as it could cause irritation, swelling and even burns! If this did happen and the client's clothes were affected, it could even discolour or lighten them too, which would also put the salon at risk of an insurance claim to replace the damaged items or even worse, initiate a compensation claim against the salon for negligence!

So that this never happens, make sure that you protect your client well. Put on a chemical-proof gown and secure into place, a clean, fresh towel around their shoulders. On top of this you should fix a plastic cape, ensuring that it is comfortable around the neck.

Barrier cream After gowning, you could add additional protection by applying a barrier cream around the client's hairline.

Protect yourself

Your salon must provide all the **personal protective equipment** (PPE) that you may need in routine daily practices. Perming involves the handling and application of chemicals, so this is one of those occasions where you must protect yourself from their caustic effects. Always read the manufacturer's instructions and follow the methods of practice that they specify. You are obliged to wear and use the PPE provided for you, these being disposable nitrile or polyvinyl gloves and a water/splashproof apron.

The Control of Substances Hazardous to Health Regulations (**COSHH**) 2003 lay out the potential risks that hairdressing chemicals can have for both you and your client. Read the manufacturer's instructions in every situation before you start, and wear the correct PPE.

Working effectively

Experienced hairdressers work in an organized way that makes the most out of the time available: You need to learn the ways in which you can optimize your time and effort too, so that your work is both productive and effective. There are a number of ways that you can make this happen.

Minimize waste Get into the habit of eliminating waste. All the resources that you use cost money and the only way that you can be more effective is to maximize your time and effort whilst minimizing the cost of carrying out your work. This can be illustrated further by thinking about what goes down the sink.

Water is the first thing that comes to mind; cold water is a costly but essential part of hairdressing. All business premises have metered water so, in principle, every shampoo and conditioning rinse can be a calculated cost. But sometimes people rinse far longer than they need to or leave taps running between shampoos and that's where the additional cost is incurred. This is made even worse if the water is hot! We know that cold water is metered; now we've got the additional cost of heating it too!

BEST PRACTICE

Remove and dispose of waste items as soon as possible. Don't leave cotton neck wool, plastic caps, etc. around at the basins. Put them into a covered bin. Wash, dry and replace perm curlers back into the trays as soon as possible.

Make the most of your time; there are always things to do in a hairdressing salon and most of them relate to preparation.

- Prepare the salon by cleaning work areas so that they are ready to receive the clients.
- Prepare the materials, look out for stock shortages and report them.
- Prepare the equipment, cleaning and washing the brushes, combs and curlers.
- Prepare the client records and get things ready for when they arrive.
- Prepare the trolleys, get the right curlers ready, make sure that the rubbers haven't perished and the end papers are at hand.

For more information on dermatitis see Unit G20, page 13.

ACTIVITY

Minimizing waste

How can you minimize wastage?
Have a look around your salon and see what things you can do to reduce the waste of resources.

Create a table for the information, recording what things you can find and how they could be used in the most effective way.

HEALTH & SAFETY

Dermatitis is an occupational hazard for hairdressers; you reduce the risk by wearing vinyl gloves when using chemicals. The gloves provide you with a guaranteed barrier against the action of harsh chemicals upon the skin.

Types of perm

For the client a perm is a major step – they will have to live with the result for several months. They may not be familiar with the range of perming solutions available so you will need to explain what the differences are and what is involved in each.

◆ Cold wave perming solutions, such as L'Oréal's Dulcia or Synchrone, are alkaline perms. These types of perm are most widely available and simplest to use with applications for all hair types and tendencies and most conditions. These solutions tend to have a pH at around 9.5 so they are a fairly strong alkali that will swell the hair and affect around 20 per cent of the disulphide bridges. They reduce the natural moisture levels within the hair and are therefore better on normal to greasy hair types. They are particularly good for achieving strong, pronounced movement and curl and therefore create lasting effects that can withstand the high maintenance of regular blow-drying, setting, etc.

◆ **Acid wave solutions** – such as Zotos's Acclaim – provide alternatives for perming when the hair is particularly delicate and needs to retain higher moisture levels or requires softer, gentler movement. They have lower pH values at around 7.5–8.5 and are therefore much gentler in the way that they work. They are suited to drier, more porous hair types too. Acid perms are two-part solutions and require the components to be mixed together just before application so that the perm is self-activated. Any residual lotion left over after application will not last and must be discarded.

◆ Exothermic perming systems – such as Zotos's Warm and Gentle – tend to be similar to acid waves in their chemical composition and therefore can have similar benefits. The only difference is that these perms need heat to be activated and will self-generate this when the two chemical parts (*reagents*) are added together, without the need for accelerators or hood dryers.

Prepare for perming and neutralizing hair

BEST PRACTICE

Contra-indications for perming

The following list indicates situations when perming should not be undertaken:

◆ when the hair is particularly porous (possibly over-lightened)

◆ when the scalp has abrasions or sensitive areas

◆ when the hair is weakened, broken or damaged

◆ when the hair is inelastic (does not have any ability to stretch and return to same length)

◆ when **incompatible chemicals** have been used on the hair (e.g. compound henna, colour restorers, etc.)

◆ when the hair has varying levels of porosity throughout the lengths (poorly coloured or lightened)

◆ when there is any evidence of physical or chemical changes on the hair or scalp and the client is unable to provide you with a full, satisfactory account of what actions have been taken

◆ when there is any evidence of scalp disease or disorder.

BEST PRACTICE

Acid and exothermic perms require the mixing of parts A and B together before the perms are applied to the curlers. This starts a chemical reaction, enabling the perm to work on the hair. Make sure that you protect yourself and your client by wearing disposable gloves and an apron and applying barrier cream and moistened cotton wool around the client's hairline, so that any drips do not cause any irritation or burning of the skin. It is advisable to check that the client is comfortable during processing and, if necessary, change the cotton wool again with more moistened cotton wool.

ACTIVITY

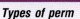

Types of perm

Many clients are uncertain about the types of perms and the effects that they will achieve. This activity will review your knowledge about the different perm types and what is involved in each.

Complete the table below.

Type of perm	Features
Cold wave	
Acid wave	
Exothermic	

Consultation

Find out your client's requirements – what they expect from perming – and determine whether this is the best solution, bearing in mind the added maintenance, care and attention needed to achieve the desired effect.

◆ Consider the style and cut, together with your client's age and lifestyle.

◆ Examine the hair and scalp closely. If there are signs of inflammation, disease or cut or grazed skin, do not carry out a perm. If there is excessive grease or a coating of chemicals or lacquer you will need to remove these by washing with a pre-perm shampoo first. Previously treated hair will need special consideration.

◆ Analyze the hair texture, condition and porosity.

◆ Carry out the necessary tests to select the correct perm lotion.

◆ Always read manufacturer's instructions carefully.

◆ Determine the types of curl needed to achieve the chosen style.

◆ If this is a regular client, refer to the records for details of previous work done on their hair.

◆ Advise your client of the time and costs involved. Summarize what has been decided to be sure there aren't any misunderstandings.

◆ Minimize combing and brushing to avoid scratching the scalp before the perm.

◆ Update the client's treatment records for future reference.

Analysis/examination It is important to make sure you choose the most suitable perm lotion, the correct processing time and the right type of curl for the chosen style. Consider the following factors.

◆ *Hair texture* – For hair of medium texture, use perm lotion of normal strength. Fine hair curls more easily and requires weaker lotion; coarser hair can often be more difficult to wave and may require a stronger lotion for resistant hair. (Although this is not true for oriental hair types.)

◆ *Hair porosity* – The porosity of the hair determines how quickly the perm lotion is absorbed. Porous hair in poor condition is likely to process more quickly than would hair with a resistant, smooth cuticle.

◆ *Previous treatment history* – 'Virgin' hair – hair that has not previously been treated with chemicals – is likely to be more resistant to perming than hair that has been treated. It will require a stronger lotion and possibly a longer processing time.

◆ *Length and density of hair* – Longer, heavier hair requires a tighter curl than shorter hair because the hair's weight will cause it to stretch. Short, fine hair may become too tightly curled if given the normal processing time.

◆ *Style* – Does the style you have chosen require firm curls or soft, loose waves? Do you simply wish to add body and bounce?

◆ *Size of rod, curler or other wave/movement former* – Larger rods produce larger curls or waves; smaller rods produce tighter curls. Longer hair generally requires larger rods. If you use very small rods in fine, easy-to-perm hair, the hair may frizz; if you use rods that are too large you may not add enough curl. To check, make a test curl before you start (see hair tests, pages 421–422).

◆ *Incompatibility* – Perm lotions and other chemicals used on the hair may react with chemicals that have already been used – for example, in home-use products. Hair that looks dull may have been treated with such chemicals. Ask your client what products are used at home, and test for incompatibility.

See the section on pre-perming treatments later in this chapter.

TOP TIP

Always record the details of the consultation/service for future reference.

TOP TIP

Some medical conditions affect the way that hair responds. For example, clients with thyroid problems may find that perms don't seem to take properly or last.

TOP TIP

Clients that have been taking health supplements such as cod liver oil over long periods of time will notice that they affect the way that the perm takes in the hair. (When cod liver oil supplements are taken, increased levels of rich oils change the properties of the hair which, ultimately, overloads the hair and results in limp curls.)

What should you find out before you start?

First of all	Things to consider
Does the client know of any reasons that would affect your choice of service?	Ask the client about their hair to find out if there are any known reasons why the service cannot continue – are there any contra-indications?
What type of perm would be best to suit their needs?	Should you be using a cold wave, acid or exothermic type of perm?
How can the desired effect be best achieved?	What type of wind should you use: conventional, brick, directional? What size curlers should you use, what curl or movement is required?

First of all	Things to consider
How long will it last?	Is perming suitable for the hair type, condition and texture?
How much will it cost?	Is perming a cost effective solution for the client?
How will it affect the hair?	Will the long-term effects be what the client expects?
Is the hair suitable for perming?	Have you tested the hair and skin beforehand to see if there are any contra-indications or hair condition issues that will affect the result?

Now consider

What are the client's expectations?	How will the perm enhance or support the style and the hair? What are the benefits for them?
What are the results of your tests?	Examine the hair: does it present any limitations for what you intend to do?
What is the hair condition like?	Are there any factors that will change the way in which perming will work on the hair? What previous information is available?
What do the client's records say?	Does this information influence the choice and perm process?
How will you show the effect to the client?	Have you got any illustrations of the finished effect?
How long will the process take?	Is there enough time to complete the effect? Has anything changed as a result of the consultation? Would this service now need to be re-booked or do you have the time to complete it still?

What contra-indications should I be looking for?

Contra-indications are	How could you find out?	How else would you know?
Skin sensitivity	By asking the client if they have ever had a reaction to hair or skin products in the past	Patch test/sensitivity test
Allergic reaction	By asking the client if they have ever had a reaction to hair or skin products in the past	Patch test/sensitivity test
Skin disorder	Ask the client if they know about any current skin disorders	Examine the scalp to see if there are any physical signs of skin abrasions, discolouration, swellings, infestation or infections
Incompatible products	If you see the results of any previous colour ask what type it was, how was it done?	Look for discolouration or unnatural colour effects on the hair, test for incompatibles
Medical reasons	Ask the client if there are any current medical reasons why perming cannot be performed	Examine the hair; look for signs of healthy active growth If there are signs of weakened, damaged, broken or missing hair; ask for more information and test for elasticity and porosity
Damaged hair	Ask the client if there are any current known reasons why the hair is in its current state/condition	Examine the hair; look for signs of healthy active growth. If there are signs of weakened, damaged, broken or missing hair, ask for more information and test for elasticity and porosity

Hair tests

◆ *Skin test* – The skin sensitivity test is used to assess the reaction of the skin to chemicals or chemical products. Some people are allergic to external contact with chemicals such as **ammonium thioglycolate** which is found in perm solutions. This can cause dermatitis or, in more severe cases, burning, permanent scarring and even hair loss.

To find out whether a client's skin reacts to chemicals in permanent colours, the following test should be carried out at least 24 hours prior to the chemical process.

Note: Skin testing is not just for new clients, it has now been found that clients can develop sensitivity to chemicals through prolonged use of the same or similar products. Therefore periodic testing for adverse reactions is essential and should be carried out routinely from time to time.

1 Clean an area of skin about 8mm square behind the ear or in the fold of the arm. Use a little spirit on cotton wool to remove the grease from the skin.

2 Apply a little of the selected perm solution to a simple dressing and apply it to the prepared area of skin.

3 Ask your client to report any discomfort or irritation that occurs over the next 24 hours. Arrange to see your client at the end of this time so that you can check for signs of reaction.

4 If there is a *positive response*, i.e. a skin reaction such as inflammation, soreness, swelling, irritation or discomfort, do not carry out the intended service. Never ignore the result of a skin test. If a skin test showed a reaction and you carried on anyway, there may be a more serious reaction which could affect the whole body.

5 If there is a *negative response*, i.e. no reaction to the chemicals, then carry out the treatment as proposed.

Warning: In recent years there have been a growing number of successful personal injury claims made against salons where the necessary precautions have not been taken.

◆ *Elasticity test* – This tests the tensile strength of the hair. Hair in good condition has the ability to stretch and return to its original length, whereas hair in poor or damaged condition will stretch and will not return to original length. This lack of elasticity will make the hair difficult to manage and maintain. A clear indication for this would be to ask the client how long their set or blow-dry lasts after it has been done. When the styling drops or can't be sustained in the hair, it is a clear indication that the hair has lost this vital attribute of elasticity. Take a single hair strand and hold firmly at either end then stretch between your fingers. If it breaks easily the cortex may be damaged and perming could be harmful.

◆ *Porosity test* – The purpose of this test is to find out how well protected the inner cortex is by the cuticle layers. Porous hair has a damaged cuticle layer and readily absorbs moisture; this presents a problem when drying, as this hair takes longer to dry and often lacks the ability to hold a style well. This can be done by taking a small section of hair and sliding from the points, back down to the roots, between your fingertips (against the natural lie of the cuticle layers). From this you can feel how rough or smooth it is. Rougher hair (as opposed to coarse hair) is likely to be more porous, and will therefore process more quickly.

◆ *Incompatibility test* – Hairdressing products are based upon organic chemistry formulations. These are incompatible with inorganic chemistry compositions and will cause damage to the client's hair. This test will identify whether **metallic salts** are present within the hair, a clear contra-indication that the perm may be carried out. Protect your hands by wearing disposable gloves. Place a small cutting of hair in a mixture of 20 parts of six per cent hydrogen peroxide and one part ammonium-based compound. Watch for signs of bubbling, heating or discolouration: these indicate that the hair already contains incompatible chemicals. The hair should not be permed, nor should it be coloured or lightened. Perming treatment might discolour or break the hair, and might burn the skin.

◆ *Pre-perm test curl* – If you are unsure about how your client's hair will react under processing you could conduct a pre-perm test curl. Sometimes this can be done on the head and in other situations where there isn't sufficient time etc. you will need to cut your sample for testing. Wind, process and neutralize one or more small sections of hair. The results will be a guide to the optimum rod size, the processing time and the strength of lotion to be used. Remember, though, that the hair will not all be of the same porosity.

◆ ***Development test curl*** – This test is always carried out after the hair has been dampened with perm solution and during the processing time. It will determine the stage of curl development so that the processing is not allowed to continue beyond the optimum. Unwind – and then rewind – rods during processing, to see how the curl is developing. If the salon is very hot or cold this will affect the progress of the perm: heat will accelerate it, cold will slow it down. When you have achieved the 'S' shape you want, stop the perm by rinsing and then neutralizing the hair.

BEST PRACTICE

Record the results

After any treatment or tests have been carried out always update the client's records immediately. These tests and the findings are critical to the client's well-being and the salon's good name. You should record the:

◆ date
◆ the test carried out
◆ development times
◆ results
◆ recommended home care or follow-up advice given.

Recording the results

Make sure that you record the details of any test that you conduct. Update the client's record card in full and immediately after you have done the test. Don't leave it until later, you might forget! These records are essential information that will be needed again and help to show that a competent service has been provided at that time.

This would be vitally important if there was a problem at some later stage, particularly if it involved any legal action taken against the salon.

Pre-perm and post-perm treatments

Matching the correct perm lotion to hair type is an essential part of the hair analysis. However, many perming solutions come in only:

◆ coloured

◆ normal or

◆ resistant formulations

And this alone will not cater for all hair conditions as the client's hair can be in at least two of these states, most of the time!

For example: How often do you see a client with coloured hair without a natural regrowth showing? Yes, only when they have just had it done!

Dry, porous hair will absorb perming solutions more readily; therefore special attention needs to be given to it. **Pre-perming treatments** are a way to combat these conditioning issues. Porous hair that is suitable for perming will have an *uneven porosity* throughout the lengths. Hair that is nearer the root will have a different porosity level to that at mid-length hair, or that of the ends. Therefore the hair's porosity levels will need to be evened out, i.e. balanced before the perm lotion is applied. This enables the hair to absorb perm lotion at the same rate, evening out the development process and ensuring that the perm doesn't over-process in certain areas. A pre-perming treatment is applied before winding on damp hair and combed through to the ends. Any excess is removed and the hair is wound as normal.

After perming and neutralizing it is also necessary to rebalance the hair's pH value back to that of 5.5. Post-perm treatments do this by removing any traces of residual oxygen from the neutralizing process.

BEST PRACTICE

Record the client's responses to your questions and the comments on how any tests affected their hair and skin.

TOP TIP

Temperature has a major impact on perming. This could be general salon temperature or by added heat from a hood dryer. In either case remember that processing times will be *reduced* considerably.

ACTIVITY

Hair tests

Complete this activity by filling in the missing information in the spaces provided

Type of test	What is the purpose of the test?	How is the test carried out?
Elasticity		
Porosity		
Incompatibility		
Development test curl		
Pre-perm test curl		

Perming and neutralizing hair

Step-by-step: Perm preparation

1 Prepare your trolley. You will need:

- ◆ rods or curlers of the chosen sizes
- ◆ end papers, for use while winding
- ◆ a tail comb and clips, for sectioning and dividing
- ◆ cotton wool strips, to protect your client
- ◆ nitrile/polyvinyl gloves, to protect your hands
- ◆ perm lotion and a suitable neutralizer (read the instructions carefully)
- ◆ a water spray, to keep the hair damp
- ◆ a plastic cap and a timer for the processing stage
- ◆ barrier cream for the hairline
- ◆ tensioning strips to bridge between curlers under the rubbers.

2 Protect your client with a gown and towels.

3 Shampoo the hair to remove grease or dirt with a pre-perming, soapless shampoo (failure to remove build-up of styling products could block the action of the perm lotion).

4 Towel-dry the hair. (Excess water dilutes the lotion, but if the hair is too dry the perm lotion won't spread evenly through the hair.)

5 If you are going to use a pre-perm lotion to help even out porosity apply it now. Make sure you have read the instructions carefully. Too much pre-perm lotion may block the action of the perm itself.

6 Check that your client's skin and clothing are adequately protected.

Winding techniques

Sectioning/sequence of winding First of all divide the hair into workable sections. This makes the hair tidier, easier to control and looks professional. Done properly, sectioning makes the rest of the process simple and quick. If it's not done well, you will have to re-section the hair during the perm, and this may spoil the overall result.

Step-by-step: Nine-section perm wind

1 Following shampooing and towel-drying, comb the hair to remove any tangles.

2 Make sure you have the tools you will need, including a curler to check the width of the section size.

3 Now divide the hair into nine sections, as follows (use clips to secure the hair as you work): divide the hair from ear to ear to give front hair and back hair

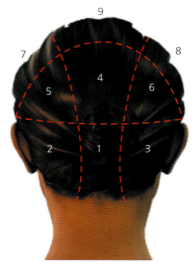

Sectioning nine-section wind

◆ divide the back hair into lower, nape hair and upper top back hair

◆ divide the front hair, approximately above the mid-eyebrow, to give a middle and two sides

◆ divide the top section along the same lines, to give a middle and two sides

◆ divide the nape section likewise, to give a middle and two sides.

Once the hair has been divided into the nine sections and firmly secured with clips you can start to wind in the perm rods. The diagram on sectioning shows these sections, the numbering refers to the order in which the sections are wound. You start winding at the occipital area down the back of the head in an organized and controlled way.

Note

The sectioning techniques for perming can be adapted and used for many other techniques. For more information on directional and brick-type winds see the section on winding techniques below.

Six-section wind The Level 2 standards always seem to insist that the learner demonstrates the nine-section wind technique. But there is another, quicker version that the salons use and that is the six-section wind.

In the diagram on the previous page, the six-section winding technique joins the zones 5 and 2, 4 and 1, and 6 and 3, to form only three rear panels at the back of the head. This means that the wind is started centrally, at the top rather than halfway down the back. This is easier to manage than the nine-section wind, although it will take a little more care in sectioning accurately.

Winding the rods into the hair Winding is the process of placing sections of hair onto a variety of rods or curlers. There are various winding techniques, designed to produce different effects, but the method is basically the same in each case. In modern perming systems you need to wind the hair finely and evenly, but without stretching the hair or leaving it in tension.

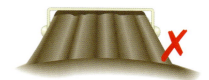

Winding: Depth section

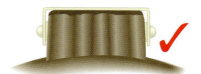

Winding: Width section

STEP-BY-STEP: WINDING

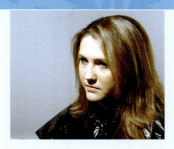

1 Before.

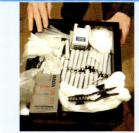

2 Make sure you have everything to hand.

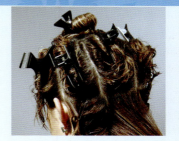

3 Divide the hair into nine secured sections or more conveniently, into six sections.

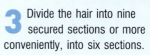

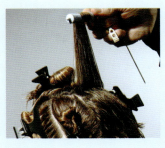

4 Start at the top, take a section no wider or deeper than the curler being put in.

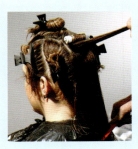

5 Wind down the curler with even tension.

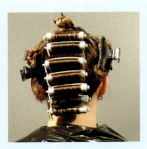

6 Position the curler so that it sits upon its own base and doesn't impede the next curler's positioning.

Continue down the back until all of the curlers have been placed, then move on to the sides.

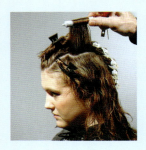

7 With the first back section wound, start the sides ensuring that the remainder hair on the top is no wider than the width of a curler.

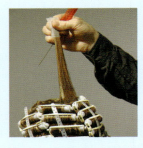

8 With the sides and back completed and bridging strips in place, finish off the top working forwards from the crown.

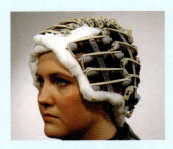

9 Apply lightly dampened cotton wool around the hairline and then apply the perm lotion to each curler.

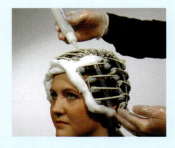

10 Apply just enough lotion to each curler so they are moisturized but not saturated. Then a plastic cap can be placed around all of the curlers for the development process.

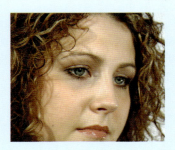

11 Finished effect.

TOP TIP

Wear gloves from the beginning if you are going to wind with lotion instead of water.

Winding techniques

Complete the chart below by explaining the effect on the hair for each of the listed winding techniques.

Draw diagrams or add pictures of the different winding techniques into the first column.

Technique	Effect that it has upon the hair
Nine-section wind	
Brick wind	
Directional wind	

Other techniques There are various winding techniques used to produce varied effects. The following are the most commonly used.

Directional winding

The hair is wound in the direction in which it is to be finally worn. This technique is suitable for enhancing well-cut shapes. The hair can be wound in any direction required, and the technique is ideal for shorter hairstyles.

Brick winding

The wound curlers are placed in a pattern resembling brickwork. By staggering the partings of the curlers, you avoid obvious gaps in the hair. This technique is suitable for short hairstyles.

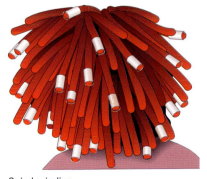

Spiral winding

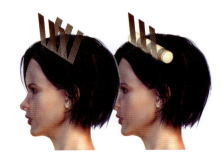

Weave winding

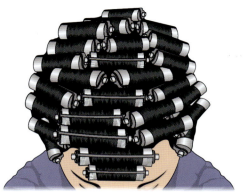

Staggered or brick winding

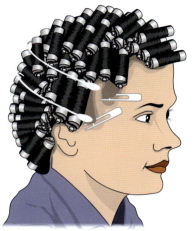

Directional Winding

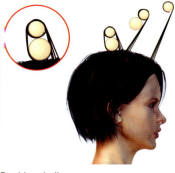

Double winding

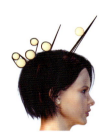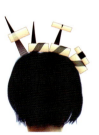

Piggyback winding

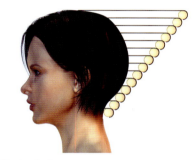

Stack winding

Perming tools and equipment

- The pin-tail comb is useful for directing small pieces of hair onto the curler. The pin-tail comb is narrower than a plastic tail comb so you can guide the wound hair around the wound section to make sure that all the hair has an even tension.

- End papers or wraps are specially made for winding perms. Very few hairdressers would consider winding without them as they ensure control of the hair when it is wound. Fold them neatly over the hair points (never bundle them). The wrap overlaps the hair points and prevents fish-hooks. For smaller or shorter sections of hair, half an end wrap is sufficient – a full one would cause unevenness. Other types of tissue may absorb the perm lotion and interfere with processing, and these are best avoided.

- Many kinds of curler are suitable for perm winding. Plastic, wood and PVC foam are amongst the commonest materials used. The manufacturer uses different colours to indicate size. The greater the diameter or the fatter the curler, the bigger the wave or curl produced. The smallest curlers are used for short nape hair or for producing tight curls. Most curlers are of smaller diameter at the centre: this enables the thinner, gathered hair points to fill the concave part evenly and neatly as the hair is wound, widening out to the shoulder of the curler as you wind closer to the head.

ACTIVITY

Try out different curlers, rods and winding shapes. Note the varied effects they produce. Practise the different curler positions for perming. Try these out on blocks or models to appreciate the differences. On a modelling block, experiment with the effects produced by different incorrect forms of winding. This will help you to recognize and avoid these effects.

Processing and development

Perm lotion may be applied before winding (**pre-damping**) or when winding is complete (post-damping). Pre-damping is used more on longer hair to ensure the solution penetrates evenly through the hair length. When pre-damping, you have to work quickly to avoid over-processing the hair. Your work should be complete within 35 minutes. Follow the manufacturer's instructions on the type of application to use. Post-damping is perhaps more convenient as the time taken in winding doesn't affect the overall processing time.

Applying the perm lotion Most modern perming systems come in individually packed perm lotions, ready for application. Others may need to be dispensed from a litre-size bottle to a bowl, before applying to the wound head using cotton wool, a sponge or a brush.

◆ Underlying hair is often more resistant to perming (e.g. at the nape of the neck), so you could apply lotion to those areas first (see the diagram on sectioning on page 424).

◆ Keep lotion away from the scalp. Apply it to the hair section, about 12mm from the roots.

◆ If post-damping, apply a small amount of the perm lotion to each rod; do not over-saturate as the lotion will flood onto the scalp and will drip on to the client. This could cause either irritation or burning on the scalp or skin.

◆ It is better to apply the lotion again once the first application has started to absorb into the hair.

◆ Don't overload the applicator, and apply the lotion gently. You will be less likely then to splash your client.

◆ If you do splash the skin, quickly rinse the lotion away with water.

Processing time Processing begins as soon as the perm lotion is in contact with the hair. The time needed for processing is critical. Processing time is affected by the hair texture and condition, the salon temperature and whether heat is applied, the size and number of curlers used and the type of winding used.

The perm needs to be checked during the development so that over-processing is avoided. The optimum processing ensures that the curl is maximized whilst there is no detrimental effect to the hair condition.

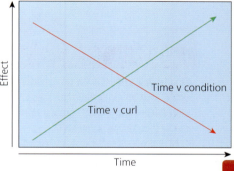

Processing time

This figure on processing time shows two intersecting lines; both have a time element, but each one has a different resultant effect. The green line has an increase in curl development over time, whereas the red line has a decrease in hair condition/damage over time. Ideally, where the two lines cross, it will denote the optimum perm processing. At this point a curl development check will show a good 'S' movement without loss of essential hair moisture and subsequent impaired condition.

Hair texture and condition

Fine hair processes more quickly than coarse hair and dry hair faster than greasy hair. Hair that has been processed previously will perm faster than virgin hair.

Temperature

A warm salon cuts down processing time; in a cold salon it will take longer. Even a draught will affect the time required. Usually the heat from the head itself is enough to activate perming systems. Wrap your client's head with a plastic cap to keep in the heat. Don't wrap the hair in towels: these will absorb the lotion and slow down the processing.

Some perm lotions require additional heat from computerized accelerators, roller balls or dryers. Don't apply heat unless the manufacturer's instructions tell you to – you might damage both the hair and the scalp. And don't apply heat unless the hair is wrapped; the heat could evaporate the lotion or speed up the processing too much.

Curlers

Processing will be quicker with a lot of small sections on small curlers than with large sections on large curlers. (The large sections will also give looser results.)

Winding

The type of winding used, and the tension applied, can also affect processing time. Hair wound firmly processes faster than hair wound slackly – in fact, if the winding is too slack it will not process at all. Hair wound too tightly may break close to the scalp. The optimum is a firm winding without tension.

Development test curl

This involves testing the curl during processing. As processing time is so critical, you need to use a timer. You also need to check the perm at intervals to see how it's progressing. If you used the pre-damping technique, check the first and last curlers that you wound. If you applied the lotion after winding check curlers from the front, sides, crown and nape:

◆ Unwind the hair from a curler. Is the 'S' shape produced correct for the size of curler used?

◆ If the curl is too loose, rewind the hair and allow more processing time. (But if the test curl is too loose because the curler was too large, extra processing time will damage the hair and won't make the curl tighter.)

◆ If the curl is correct, stop the processing by rinsing.

BEST PRACTICE

Always read the manufacturer's instructions carefully before applying the lotion.

HEALTH & SAFETY

Don't pack curlers with dry cotton wool. This absorbs the perm lotion; it also keeps it in direct contact with the skin, causing irritation.

Remember to use a barrier cream across the hairline. Don't let barrier cream get on the hair, however, as it will prevent the lotion from penetrating into the hair.

ACTIVITY

Preparing and planning for perming

Making the right preparations and taking appropriate action is an essential part of any hairdressing service. Complete the table below to review this chapter.

Task	How do you do this?	Why do you do this?
Prepare materials		
Prepare the client		
Prepare yourself		
Update records		

Neutralizing

Introduction

The successful outcome of a perm is dependent on the correct processing and the way the hair is rebalanced during the action of neutralizing.

In this section we will look at:

◆ the principles of neutralizing perms

◆ how neutralizing works

◆ choosing a neutralizer

◆ neutralizing techniques

◆ what to do after perming.

Rebalancing the hair Neutralizing is the process of fixing the curl or movement into the hair, whilst returning the hair back to a balanced chemical state. An industry term, 'neutralizing' is a little misleading. In chemistry, a 'neutral' chemical condition is neither acidic nor alkaline (pH 7.0).

Conversely, during the hairdressing treatment of 'neutralizing', the previously processed hair is returned to the skin's healthy, slightly acidic natural state of pH 4.5–5.5. Rebalancing the pH value of the hair is essential for maintaining hair in good condition, if the hair is not rebalanced the hair will be dry, porous and the perm will be very difficult to manage afterwards.

How neutralizing works As described earlier, perm lotion acts on the keratin in the hair. The strongest bonds between the polypeptides are the disulphide bridges. Perm lotion breaks some of these, allowing the keratin to take up a new shape. This is how new curls can form.

What neutralizing does is to make new disulphide bridges. If you didn't neutralize the hair it would be weak and likely to break, and the new curls would soon fall out.

Neutralizing is an oxidation process – a process that uses oxidizing agents such as hydrogen peroxide.

Choosing a neutralizer

Manufacturers of perm lotions usually produce matching neutralizers. These are designed to work together. Always use the neutralizer that matches the perm lotion you've used. As most perms are individually packed, you will find a perm lotion and neutralizer in the box.

A neutralizer may be supplied as an emulsion cream, foam or a liquid. Always follow the manufacturer's instructions. Some can be applied directly from the container; others are applied with a sponge or a brush.

Neutralizing technique

Neutralizing follows directly on from perming. Imagine that you have shampooed, dried and wound the hair. The hair is now perming, and you are timing the perm carefully and making tests to check whether it is complete. You will also be reassuring the client that they have not been forgotten! As soon as the perm is finished, you need to be ready to stop the process immediately.

Preparation

1 Gather together the materials you will need.

2 Make sure there is a wash basin free, this makes it easier for you to keep chemicals away from the client's eyes.

3   Put on your disposable gloves.

First rinsing

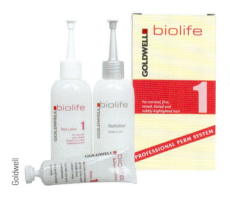

Goldwell

1 As soon as the perm is complete, move your client immediately to the back wash basin. Make sure they are comfortable.

2 Carefully remove the cap. The hair is in a soft and weak stage at this point, so don't put unnecessary tension on it. Leave the curlers in place.

3 Run the water. You need an even supply of warm water. The water must be neither hot nor cold as this will be uncomfortable for the client. Hot water will also irritate the scalp and could burn. Check the pressure and temperature against the back of your hand. Remember that your client's head may be sensitive after the perming process.

4 Rinse the hair thoroughly with the warm water. This may take about five minutes or longer if the hair is long. It is this rinsing that stops the perm process – until you rinse away the lotion, the hair will still be processing. Direct the water away from the eyes and the face. Make sure you rinse *all* the hair, including the nape curlers. If a curler slips out, gently wind the hair back onto it immediately.

Applying neutralizer

1 Make sure your client is in a comfortable sitting position.

2 Blot the hair thoroughly using a towel (you may need more than one). It may help if you pack the curlers with cotton wool.

3 When no surplus water remains, apply the neutralizer. Follow the manufacturer's instructions. These may tell you to pour the neutralizer through the hair, or apply it with a brush or sponge, or use the spiked applicator bottle. Some foam neutralizers need to be pushed briskly into the hair. Make sure that neutralizer comes into contact with all of the hair on the curlers.

4 When all the hair has been covered, time the process according to the instructions. The usual time is five to ten minutes. You may wrap the hair in a towel or leave it open to the air – follow the manufacturer's instructions.

5 Gently and carefully remove the curlers. Don't pull or stretch the hair. It may still be soft, especially towards the ends, and you don't want to disturb the curl formation.

6 Apply the neutralizer to the hair again, covering all the hair. Arrange the hair so that the neutralizer does not run over the face. Leave for the time recommended, perhaps another five to ten minutes.

BEST PRACTICE

When applying a conditioner apply to the palms of the hands first and gently work the conditioner through the hair. Do not massage the scalp or pull or comb the hair as it may soften the newly formed curl.

Second rinsing

1 Run the water, again checking temperature and pressure.

2 Rinse the hair thoroughly to remove the neutralizer.

3 You can now treat the hair with an after-perm (anti-oxidant) or conditioner. Use the one recommended by the manufacturer of the perm and neutralizer, to be sure that the chemicals are compatible.

Perm aids or conditioner and balanced conditioners (anti-oxidants) help neutralize the effect of the chemical process by helping to restore the pH balance of the hair to pH 4.4–5.5 and smooth down the hair cuticle improving the hair's look, feel, comb-ability and handling.

After neutralizing At the end of the neutralizing process, you will have returned the hair to a normal, stable state.

◆ The reduction and oxidation processes will have been completed.

◆ The hair will now be slightly weaker – fewer bonds will have formed than were broken by the perm.

◆ Record any hair or perm faults on the client's record card. Correct faults as appropriate.

◆ Under-neutralizing – not leaving neutralizer on for long enough – results in slack curls or waves.

◆ Over-oxidizing – leaving the neutralizer on too long or using oxidants that are too strong – results in weak hair and poor curl.

The hair should be ready for styling, blow-drying or setting.

After the perm

1 Check the results of perming.

◆ Has the scalp been irritated by the perm lotion?

◆ Is the hair in good condition?

◆ Is the curl even?

2   Dry the hair into style.

- Depending on the effect you want, you may now use finger-drying, hood-drying or blow-drying technique.

- Treat the hair gently as the hair may take a few washes to settle in. If you handle it too firmly the perm may relax again.

3   Advise the client on how to manage the perm at home.

- The hair should not be shampooed for a day or two.

- The manufacturer of the perm lotion may have supplied information to be passed to the client

- Discuss general hair care with your client.

4   Clean all tools thoroughly so that they are ready for the next client.

5   Complete the client's record card.

- Note details of the type of perm, the strength of the lotion, the processing time, the curler sizes and the winding technique.

- Record any problems you have had. This information will be useful if the hair is permed again.

Perming faults and what to do about them

Fault	Action now	Possible cause	In future
The perm is slow to process	Increase warmth but do not dry out; check the winding tension and the number of curlers	Winding was too loose The curlers were large, or too few were used The wrong lotion was used The sections were too large The salon is too cold Lotion was absorbed from the hair Too little lotion was used	Wind more firmly or use smaller curlers Use smaller curlers and more of them Double-check labels on bottles Take smaller sections The temperature should be comfortable Don't leave cotton wool on the hair Don't skimp on the lotion or miss sections
The scalp is tender, sore or broken	Seek advice from a qualified first-aider	The curlers were too tight The wound curlers rested on the skin Lotion was spilt on the scalp There was cotton wool padding soaked with perm lotion between the curlers The hair was pulled tightly The perm was over-processed	Don't apply too much tension when winding Curlers should rest on the hair Keep lotion away from the scalp Renew the cotton wool as necessary or don't use it Don't overstretch it Time perms accurately

Fault	Action now	Possible cause	In future
There are straight points or roots	Re-perm, if the hair condition permits*	The curlers or sections were too large	Take sections no longer or wider than the curler used
		Sections were overlooked	Check that all hair has been wound
		Too few curlers were used	Put curlers closer together
		The winding was too loose	Be a little firmer next time
		Lotion was applied unevenly	Take care to apply it evenly
There are fish-hooks	Remove by trimming the ends	The hair points were not cleanly wound	Comb the hair cleanly
		The hair points were bent or buckled	Place hair sections evenly on to the curlers
		The hair was wrapped un-evenly in the end papers	Curl from the hair points
		Winding aids were used incorrectly	Take more care; practise winding
Hair is broken	Nothing can be done about the broken hair. After discussion with your senior or trainer, condition the remaining hair	The hair was wound too tightly	Wind more loosely next time
		The curlers were secured too tightly	Secure them more loosely next time
		The curler band cut into the hair base	Keep it away from the hair base
		The hair was over-processed	Follow the instructions more carefully
		Chemicals in the hair reacted with the lotion	Test for incompatibility beforehand
The hair is straight	Re-perm, if the hair condition permits*	The wrong lotion was used for hair of this texture	Choose the lotion more carefully
		The hair was under-processed	Time perms accurately
		The curlers were too large for the hair length	Measure the curlers beforehand
		The neutralizing was incor-rectly done	Follow the instructions more carefully
		Rinsing was inadequate	Rinse more thoroughly
		Conditioners used before perming were still on the hair	Prepare the hair more carefully
		The hair was coated and resistant to the lotion	Check for substances that block the action of perm lotion, shampoo if necessary
The hair is frizzy	Cut the ends to reduce the frizziness	The lotion was too strong for hair of this texture	Assess texture correctly; select suitable lotions; read manufacturer's instructions
		The winding was too tight	Practise and experiment to avoid this
		The curlers were too small	Choose more suitable curlers
		The hair was over-processed	Time perms accurately
		The neutralizing was incor-rectly done	Follow the instructions more carefully
		There are fish-hooks	Avoid bending hair points when winding

Fault	Action now	Possible cause	In future
The perm is weak and drops**	Re-perm, if the hair condition permits*	Lotion was applied unevenly	Apply lotion more evenly
		The neutralizer was dilute	Follow the instructions more carefully
		Neutralizing was poorly done	Be more careful
		The hair was stretched while soft	Handle the hair gently
		The curlers or sections were too large	Use more curlers
Some hair sections are straight	Re-perm if the hair condition permits*	The curler angle was wrong	Wind correctly
		The curlers were placed incorrectly	Wind correctly
		The curlers were too large	Use smaller curlers
		Sectioning or winding was done carelessly	Practise before perming again
		Perm lotion or neutralizer was not applied correctly	Make sure that all curlers get the correct application of chemicals
The hair is discoloured		Metallic elements or compounds present	Test for incompatibility
Unknown/unexpected result	Seek assistance from a senior operator/follow their instructions		Learn from this experience and modify your process accordingly

*Don't re-perm the hair unless its condition is suitable. For example, you should not re-perm if the hair is over-processed. Conditioning treatments and/or cutting may help. Discuss the problem with a senior or your trainer.

**Before attempting to correct this fault make sure that the hair is not over-processed. Dampen the hair to see how much perm there is.

Provide aftercare advice

Clients need your help to look after their hair at home; you need to give them the right advice so that they can make the most of their new perm and style between visits.

Remember to tell them how a new perm needs particular care in the way that it is handled and that stretching during styling will weaken the result and could even cause the perm to fail prematurely.

You should tell them what sorts of products they could use that would benefit the condition and manageability of their hair. You should also make a point of telling them what they should avoid, as some products will work against the new perm.

Explain the benefits of maintaining their hair in good condition, as hair in good condition is easier to manage, it lasts longer, looks better and is noticeable to everyone else as well.

Finally, if you would like to see more information on aftercare advice, see Units GH8 Shampoo, condition and treat the hair and scalp (pages 138–163), and GH12 Cut hair using basic techniques (pages 266–299).

SUMMARY

Remember to:

✓ prepare clients correctly for the services you are going to carry out

✓ check the results of any tests that have been undertaken

✓ put on the protective wear available for perming and neutralizing

✓ listen to the client's requirements and discuss suitable courses of action

✓ adhere to the safety factors when working on clients' hair

✓ keep the work areas clean, hygienic and free from hazards

✓ promote the range of services, products and treatments within the salon

✓ clean and sterilize the tools and equipment before they are used

✓ apply the science aspects you have learnt relating to perming and neutralizing hair

✓ work carefully and methodically through the chemical processes

✓ time the development of any chemical processes carefully

✓ communicate what you are doing with the client as well as your fellow staff members

✓ record the processes in the client's treatment history.

Knowledge Check

Project 1

For this project you will need to collect and test a range of hair samples.

Over a period of time, collect and fix together a variety of different hair samples.

You will need to create three batches of:

◆ grey/white hair

◆ coloured hair

◆ double processed hair

◆ lightened hair

◆ previously permed hair

◆ natural virgin hair.

For each type, record the differences in tendency, texture and condition.

Use a little perm lotion in each scenario.

1 Perm your first batch of samples with the correct/matched lotion for the correct length of development time with a medium size curler.

2 After you have rinsed and neutralized each one, note any changes in tendency, texture and condition in your portfolio.

3 Repeat the process again with a second batch of samples using:

◆ lotion for coloured hair on the grey/white hair

◆ normal lotion on the coloured or lightened and double processed hair

◆ resistant lotion on the previously permed and virgin hair.

Now record your findings again after over-processing the samples and see the differences.

Note: Keep your third batch for a later project with neutralizing.

Project 2

Use the remainder of your hair samples from project 1.

Perm them and prepare them, ready for neutralizing.

Try out different ways of neutralizing. Note the different effects produced and record them for your portfolio. Carry out this project in the following ways:

1 Without rinsing the hair sample, apply the neutralizer and time as directed by the instructions. What are the effects produced when the hair is still wet and the effects when it has been dried?

2 Using another permed hair sample, rinse the hair but do not apply any neutralizer. What are the effects produced when the hair is still wet and the effects when it has been dried?

3 On the third sample, leave out both rinsing and neutralizing phases. What are the effects produced when the hair is still wet and the effects when it has been dried?

4 Rinse and neutralize the fourth sample as directed by the perm manufacturer. What are the effects produced when the hair is still wet and the effects when it has been dried?

5 Retain these samples and compare the results when the hair has dried out. Then check again after 12, 24 and 48 hours

6 List and try out different types of neutralizer, with varying times of application. Compare the results.

7 Repeat these experiments using hair of different textures. Make sure that you have a correctly permed and neutralized sample with which to compare your results.

ASSESSMENT OF KNOWLEDGE AND UNDERSTANDING

A selection of different types of questions to check your knowledge.

Q1 A development test _____ will identify when optimum movement is achieved.   Fill in the blank

Q2 Cold wave perms are usually post-dampened.   True or false

Q3 Which of the following factors are likely to be affected by perming?   Multi selection

Elasticity	☐ 1
Natural colour	☐ 2
Thickness	☐ 3
Texture	☐ 4
Porosity	☐ 5
Abundance	☐ 6

Q4 Neutralizers contain hydrogen peroxide.   True or false

Q5 Which of the following chemical bonds are permanently rearranged during perming?   Multi choice

Salt bonds	○ a
Hydrogen bonds	○ b
Disulphide bonds	○ c
Oxygen bonds	○ d

Q6 Time and temperature have a direct impact upon perm development.   True or false

Q7 Which of the following tests are *not* applicable to perming?   Multi selection

Strand test	☐ 1
Incompatibility test	☐ 2
Peroxide test	☐ 3
Porosity test	☐ 4
Elasticity test	☐ 5
Skin test	☐ 6

Q8   The rearrangement of chemical bonds takes place within the _____.   Fill in the blank

Q9   The chemical compound responsible for modifying the hair's structure   Multi choice
during the perming stage is?

Hydrogen peroxide	○ a
Ammonium hydroxide	○ b
Ammonium thioglycolate	○ c
Oxygen	○ d

Q10   Smaller perming rods produce tighter curl effects.   True or false

Appendix 1: Health and safety legislation

This section will provide you with an outline of the main health and safety regulations that affect hairdressers and their work. The Health and Safety at Work Act 1974 is the legislation that covers a variety of safe working practices and associated regulations. You do not need to know the contents of this Act, but you should at least be aware of the existence of relevant regulations made under its provisions. They cover the following aspects at work:

- management of safety at work (assessing risk in the workplace)
- safe equipment and systems of work
- protective equipment
- handling chemicals and substances
- electricity
- first-aid
- handling and moving objects
- fire precautions.

HSE information

Go online for more information at www.hse.gov.uk and www.hsedirect.gov.uk

The Management of Health and Safety at Work Regulations 1999

The main regulation requires the employer to appoint competent personnel to conduct risk assessments for the health and safety of all staff working on the premises as well as other visitors to the business premises. Staff must be adequately trained to take appropriate action, eliminate or minimize any risks. Other regulations cover the necessity to set up procedures for emergency situations, reviewing the risk assessment processes. In salons where five or more people are employed, there is the added obligation to set up a system for monitoring health surveillance, should the risk assessments identify a need.

The main requirements for management of health and safety are:

- identifying any potential hazards
- assessing the risks which could arise from these hazards identifying who is at risk
- eliminating or minimizing the risks

◆ training staff to identify and control risks

◆ regular reviewing of the assessment processes.

The Workplace (Health, Safety and Welfare) Regulations 1992

These regulations supersede the Offices, Shops and Railway Premises Act 1963 (OSRPA) and cover the following workplace key points:

◆ maintenance of the workplace and the equipment in it

◆ ventilation, temperature and lighting

◆ cleanliness

◆ sanitary and washing facilities

◆ drinking water supply

◆ rest, eating and changing facilities

◆ storage of clothing

◆ glazing

◆ traffic routes

◆ work space.

Amendments and additions in this regulation provide new requirements for employers with particular attention for glazed areas such as windows and doors, etc. Any transparent and translucent partitions must be made of safe materials and if they could cause injury to anyone, they should be appropriately marked. Other amendments have particular rules for rest rooms and rest areas. These must include suitable alternative arrangements to protect non-smokers from the effects caused by tobacco smoke and suitable rest facilities for any person at work who is either pregnant or a nursing mother.

The Health and Safety (First-Aid) Regulations 1981

The Health and Safety (First-Aid) Regulations 1981 require the employer to provide adequate and appropriate equipment, facilities and personnel to enable first-aid to be given to their employees if they are injured or become ill at work.

The minimum first-aid provision on any work site is:

◆ a suitably stocked first-aid box

◆ an appointed person to take charge of first-aid arrangements

It is also important to remember that accidents can happen at any time. *First-aid* provision needs to be available at all times people are at work.

The Personal Protective Equipment (PPE) at Work Regulations 1992

These relate to the requirement of employers to provide suitable and sufficient protective clothing and equipment for all employees to use. The PPE Regulations 1992 require managers to make an assessment of the processes and activities carried out at work and to identify where and when special items of clothing should be worn. In hairdressing environments, the potential hazards and dangers revolve around the task of providing hairdressing services – that is, in general, the application of hairdressing treatments and associated products.

Potentially hazardous substances used by hairdressers include:

◆ acidic solutions of varying strengths

◆ caustic alkaline solutions of varying strengths

◆ flammable liquids, which are often in pressurized containers, vapours and dyeing compounds.

There are also potentially hazardous items of equipment and their individual applications, such as:

◆ electrical appliances

◆ heated/heating instruments

◆ sharp cutting tools.

All these items require correct handling and safe usage procedures, and for several of them this includes the wearing of suitable items of protective equipment.

Control of Substances Hazardous to Health Regulations 2003 (COSHH)

Hairdressing employers are required by law to make an assessment of the exposure to all the substances used in their salon that could be potentially hazardous to themselves, their employees and other salon visitors, who may be affected by the work activity. The purpose of COSHH regulations is to make sure that people are working in the safest possible environment and conditions.

A substance is considered to be hazardous if it can cause harm to the body. It only presents a risk if it is:

◆ in contact with the skin or eyes

◆ absorbed through the skin or via the eyes (either directly or from contact with contaminated surfaces or clothing)

◆ inhaled (breathed in from the atmosphere)

◆ ingested via contaminated food or fingers

◆ injected

◆ introduced to the body via cuts and abrasions.

Cosmetic Products (Safety) Regulations 1989

These regulations lay down the recommended volumes and percentage strengths of different hydrogen-based products. The strength will vary depending on whether it has been produced for professional or non-professional use. It is important that the manufacturer's guidance material and current legislation is checked when using or selling products.

Health and Safety (Information for Employees) Regulations 1989

The regulation requires the employer to make available/display to all employees, notices, posters and leaflets either in the approved format or those actually published by the HSE.

The Health and Safety (Display Screen Equipment) Regulations 1992

These regulations cover the use of computers and similar equipment in the workplace. Although not generally a high risk, prolonged use can lead to eye strain, mental stress and possible muscular pain. As more hairdressing salons use information technology and computers this is becoming a major consideration for hairdressing employees.

It is the employer's duty to assess display screen equipment and reduce the risks that are discovered. They will need to plan the scheduling of work so that there are regular breaks or changes in activity and provide information training for the equipment users. Computer users will also be entitled to eyesight tests which will be paid for by the employer.

Manual Handling Operations Regulations 1992

These regulations apply in all occupations where manual lifting occurs. They require employers to carry out a risk assessment of the work processes and activities that involve lifting. The risk assessment should address detailed aspects of the following:

- any risk of injury
- the manual movement that is involved in the task
- the physical constraints the loads incur
- the work environmental constraints that are incurred

◆ the worker's individual capabilities

◆ steps and/or remedial action to take in order to minimize the risk.

Provision and Use of Work Equipment Regulations (PUWER) 1998

These regulations refer to the regular maintenance and monitoring of work equipment. Any equipment, new or second-hand, must be suitable for the purpose that it is intended. In addition to this they require that anyone using this equipment must be adequately trained.

Electricity at Work Regulations 1989

This requires employers to maintain electrical equipment in a safe condition and to have them checked by a suitably qualified person (PAT tested). A written record of testing must be kept and made available for inspection. It is the employees' responsibility to report any known faulty equipment to their employer or supervisor. The following information must be kept:

◆ the electrician's/contractor's name, address contact details

◆ an itemized list of salon electrical equipment along with serial number (for individual identification)

◆ the date of inspection

◆ the date of purchase/disposal.

The Reporting of Injuries, Diseases and Dangerous Occurrences Regulations 1995 (RIDDOR)

Under these regulations there are certain diseases and groups of infections that, if sustained at work, are notifiable by law. So if any employees suffer a personal injury at work which results in one of the following:

◆ death

◆ major injuries including; fractures, (not fingers and toes) amputation, dislocation, loss of sight and other eye injuries

◆ more than 24 hours in hospital

◆ an incapacity to work for more than seven days.

they must be reported to the appropriate authority.

Appendix 2: Infections, accidents and emergencies

Preventing infection

A warm, humid salon can offer a perfect home for disease-carrying bacteria. If they can find food in the form of dust and dirt, they may reproduce rapidly. Good ventilation, however, provides a circulating air current that will help to prevent their growth. This is why it is important to keep the salon clean, dry and well aired at all times – and this includes clothing, work areas, tools and all equipment.

Some salons use sterilizing devices as a means of providing hygienically safe work implements. 'Sterilization' means the complete eradication of living organisms. Different devices use different sterilization methods, which may be based on the use of heat, radiation or chemicals.

Chemical sterilization/disinfection

Chemical disinfectants are widely used within salons and barber shops, and you should only handle them when wearing gloves. These solutions are hazardous to health and should not come into contact with the skin. The most effective form of disinfecting is achieved by the total immersion of the contaminated implements into a bath of fluid, e.g. Barbicide™

Disinfectants reduce the probability of infection and are widely used in general day-to-day salon cleaning/maintenance. Antiseptics are used specifically for treating wounds.

Ultraviolet radiation

Ultraviolet (UV) cabinets may be utilized to store previously sterilized or disinfected tools and equipment.

Autoclaves

The autoclave provides a very efficient way of sterilizing using heat. It is particularly good for metal tools although the high temperatures are not suitable for plastics such as brushes and combs. Items placed in the autoclave take around 20 minutes to sterilize. (Check with manufacturer instructions for variations.) Autoclaves must be regularly checked by a competent person under the Pressure Systems Safety Regulations 2000.

Fire

Faulty or badly maintained electrical equipment, such as hand dryers or hood dryers, may malfunction and overheat, or even catch fire! However, annual PAT testing has reduced this risk, as this process is meant to spot early deterioration of leads, plugs and faulty appliances. Your salon will have set fire safety procedures, and these must always be followed.

Your salon premises will have been assessed for fire risk and will have a written policy, if five or more people are employed there. The fire risk assessment will take into account all other people on the premises, clients and visitors as well as others, if other firms and businesses occupy other parts of the building.

Emergency evacuation

All premises must have a designated means of escape from fire. This route must be kept clear of obstructions at all times and during working hours the fire doors must remain unlocked. The escape route must be easily identifiable, with clearly visible signs. In buildings with fire certificates, emergency lighting must be installed. These lighting systems automatically illuminate the escape route in the event of a power failure.

In the event of fire breaking out the main consideration is to get everybody out:

◆ *Raising the alarm* – Anyone discovering a fire must immediately raise the alarm by operating the nearest alarm. Staff and customers must be warned, and the premises must be evacuated.

◆ *On hearing the alarm* – All people must exit the building via the designated fire exits and proceed to the designated assembly point. Doors should be closed on exiting the building and designated staff may assist the less able.

◆ *Assembly point(s)* – Everyone must remain at the assembly point, away from danger whilst awaiting further instruction.

◆ *Call the fire brigade* – After exiting the building, call the emergency services. Dial 999, ask the operator for the fire service, and give your telephone/mobile number. Wait for the transfer to the fire service and then tell them your name and the address of the premises that are on fire. Do this even if you believe that someone else has already phoned.

Firefighting

Under the Regulatory Reform (Fire Safety) Order 2005, all premises are required to have firefighting equipment, which must be suitably maintained in good working order. However, *only* those people with adequate training can attempt to put a fire out.

Fire safety training

It is essential for staff to know the following fire procedures:

◆ fire prevention

◆ raising the alarm

◆ evacuation during a fire

◆ assembly points following evacuation.

Training must be given to new members of staff during their induction period and this training must be regularly updated for all staff, and fire drills must be held at regular intervals.

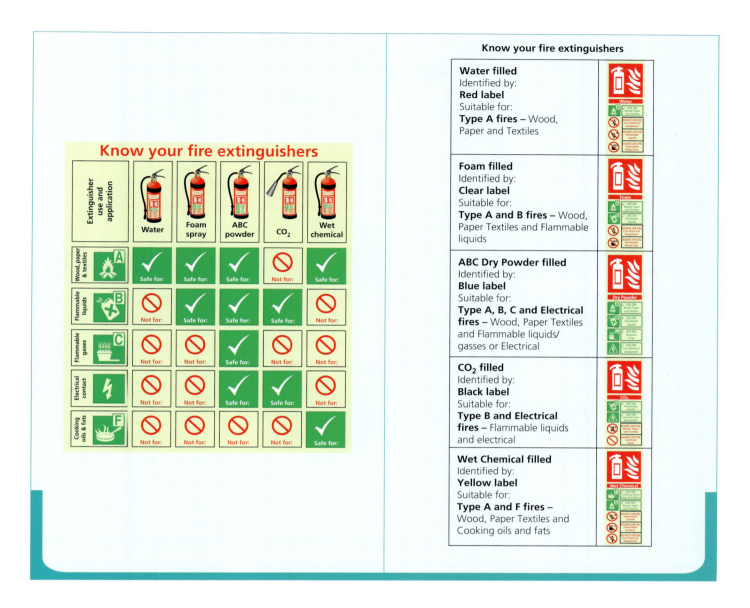

Fire blankets   Fire blankets are made of a fire resistant material. They are useful for smothering a small fire such as wrapping around a person whose clothing is burning. They will put out flames by starving the fire of oxygen, so they should not be flapped about as this will fan the flames, they should be in close contact with the fire in order to work.

Sand   A small bucket of sand is useful for soaking up liquids which could be a source for a fire such as cooking oil or fats.

Accidents (first aid)

The Health and Safety (First Aid) Regulations 1981 require the employer to provide equipment and facilities which are adequate and appropriate for providing first aid. In the event of an accident the 'Appointed Person' should be notified. This person takes control in these situations and will, if necessary, call an ambulance. There is also an appointed first aider who is qualified to administer first aid within the salon.

What is an Appointed Person?   An Appointed Person is someone who:

◆ takes charge if someone is injured or falls ill including calling an ambulance if required

◆ looks after the first aid equipment, e.g. restocking the first-aid box.

They should not attempt to provide first aid unless they have received appropriate training

Every salon must have a first-aid kit in accordance with the regulations and, in the event that materials have been used, they must be replaced as soon as possible. All accidents and emergency aid given within the salon must be documented in the accident book.

Minimum contents of a typical first-aid box

1	first-aid guidance notes (HSE leaflet *Basic Advice on First Aid at Work*)
20	individually wrapped sterile adhesive dressings
2	sterile eye pads
4	individually wrapped sterile triangular bandages
6	safety pins
6	medium size (12cm × 12cm approx) sterile unmedicated dressings
2	large size (18cm × 18cm approx) sterile unmedicated dressings
1	pair of disposable gloves

What is a first aider?   A first aider is someone who has undergone a training course in administering first aid at work and holds a current first aid at work certificate. A first aider can undertake the duties of an appointed person. (Lists of approved first-aid training organizations in your area are available from HSE.)

Recording accidents and illness   All accidents must be recorded in the accident book. The recording system should always be kept readily available for use and inspection. When you are recording accidents, you will need to document the following details:

◆ date, time and place of incident or treatment

◆ name and job of the injured or ill person

◆ details of the injury or of the ill person and what treatment given

◆ what happened to the person immediately afterwards (e.g. went home, or went to hospital) were they taken in an ambulance

◆ name and signature of the person providing the treatment and record entry.

Under the Reporting of Injuries, Diseases and Dangerous Occurrences Regulations 1995 major occurrences of injury or disease need to be reported more information is available online at http://www.hse.gov.uk/riddor/index.htm.

General guidance on first aid   The following basic information is available in leaflet form from HSE, ISBN 0 7176 1070 5 in priced packs of 20.

HEALTH & SAFETY

You should not attempt to give anything more than basic first aid!

What to do in an emergency

Priorities

Your priorities are to:

- assess the situation – do not put yourself in danger
- make the area safe
- assess all casualties and attend first to any unconscious casualties
- send for help – do not delay.

Check for a response

Gently shake the casualty's shoulders and ask loudly, 'Are you all right?' If there is no response, your priorities are to:

- shout for help
- open the airway
- check for normal breathing
- take appropriate action.

Unconsciousness

In most workplaces expert help should be available fairly quickly, but if you have an unconscious casualty it is vital that their airway is kept clear. If you cannot keep the airway open as described here, you may need to move the casualty into the recovery position. *The priority is an open airway.*

A = Airway

To open the airway:

- place your hand on the casualty's forehead and gently tilt the head back
- lift the chin with two fingertips.

B = Breathing

Look, listen and feel for normal breathing for no more than ten seconds:

- look for chest movement
- listen at the casualty's mouth for breath sounds
- feel for air on your cheek.

If the casualty *is* breathing normally:

◆ place in the recovery position

◆ get help

◆ check for continued breathing.

If the casualty is *not* breathing normally:

◆ get help

◆ start chest compressions (see CPR).

C = CPR

To start chest compressions:

◆ lean over the casualty and with your arms straight, press down on the centre of the breastbone 4–5cm, then release the pressure

◆ repeat at a rate of about 80 times a minute

◆ after 30 compressions open the airway again

◆ pinch the casualty's nose closed and allow the mouth to open

◆ take a normal breath and place your mouth around the casualty's mouth, making a good seal

◆ blow steadily into the mouth while watching for the chest rising

◆ remove your mouth from the casualty and watch for the chest falling

◆ give a second breath and then start 30 compressions again without delay

◆ continue with chest compressions and rescue breaths in a ratio of 30:2 until qualified help takes over or the casualty starts breathing normally.

Wounds and bleeding

Open wounds should be covered – *after you have put on sterile gloves*. Apply a dressing from the first-aid box over the wound and press firmly on top of it with your hands or fingers. The pad should be tied firmly in place. If bleeding continues another dressing should be applied on top. *Do not remove the original dressing*. Seek appropriate help.

Severe bleeding

If there is severe bleeding:

◆ apply direct pressure to the wound;

◆ raise and support the injured part (unless broken);

◆ apply a dressing and bandage firmly in place.

Minor injuries
Minor injuries, of the sort which the injured person would treat themselves at home, can be treated from the contents of the first-aid box. The casualty should wash their hands and apply a dressing to protect the wound and prevent infection. In the workplace special metallic and/or coloured or waterproof dressings may be supplied according to the circumstances. Wounds should be kept dry and clean.

Broken bones and spinal injuries   If a broken bone or spinal injury is suspected, obtain expert help. Do not move casualties unless they are in immediate danger.

Burns   Burns can be serious – if in doubt seek medical help. Cool the part of the body affected with cold water until the pain is relieved. Thorough cooling may take ten minutes or more but this must not delay taking the casualty to hospital.

Certain chemicals may seriously irritate or damage the skin. Avoid contaminating yourself with the chemical. Treat in the same way as for other burns but flood the affected area with water for 20 minutes. Continue treatment even on the way to hospital, if necessary. Remove any contaminated clothing which is not stuck to the skin.

Eye injuries   All eye injuries are potentially serious. If there is something in the eye, wash out the eye with clean water or sterile fluid from a sealed container, to remove loose material. Do not attempt to remove anything that is embedded in the eye.

If chemicals are involved, flush the eye with water or sterile fluid for at least ten minutes, while gently holding the eyelids open. Ask the casualty to hold a pad over the injured eye and send them to hospital.

Suggested numbers of first aid personnel   Here is a guide to the numbers of first aiders you should have, however the onus is on the employer to undertake a risk assessment to determine the requirements.

Category of risk	Number employed at one location	Suggested number of first aid personnel
Low risk:	Fewer than 50	At least one Appointed Person
shops, offices	50–100	At least one first aider
	100+	One additional first aider for every 100 people employed

Special hazards

Electrical and gassing accidents can occur in the workplace. You must assess the danger to yourself and not attempt assistance until you are sure it is safe to do so. If the casualty has stopped breathing and you are competent to give artificial ventilation and cardiac resuscitation, do so. Otherwise send for help without delay.

Useful addresses and websites

Business

Arbitration, Conciliation and Advisory Service (ACAS)

Acas National (Head Office)
Euston Tower
286 Euston Road
London
NW1 3JJ
Tel: 08457 38 37 36
www.acas.org.uk
Call the Helpline on 08457 47 47 47
Monday–Friday, 8am–8pm and Saturday, 9am–1pm

Hairdressing Employers Association (HEA)

10 Coldbath Square
London
EC1R 5HL
Tel: 020 7833 0633

Training & Education

Hairdressing and Beauty Industry Authority (HABIA)

Oxford House
Sixth Avenue
Sky Business Park
Robin Hood Airport
Doncaster
DN9 3GG
Tel: 0845 2 306080
Fax: 01302 774949
www.habia.org

Association of Colleges (AOC)

2-5 Stedham Place
London
WC1A 1HU
Tel: 020 7034 9900
Fax: 020 7034 9950

City and Guilds (C&G)

1 Giltspur Street
London
EC1A 9DD
Tel: 020 7294 2800
www.city-and-guilds.co.uk

Department for Education and Skills

http://www.education.gov.uk/

Lifelong Learning

www.direct.gov.uk/NationalCareersService

The Institute of Trichologists

107 Trinity Road
Upper Tooting
London
SW17 7SQ
Tel: 0845 604 4657
www.trichologists.org.uk

Vocational Training Charitable Trust (VTCT)

Third Floor
Eastleigh House
Upper Market Street
Eastleigh
Hampshire
SO50 9RD
Tel: +44 (0) 2380 684 500
Fax: 02380 651493
www.vtct.org.uk

World Federation of Hairdressing and Beauty Schools

PO Box 367
Coulsdon
Surrey
CR5 2TP
Tel: 01737 551355

Further Education and 6th Form Colleges in the UK

FIND FE

(A website listing all FE colleges in England, Wales, Scotland and N. Ireland)

http://findfe.com/

Publications/Fashion forecasting

Hairdressers Journal International (HJ)

Quadrant House
The Quadrant
Sutton Surrey
SM2 5AS
Tel: 020 8652 3500
www.hji.co.uk

Creative Head

21 The Timberyard
Drysdale Street
London
N1 6ND
Tel: 020 7324 7540
Fax: 020 7739 7789
www.creativeheadmag.com

Runway Magazine

http://www.runwaybeauty.com/

Black Beauty and Hair

Culvert House
Culvert Road
London
SW11
Tel: 020 7720 2108
www.blackbeautyandhair.com

Trade associations

British Association of Beauty Therapy and Cosmetology Limited (BABTAC)

Ambrose House
Meteor Court
Barnett Way
Barnwood
Gloucester
GL4 3GG
www.babtac.com

Commission for Racial Equality

Elliot House
10–12 Allington Street
London
SW1E 5EH
Tel: 020 7828 7022
www.civicus.org

Cosmetic, Toiletry and Perfumery Association (CTPA)

Josaron House
5–7 John Princes Street
London
W1G 0JN
Tel: 020 7491 8891
www.ctpa.org.uk
www.thefactsabout.co.uk

Fellowship for British Hairdressing

Bloxham Mill
Barford Road
Bloxham
Banbury
Oxon
Tel: 01295 724579
www.fellowshiphair.com/

Freelance Hair and Beauty Federation

FHBF Head Office
The Business Centre
Kimpton Road
Luton
Beds
LU2 0LB
www.fhbf.org.uk

The Hairdressing and Beauty Suppliers Association

Greenleaf House
128 Darkes Lane
Potters Bar
Hertfordshire
EN6 1AE
Tel: 01707 649499
Fax: 01707
www.hbsa.uk.com

The Hairdressing Council (HC)

30 Sydenham Road
Croydon
CR0 2EFT: 020 8771 6205
www.haircouncil.org.uk

Health and Beauty Employers Federation (part of the Federation of Holistic Therapists)

18 Shakespeare Business Centre
Hathaway Close
Eastleigh Hampshire
SO50 4SR
www.fht.org.uk

Incorporated Guild of Hairdressers, Wigmakers and Perfumers

Langdale Road
Barnsley
South Yorkshire
S71 1AQ
Tel: 01226 786 555
Fax: 01226 731 814

National Hairdressers' Federation (NHF)

One Abbey Court
Fraser Road
Priory Business Park
Bedford
MK44 3WH
www.the-nhf.org
Tel: 01234 831965 or 0845 345 6500

Legal and regulatory

Health and Safety Executive

Publications
PO Box 1999
Sudbury
Suffolk
CO10 6FS
(HSE) Infoline
Tel: 0845 345 0055
www.hse.gov.uk

Equal Opportunities Commission

Tel: 0845 604 6610

Union of Shop, Distributive and Allied Workers (USDAW)

188 Wilmslow Road
Fallowfield
Manchester
M14 6LJ
Tel: 0161 224 2804/249 2400

Glossary

Abrasion Broken, damaged skin (grazed)

Absorption The act of taking up or taking in water, e.g. a sponge absorbs water

Accelerator A machine that produces radiant heat (infrared radiation) which can speed up chemical hair processes such as colouring or conditioning

Accessories (hair) See ornamentation

Accident book A record of accidents within the workplace required by health and safety law. Incidents in the accident book should be reviewed to see where improvements to safe working practices could be made

Acid conditioner A conditioner which has an acidic pH and helps to restore the hair's natural pH

Acid mantle The layer of acidity maintained on the skin's surface which gives the skin slightly antiseptic properties

Acid wave solutions Milder type of perm solution

Acid wave These lotions provide alternatives for perming when the hair is particularly delicate and needs to retain higher moisture levels or requires softer, gentler movement. They have lower pH values at around 6–7 and are therefore much gentler in the way that they work

Acid A substance that gives hydrogen ions in water and produces a solution with a pH below 7

Acne A condition causing spots to appear normally seen around the face, cheeks and mouth due to the overproduction of sebum from the sebaceous glands

Activator A chemical used in bleaches or some perm lotions to start or boost its action

Acute Sharp, severe or having pronounced symptoms

Added hair A general term that covers the addition of hair pieces, wefts and extensions

African type hair Any hair type, which is tightly or loosely coiled, resembling black African hair

Aftercare advice Recommendations given to the client following a service to maintain the finished result and enable the benefits to be continued at home

Albinism A condition of the hair and skin where there is an absence of pigment

Alkaline A substance or compound having the qualities of an alkali

Allergic reaction A bodily reaction disclosing intolerance to a substance/chemical

Allergy A sensitivity and possible intolerance to certain products, chemicals or compounds

Aloe vera (shampoo ingredient) A popular, mild natural base ideal for healthy hair and scalps that can be used on a frequent basis

Alopecia areata Small circular patches of baldness, which eventually grow back, or move to other areas

Alopecia totalis A term referring to the total lack of hair on the body

Alopecia A general term covering a wide range of thinning or bald hair

Alpha keratin Hair in its natural state, prior to styling, i.e. the state the hair is in before stretching and setting it into a new shape

Ammonia A strong smelling gas that is very soluble in water. An alkaline component of many high lift colours and ammonium based compounds found in bleach lighteners

Ammonium thioglycolate An active, alkaline substance in perm lotions that reacts with the disulphide bonds

Anagen The stage of hair growth during which the hair is actively growing

Anatomy The science of the structure of organic bodies

Anchor A beard shape that resembles an anchor from the centre of the bottom lip and around and up the chin

Anti-dandruff treatment A shampoo or conditioning treatment that is used to combat dandruff

Anti-oxidant (conditioner) A conditioner that stops the oxidation process of chemical services

anti-oxidizing treatment A treatment for removing excess oxygen from the hair after a chemical process

Antiseptics Substances that reduce the growth of micro-organisms that cause disease

Apocrine gland A type of sweat gland attached to the hair follicles in the armpits, pubic regions and nipples

Appointment system A system of organizing the volume of work (client services or treatments) undertaken by a salon. This may be completed manually or by a computerized system

Appointment An arrangement made for a client to receive a service on a particular date and at a particular time

Appraisal A process of reviewing work performance over a period of time and planning future work objectives

Arrector pili (muscle) The muscles that are attached to the walls of the follicle and, when contracted, raise the hair upright forming 'goose bumps'

Artificial colour Any form of colour that is not a naturally occurring pigment. This is also called synthetic colour

Ash/ashen tones Hair colour shades that contain blue, violet tones producing 'cooler' effects

assessments An evaluation or judgement of input, value and/or attainment

Astringent A substance which causes contraction and is applied after shaving to close the pores

Asymmetrical Unevenly balanced, without an equal distribution of hair on either side

attachments A term referring to different sizes of clipper attachments / grades

Autoclave A device for sterilizing items in high temperature steam

Avant garde A genre of fashion that is considered progressive or exaggerated

Awarding organization An approved examining body such as City and Guilds, VTCT, Edexcel, OCR, who define the examinations and assessment processes and conduct the certification administration.

Backcombing/backbrushing Pushing hair back to bind or lift the hair using a comb or brush

Backwashes Wash basins where the client reclines backwards so that the neck rests in the basin

Bacteria A tiny organism that can only be seen under a microscope

Balance When equal or appropriate proportions create symmetry

Baldness The loss of hair

Barber's itch An infection of the hair follicles in the beard area of the face. Shaving makes it worse. Common Name **Folliculitis**

barbering comb A comb that has a tapered body (narrower at one end from the other)

Barbicide™ A commonly used disinfectant for hygienically preparing tools

Barrel curls A long hair dressing where wefts of hair are moulded into cylindrical shapes with an open centre. These are gripped into position and produce a chic, classic effect, popular for bridal work

Barrier cream A cream that protects the skin against harmful moisture or infection

Baseline A cut section of hair which is used as a cutting guide for following sections of hair. The baselines will determine the perimeter of the hairstyle, or part of the style, and may take different shapes according to the effects required

BD Appointment abbreviation for blow-dry

Beard and moustache shaping For a beard: shaping the facial hair shape around the mandible (jaw-line). For a moustache: shaping any facial hair worn above the upper lip

Benefits Aspects that influence potential purchasers about the ways in which the functions of products or services may provide advantages for them

Beta keratin The state the hair is in after it has been stretched and set into a new shape. See also alpha keratin

Bleach A hairdressing product that dissolves/removes natural colour pigments from hair. It is available in powder, cream and oil forms

blend area The area within a layered haircut that joins two differing lengths

Blending A technique for mixing different colours of hair extension fibres to create more naturally occurring effects, multi-toned effects and highlighted effects

Blunt cutting Cutting sections of hair straight across (parallel) while holding the hair between the index and middle finger

Body language Non-verbal communication provided by gestures, expressions and mannerisms that reveals the way a person is thinking or feeling

Body odour (BO) The result of poor personal hygiene and lack of regular washing

Booster An activator or colour development accelerator

Braid Another name for a plait or plaiting

braiding band A professional type of band for securing hair without causing damage

Brick wind A technique of winding rods into the hair so that there aren't any uniform divisions or 'roller marks' after the perm is finished. When the hair has been wound in this formation it looks like a brick wall

brush out The process of dressing hair out after drying a set

Camomile (shampoo ingredient) The best ingredient for use on oily scalps as it has a natural lightening effect

Cane rows An effect created by multiple rows of scalp plaits that follow the contour of the head. Also known as cornrows

Canites Grey/white hair

Capillary A small 'hair-like' filament or tube, e.g. blood capillaries. These are the narrowest parts of the blood circulatory system that provide nourishment to the dermal papilla

Catagen The stage of hair growth during which the hair stops growing, but the hair papilla is still active

Caustic A very irritant substance, capable of burning or destroying tissue

CBD Appointment abbreviation for cut and blow-dry

Charge cards A form of payment where the complete amount of credit spent must be repaid by the cardholder each month to the card company

Chemical reaction A process of two or more chemicals combining to create a different substance

Chemically treated hair Hair that has been permed, coloured, bleached or relaxed

Cheques An alternative form of payment to that of using cash

Chignon A long 'hair-up' style forming a 'classic' knotted effect

Chipping A cutting technique where the points of the scissors are used to 'chip' in to sections of hair, removing small chunks to create texture

Cicatricial alopecia Baldness due to scarring of the skin arising from chemical or physical injury. The hair follicle is damaged and permanent baldness results

Clarifying shampoo Strong, deep acting shampoo often used prior to chemical services to remove the build-up of styling products and dirt

Cleanser Removes dead skin cells, sebum and debris from the skin

clip-on extension Pre-coloured wefts of hair that have clips or combs attached to them so that they can be affixed to the hair

Client Care A way of providing a service to customers that promotes goodwill, comfort, satisfaction and interest. Maintaining goodwill ultimately results in regular repeated business

Client consultation A service usually provided before the client has anything done to their hair to find out what the client wants, identify any styling limitations, provide advice and maintenance information and formulate a plan of action

Clip-on hair extensions Pre-coloured wefts of hair that have clips or combs attached to them so that they can be affixed to the hair

Clipper over comb A technique of cutting hair with electric clippers, using the back of the comb as a guide. This technique is often used on very short hair and hairline profiles

clipper-grade attachments See attachments

Clippers Hair clippers are a mechanical cutting device operated by mains electricity or battery power. The cutting parts are created by two parallel blades with serrated teeth. The hand holds the direction of the clippers and subsequently, the cut. Hair is trapped within the teeth and the upper, moving blade oscillates back and forth to cut away all the hair that is exposed

clockspring curl A pincurl with a closed centre

Closed questions Simple questions that only require a 'yes' or 'no' response

Club cutting The most basic and most popular way of cutting sections of hair straight across (parallel) while holding the hair between the index and middle finger

Coarse hair A texture of hair where the individual thickness of the hair is greater than that of fine or medium types. Coarser hair has more layers of cuticle than those on finer types

Coconut (shampoo ingredient) Coconut contains an emollient which helps dry hair to regain its smoothness and elasticity

Cohesive setting The wetting, moulding and drying of hair into a stretched position. See also alpha keratin

Col (Rt or Fh) Appointment abbreviation for colouring, either root application or full head

Cold wave lotions These are alkaline perms and are the most widely available and simplest to use with applications for all hair types and tendencies and most conditions. These solutions tend to have a pH at around 9.0 so they are a fairly strong alkali that will swell the hair and affect around 20 per cent of the disulphide bridges

colour accelerator An item of equipment for speeding-up the development of a colour

Colour correction An overarching term that encompasses a variety of colouring problems and processes, such as removing artificial colour, removing or correcting banded colour and re-colouring hair that has been lightened back to a depth and tone similar to the hair's natural pigmentation

Colour stripper A colouring product that is specially formulated to reduce the size of synthetic or artificial pigments within a client's hair and therefore removing depth and tone from previously coloured hair

Colour test A diagnostic test to find out if a colour is suitable and/or achievable. It can be done by taking a test cutting or by applying colour on a small section of hair on the head

Colour wheel (used during colour consultation) A diagram made up of colours that provides an at-a-glance, visual aid for showing complementary colours and opposite, neutralizing tones

Colouring products Any products associated with the selection, preparation, application, and modification of hair colour, by artificial means

Communication Good communication is essential for establishing good customer service. We demonstrate this by listening to the client's requests, hearing and acting on what they are saying and always responding to clients in a polite but positive way

Compatible Able to mix without an unwanted reaction

Compound henna   A mixture of vegetable henna and mineral elements that produce an incompatible hair dye. A contra-indication to all oxidation processes

Concave   When referring to this in cutting terms, a concave shape has a perimeter that creates a curved shape which is higher at the centre rather than lower (i.e. convex)

Conditioner   A product that can be used to treat the hair or scalp, such as surface conditioners, penetrating conditioners, scalp treatments and leave-in conditioners

confidential information   Private or personal information, not intended for general discussion. May include personal aspects of conversations with clients or colleagues, contents of client records, client and staff personal details

Confidentiality   Client confidentiality is a discrete and professional way of handling client information without disclosing private matters to other staff or personnel

Consumer Protection Act (1987)   Legislation protecting customers from unlawful sales practices and mishandling of personal information. The Act safeguards the consumer from products that do not reach reasonable levels of safety

Contact dermatitis   A skin disorder caused by intolerance of the skin to the direct contact with a particular substance or a group of substances. On exposure to the substance the skin quickly becomes irritated and an allergic reaction occurs

Contagious   Communicable or transmissible (infectious)

Contaminate   To infect with germs

Continuing Professional Development (CPD)   A title given to a process of updating knowledge and experience on a continuous basis within a particular vocational sector

Contra-indication   A limiting factor that affects the original/proposed plan of action, possibly allowing a treatment or service to continue, if and only when, specific conditions are met. In some cases a contra-indication will stop a proposed service altogether

Contrasts   A marked difference, e.g. between colours, say black and white

controllers   A booster or activator for a colour or bleach\

Convex   When referring to this in cutting terms, a convex shape has a perimeter that creates a curved shape which is lower (dips) at the centre. See also concave

Cornrows/cornrowing   A styling effect created by plaiting hair into small three stem plaits close to the scalp. Several cornrows produce linear or curved designs across the head

Corrosive   A substance that destroys organic tissue by chemical means

Cortex   The inner part of the hair where hairdressing chemical processes change or modify the natural hair, i.e. where permanent colour is deposited and where perms make physical changes to the hair

COSHH   An abbreviation for Control of Substances Hazardous to Health. COSHH safety regulations affect the way in which chemicals are handled at work. These health and safety regulations are created for your safety and must be adhered to

Cross-check   A final checking technique for assessing the continuity and accuracy of the haircut. Where you find an imbalance in weight, or extra length that still needs to be removed, it provides you with the opportunity to remove it in order to create the perfect finish

Cowlick   A hair growth pattern that appears at the front hairline where strong movement makes part of the hair stand away from the rest. This limits styling options and can be made worse by removing weight and length

Credit card   An alternative form of payment to using cash. These cards are held by those who have a credit account where there is a pre-arranged borrowing limit

Cross checking   A final checking technique for assessing the continuity and accuracy of the haircut. Where you find an imbalance in weight, or extra length that still needs to be removed, it provides you with the opportunity to remove it in order to create the perfect finish

cross-infection   A way of passing infection from one person to another

Curtain rail   A narrow band of hair that is left around the jaw-line

Customer care/Client care   A way of providing a service to customers that promotes goodwill, comfort, satisfaction and interest. Maintaining goodwill ultimately results in regular repeated business

Cuticle   The outer protective layers of the hair that produce an overlapped effect (like tiles on a roof)

Cutting angle   The angle at which the scissors, razor etc. cuts the hair

Cutting comb   A type of comb that is between 12–20cms long. It is used for general cutting and is rigid and parallel throughout its length or it is used for barbering and is tapered and more flexible. Most cutting combs have two different teeth patterns; one end finer with closer teeth for precision work or finer hair and the other end coarser with wider apart teeth for coarser hair and detangling

D/C   Appointment abbreviation for dry cutting

Dandruff   A commonly occurring skin dysfunction where there is an over-production of epidermal cells. White scaling flakes are shed from the scalp and can be seen on the shoulder area of darker apparel. Dandruff is not contagious

Data Protection Act (1988)   Legislation designed to protect the client's right to privacy and confidentiality. See also confidentiality

Database   An archive or repository of information held on a computer, relating to business records including client and staff names, sales, products, etc

Debit card   A method of payment where the card authorizes immediate debit of the cash amount from the client's account

Debris   A polite term referring to loose material that needs to be cleared away after different forms of styling, e.g. hair fragments, bands, glue, etc

Defining crème   A finishing product which gives control to unruly hair

Defining wax   A finishing product that provides textural effects to short or long hair when used throughout the ends of the hair

Demonstrate   Display and explain a physical instruction

Denman brush   A parallel, flat brush with removable cushioned bristles. It is used for general brushing, detangling hair before shampooing and drying straight hair of any length

Density   The amount of hair follicles that populate a particular area of the skin or scalp

Deodorant   A substance that removes or conceals offensive odours

Depth   The term used to describe the lightness or darkness of hair

Dermatitis   A form of eczema which results in a red, sore, hot and itchy rash, usually between the fingers. This is known to be caused by contact with hairdressing chemicals and solutions. The condition is avoided by the wearing of PPE (such as disposable vinyl gloves)

Dermatologist   A (qualified) medical specialist for skin conditions

Dermis   The lower layers of newer skin below the outer epidermis

Detergent   A cleansing agent found in many washing materials and virtually all shampoos. It has a 'polar' molecule structure, where one end is attracted to dirt and grease and the other to water. When it comes into contact with dirt, it surrounds it and lifts it away from a surface, forming an emulsion

developer   Another name for hydrogen peroxide

Development test curl   The checks made during processing to see if the hair has reached its optimum curl/movement

Dexterity   The skill and ease of using the hands

Diffuser   An attachment for a blow-dryer which suppresses and disperses the blast of hot air and turns it into a multidirectional diffused heat

Directional wind   A technique of winding rods in the direction in which it is to be finally styled so that, when finished, the hair will move in a particular direction

disciplinary procedures   An action taken by an employer to correct serious performance issues

Discolouration   An incongruent colour effect which can result from poor colour application, incorrect colour choice or can even indicate the presence of incompatibles

Disconnection   An area within a haircut where a continued style line is broken or disjointed. A deliberate and distinct difference exists creating two levels within the layering patterns or perimeter baselines

Disease   An abnormal condition affecting the body of an organism

Disentangling   The process of removing tangles and knots from hair. It is usually carried out with a wide toothed brush or detangling comb

Disinfectant   A chemical agent that will kill most germs and bacteria (unlike sterilization which kills 100 per cent of germs and bacteria) A typical example would be Barbicide®

Disulphide bonds   The chemical bonds within the hair that are permanently rearranged during perming, relaxing and neutralizing

Double booking   An error in the appointment system where clients' bookings overlap

double brushing   A technique of using 2 brushes during brushing out

Double crown   A common hair growth pattern which appears as two whorls of hair at, or around, the crown area. This feature limits styling options and will dictate how short and the direction of how the hair can be worn

Dressing   The process of achieving finish to previously set hair

Dry hair   A condition in which the hair loses natural moisture levels affecting the handling, maintenance and style durability. It is often as a result of chemical treatments or heat styling

Dry wax   A non-greasy finishing product that provides textural effects to short or long hair when used throughout the ends of the hair

Eczema   A skin condition which appears as a reddening of the skin accompanied with itching and sometimes inflammation. It is thought to be associated with stress although one of its forms, dermatitis, can be triggered by contact with chemicals. See also dermatitis

Effective communication   Professional communication that is not ambiguous and provides clear instruction or information

Effectiveness   The quality of output achieved in a work setting

Effleurage   A light stroking massage movement applied with either the fingers or the palms of the hands and used during shampooing and conditioning

Elasticity test   A test to check the hair's ability to stretch and return to its normal length. This is a good indicator of the hair condition and strength of the internal structure of the hair

Electricity at Work Regulations (1989)   These regulations state that electrical equipment in the workplace should be tested every 12 months by a qualified electrician. The employer must keep records of the equipment tested and the date it was checked

Emphasis   The creation of focus in a hair design that draws the eye first before it travels to the rest of the design

Emulsify   In colouring terms, the process of adding a little water to the processed hair in order to loosen the colour from the hair, without adding detergent, before shampooing

End papers   Protective, paper wrapping, used around the points of the wound sections during perming to reduce/ eliminate the risk of 'fish hooks', i.e. buckled ends

Enquiry   A question presented by clients or business contacts to find out more information

Epidermis   The older, upper, protective layers of skin that constantly migrate towards the surface

Epilation   The extraction of hair

Equality and Human Rights Commission (EHRC)   An independent, UK advocate for equality and human rights

Ethmoid bone   The bone that lies between the eye sockets

Eumelanin   Naturally occurring dark brownish or black pigments within the cortex of the hair

Evacuation procedures   The arrangements made by the salon for emergency purposes, e.g. exit routes, assembly points, etc

Exfoliation   The removal or shedding of a thin outer layer of skin from the epidermis. This is done by using a gentle abrasive substance to remove the surface skin

Exothermic perms   These perming lotions tend to be similar to acid waves in their chemical composition and therefore can have similar benefits. However, they need heat in order to work and this is self-generated when the perm is mixed together before applying to the hair/curlers

Face or facial shapes   The size and shape of the facial bone structure. Face shapes include oval, round, square, heart, diamond, oblong and pear

Fading (colour reference)   The loss of intensity of coloured hair due to harsh treatment, heat styling, wrong shampoos or environmental damage

Fading (cutting reference)   A method of blending one graduated, layered area 'seamlessly' to another, within a haircut. Or graduating very short layers out and on to the skin, e.g. classic men's barbering where short hair is faded out on to the neck

Feathering   A cutting term relating to a tapered or tapering effect

Features   The aspects of a product or service that state its functions, i.e. what it does

Finger waves   The process of moulding or styling hair in a pattern of alternating waves, using the fingers and a comb

finger-drying   A technique of drying hair using the fingers

Fish hooks   A term used to describe the buckling at the points of the hair, due to incorrect winding during perming or styling

Fish tail plait (herringbone plait)   A four strand plait which is achieved by crossing four pieces of hair over each other to create a 'herringbone' look

Flat brush   A type of brush that has a handle that extends to the brush head with a flat and not curved profile. Flat brushes and paddle brushes are used for general brushing

flat clips   Clips that can hold hair with the minimum of displacement

Flat twists   Where the hair is twisted and rolled by hand, flat to the scalp

Follicle   A 'tube-like' indentation within the skin from which the hair grows

Folliculitis   Inflammation of the hair follicles which may be caused by bacterial infection

Fragilitas crinium   The technical term which is commonly known as split ends

Franchise   A business which is licensed to operate under the branding and reputation of another

Freehand cutting   A cutting technique carried out without holding the hair. This is usually to compensate for the natural fall of hair, e.g. cutting a fringe

Freehand   Refers to a cutting technique where the hair is cut without holding and is cut with natural fall, e.g. fringes

French plait   A three-strand plait that starts, centrally, near the front hairline and continues closely to the scalp to the nape and continues as a freely hanging plait beyond. This is also known as Congo plait or Guinea plait

French pleat   A method of styling longer hair into a vertical roll positioned at the back of the head

Friction (massage technique)   A firm, vigorous rubbing massage technique made by the fingertips and used during shampooing

Frontal bone   The bone that forms the forehead

Full head application (of colour or bleach)   A colouring technique that requires a sequence of applications to the mid-lengths, ends and regrowth area

Furunculosis   Raised, inflamed, pus-filled spots giving irritation, swelling and pain

Germinal matrix   The living part of the hair root where nutrients, carried in the blood supply, are converted into keratin (making hair and skin)

Goatee   A narrow beard which circles the mouth and chin

Good customer service   A positive style of service that maintains a client's goodwill

Grade   Attachment combs for clippers that provide a range of different, predefined cutting lengths

Graduation A cutting technique that is created by a sloping variation which joins longer hair that over-falls shorter hair in one continuous, blended, cutting angle

Greasy hair A condition caused by the over-production of natural oils, i.e. sebum, which exudes from glands within the scalp onto the surface and eventually the hair

Grievance A cause for concern or complaint

Grips and hair pins A variety of metal or plastic items for securing the hair into position

gross misconduct An act or event at work that may lead to instant dismissal (i.e. without any disciplinary process or procedure) (e.g. theft)

Guideline The first or starting section of hair that is held and cut to the required length and then used as a template for the following sections.

'Habia' Habia is part of the Consumer Services Industry Authority (CSIA) and is the standards setting body responsible for National Occupational Standards in hairdressing and beauty therapy

H/L FH or HL ½H Appointment abbreviation for full head or half head highlights

Hair bulb The lower club-shaped part of the hair that is attached to the germinal matrix

Hair clay/putty A thick paste-like styling product

Hair colour The resultant effect from two colour aspects within the hair. These are depth (the lightness or darkness of a colour) and tone (the degree of red, gold, ash, etc.)

Hair extensions Pieces of artificial or natural hair that are added, either temporarily or for a longer period, to a client's natural hair to provide instant length, volume or movement

Hair gel A firm hold, wet look styling product

Hair growth patterns These are double crown, widow's peak, cow lick, nape whorl, natural parting and regrowth

Hair shaft The portion of hair that projects above the epidermis

hair strengtheners A restructuring hair conditioner

Hair tendency Refers to a hair's straightness, wave, body or curl

Hair tests There are a number of tests that can be carried out prior to a service to help evaluate the effects of processing upon the hair. These tests could reveal contra-indications to services or provide information on how the hair can be processed under certain conditions, e.g. porosity test, elasticity test, pull test, etc

Hair texture Refers to the thickness or thinness of individual hairs, either coarse, medium or fine

Hair varnish A thick, glossy, water resistant styling product

hair whorls A circulatory hair growth pattern

hair-ups A term referring to a variety of dressed hair effects that are secured with clips, pins or ornamentation

Hairdressing and Beauty Industry Authority (HABIA) HABIA is part of the Consumer Services Industry Authority (CSIA) and is the standards setting body responsible for National Occupational Standards in hairdressing and beauty therapy

Hairspray A fixative originally derived from shellac, now made from water soluble compounds and is also known as lacquer

Halitosis Bad breath

Hard water Water containing minerals which do not easily lather. Hard water contains magnesium and calcium salts

Harmony The creation of unity in a design. It is the most important of the art principles and holds all the elements of the design together

HASAWA The abbreviated term referring to the Health and Safety at Work Act (1974)

Hazard Something with a potential to cause harm

Head lice An infestation of animal parasites. A very contagious contra-indication. The trichological term for head lice is pediculosis capitis

Health and Safety (First Aid) Regulations (1981) Legislation that states that workplaces must have appropriate and adequate first-aid provision

Health and Safety at Work Act (1974) Legislation that lays down the minimum standards of health, safety and welfare requirements in all workplaces

Heat protection spray Used in conjunction with electrically heated styling tools. The product laminates the outer layer of the hair so that it is protected from the damaging effects of heat

Heated rollers Used for dry setting techniques. These are electrically heated rollers that are used as an alternative to wet setting. Heated rollers produce softer results than wet setting

Heated tongs An item of heat styling equipment that provides movement, lift, volume, waves or spiralled curls on dry hair

Henna A natural colourant derived from the Lawsonia plant. Its leaves are mixed with water to create a red hair dye

Herpes simplex The scientific name for cold sores

Highlight cap A technique for highlighting hair where small sections or wefts of hair are drawn through a close fitting 'rubberized' cap and coloured or lightened. A convenient option for people who have a sensitivity to colouring and cannot have colour applied by other means

Highlights/Hi-lites A term for a very popular partial colouring technique, where small sections of natural hair are isolated (with foil, wraps, meche, etc.) and coloured or lightened to give a multi-toned effect

HL or H/L Appointment abbreviation for highlighting

HL T sect Appointment abbreviation for highlight, top and sides only

Holding angle The angle at which the hair is held out from the head when completing a haircut

Holding tension The even pressure applied to a section of hair when it is held ready for cutting

Hood dryer An electrical item that applies dry heat to the head by sitting beneath it. The heat is adjustable and the timer can be pre-set to enable previously wet set hair to be dried

Hot towels These towels are heated and used in barbering for shaving services

Humectant A hygroscopic substance attracting water or locking moisture into the hair

Humidity The level of moisture in the air

hydrogen bonds The weak linkages (between polypeptide chains) in hair that enable it to hold a hairstyle

Hydrogen peroxide An oxidizing agent used in many hairdressing processes. It readily gives off oxygen in chemical reactions, developing or processing colours, lighteners, etc

Hydrophilic A term used in reference to the 'polar' detergent molecule. The hydrophilic end is attracted to water

Hydrophobic Molecules that tend to be non-polar and, thus, prefer other neutral molecules and non-polar solvents. Hydrophobic molecules in water often cluster together, forming micelles. Water on hydrophobic surfaces will exhibit a high contact angle

hygroscopic Absorbing moisture

ICC (International Colour Chart) system A tabular system for identifying hair colours made by different manufacturers by their depth and tone

Immersed Dipped into a liquid

Impetigo A very contagious bacterial infection of the epidermal layers of the skin. It is usually identified as large brownish scabs around the mouth and cheeks. This contra-indication must be referred to a GP

Incompatibility test A method of testing hair to see if previous chemical treatments are compatible with those used with professional salons

Incompatibility Refers to incompatible chemistry. When 'inorganic' compounds are present within the hair, for example colour restorers, 'Just for

Men' or compound henna. They will be incompatible with organic based chemicals made from carbon, hydrogen and oxygen (e.g. hydrogen peroxide)

incompatible chemicals Causing a chemical reaction on mixing; as between a chemical being added to the hair and another chemical already on the hair

Incompatible products Chemicals that will not work together

Incompatible Causing a chemical reaction on mixing; as between a chemical being added to the hair and another chemical already on the hair

Individual learning plan (ILP) A specific program or strategy of education or learning that takes into consideration an individual student's strengths and weaknesses

Infection The communication of disease from one body to another. An infection is the colonization of a host organism by a parasite species

Inflammation Inflammation is a process by which the body's white blood cells and chemicals protect us from infection and foreign substances such as bacteria and viruses

Influencing factors Anything which could affect the hairdressing service

Ingrown hair A painful condition where a build-up of skin occurs at the upper end of the hair follicle, causing the hair to grow under the surface of the skin

Inversion A term used in cutting to describe a 'V' shape within a layering pattern or perimeter outline

Irritant An agent that induces irritation.

introductory discounts A sales strategy for stimulating repeated purchases of a newly introduced product or service (e.g. a new conditioning range)

Job description A documented set of written details pertaining to a person's specific job role, duties and responsibilities

Jojoba (shampoo ingredient) A natural base better on normal to drier hair types.

Knots The effect produced when long hair is wound, positioned and secured to take on a tied or knotted rope-like effect.

Lacquer A fixative originally derived from shellac, now made from water soluble compounds and commonly known as hairspray

Layering (layered cut) A cutting technique carried out on either short or long hair to produce a multi-length effect

Legal requirements The laws affecting the way businesses are operated, how the salon or workplace is set up and maintained, people in employment and the systems of working which must be maintained

Legislation Laws created by parliament

Lemon (shampoo ingredient) Contains citric acid ideal for oily scalp types or for removing product build-up

Lighteners Products that remove natural tone from the hair such as bleach or high lift colour

limits of your own authority The extent of your responsibility, say at work

Linear patterns Patterns created from either straight or curving lines or a combination of both

Lip-linemoustache A narrow lined moustache

Long facial shape An outline perimeter facial shape that has proportions that are longer from the forehead to the chin than from ear to ear

Male pattern alopecia/Male pattern baldness (MPB) A type of alopecia caused by sensitivity to androgens (male hormones)

Manual Handling Operations Regulations (1992) Legislation requiring employers to carry out a risk assessment of all activities which involve manual handling (lifting and moving objects) with the aim being to prevent injury due to poor working practice

Manufacturer's instructions Stated guidance issued by manufacturers or suppliers of products or equipment, concerning their safe and efficient use

Materials A variety of items other than tools and equipment for carrying out work including colouring packets, foils, wraps, meche, etc

Medicated shampoo Helps to maintain the normal state of the hair and scalp. Medicated shampoo contains antiseptics such as juniper or tea tree oil

Medulla The central part of the hair that is only found in coarser hair types

Melanin The hair pigments eumelanin, pheomelanin, and trichosiderin are collectively known as melanin

Merchandising The planning, promotion and presentation of a product to a target market

Metallic dye A hair colour containing metallic salts

metallic salts A range of compounds (e.g. Lead acetate) used in colour restorers/progressive dyes

Mexican moustache A moustache following the line of the upper lip and extending around and down towards the chin

Micro-organisms Living organisms bacteria, etc. of microscopic size

Mini clippers A smaller, usually battery operated clipper for use around facial hair and necklines

Mint (shampoo ingredient) A natural base suited to normal to slightly oily scalps, often used as a frequent use shampoo

Modelling block A training head or modelling head that can be used to practise hairdressing techniques and styling effects

Monilethrix The technical term that describes a rare condition that under a microscope looks like the hair is 'beaded', i.e. thicker and thinner areas of hair along the hair shaft due to uneven cellular production

Mood board A collection of ideas themes, textures, colours, etc. that form the basis of a design plan, e.g. a competition mood board

Moulding clay A dual purpose product for styling or finishing that bonds the hair with a firm hold. It is used on most hair lengths to give a firm textural bond

Movement The direction that the hairs take, individually and collectively, which affects the overall style

Multi-buys E.G. Buy one get one free (BOGOF). Any offer that encourages the customer to buy at least one product by getting something else at an attractive discount or deal

Nape whorls A hair growth pattern which affects shorter, cut hairstyles. The nape hair grows inwards, towards the centre of the back, rather than downwards. This is a limiting factor for some hairstyles

Nape The back (posterior) part of the neck

National Occupational Standards (NOS) The standards defined by an industry for different levels of ability covering all the tasks and processes involved in the industrial sector

Natural hair Hair that still has its original, natural structure

Neck brush A small hand brush with very flexible bristles for clearing debris away from the client's face, neck, etc. during and after styling

Neck wool A continuous 'sausage-like' length of cotton wool used during perming (and other services) to protect the client from spillages and debris

Nine-section wind A classic technique for perming that starts by sectioning and securing the hair into nine, pre-defined workable areas

Non-verbal communication See body language

NVQ An abbreviation for National Vocational Qualifications. These are job ready qualifications at a range of different levels.

Oblong An outline perimeter facial shape that has proportions that roughly resemble an oblong shape

Oblong facial shape An outline perimeter facial shape that has proportions that roughly resemble an oblong shape

Occipital bone The protruding part at the back of the head (cranium) that provides contour and shaping to shorter cut layered hairstyles

Oil (shampoo ingredient) Can contain a range of natural bases such as pine, palm and almond. These are used to smooth and soften drier hair and scalps

oil or gel lightener A type of lightener

Oily scalp A condition caused by the over-production of natural oils, i.e. sebum, which exudes from glands within the scalp on to the surface and eventually the hair affecting its handling, maintenance and style durability

One-length haircut A cutting technique where all the hair is cut with the natural hair fall to produce a one-length effect, i.e. the classic 'bob'

Open or 'cut throat' style razor A razor that has a fixed, rigid blade that folds into its handle for safety. The blade is kept keen (sharp) by regular stropping and honing. The razor must be sterilized before each use

Open questions A style of question that requires a full response (E.g. questions starting with 'How' 'Where' 'When' etc.)

Organic A substance that contains the chemical element carbon and relates to living (or once living) sources

Ornamentation The term refers to the accessorizing of hair with enhancements, e.g. jewellery, beads, ribbons, tiaras, decorative pins/grips, etc

Outlines The shapes created by the perimeter of nape and front hairlines

Oval An outline perimeter facial shape that has proportions that roughly resemble an oval or elliptical shape

Oval facial shape An outline perimeter facial shape that has proportions that roughly resemble an oval or elliptical shape

Over-processing A state where the normal, safe tolerances are exceeded

Overbooking Making more appointments than are physically possible to deliver within a set timescale

Oxidation A chemical reaction where oxygen is added to a substance or compound during the chemical process

oxymelanin Natural pigments that have been oxidised

Paddle brushes A wide backed, flat brush

Papilla The lower part of the follicle where living cells migrate upwards producing hair growth

Para-dyes A shortened reference to para-phenalinediames

PPD A dye compound found in many permanent colours

Para-phenylenediamine (PPD) A dye compound found in many permanent colours

paraphenylenediamine A colour compound found in some hair colours

Parasite An animal or vegetable living upon or within another organism

Parietal bone The two bones that form the sides of the cranium

Partial colouring A term that applies to areas of the head and could include techniques such as slices, block colour, polishing/shoe shining, woven or pull through highlights and lowlights, etc

Patch test/sensitivity test See skin test

Pediculosis capitis The trichological term for the head louse. An infestation of animal parasites. A very contagious contra-indication

Pencil moustache A narrow shape following the natural line of the upper lip

Penetrating conditioner A name given to a group of deeper acting conditioners that work on the inner cortex of the hair

perm solution The first part of a permanent wave system which chemically modifies the hair's inner structure

perm solutions A range of solutions that will modify the hairs internal structure

Permanent colours A penetrating colour product that adds synthetic pigments to natural hair until it grows out

Perming (permanent wave) A two-part system for adding movement to hair by chemical means

Personal development plan An on-going action plan for self-improvement that defines personal objectives or targets set over a period of time and often reviewed during an appraisal

Personal presentation Professional personal presentation can refer to personal health and hygiene, the use of personal protective equipment, clothing and accessories suitable for salon work

Personal protective equipment (PPE) This health and safety term refers to all of the items of personal equipment that are supplied by the employer for employees' safety such as gloves, aprons, etc

Personal Protective Equipment at Work Regulations (1992) Legislation requiring employers to identify, through risk assessment, those activities which require special protective equipment to be worn or used. Instruction should be provided on how the personal protective equipment should be used or worn in order to be effective

personal targets The performance targets that are set out during an appraisal

Petrissage A slower circulatory kneading massage movement of the skin that lifts and compresses underlying structures of the skin. This movement is generally used for a scalp massage when applying conditioner

pH balance The natural acid mantle of skin and hair at pH 5.5

pH level A measurement of a solution that denotes whether it is alkaline (pH 8–14), or acid (pH 6–1). A neutral solution is pH 7

pH The presence of positive hydrogen ions with a compound which denotes its levels of acidity or alkalinity

Pharaoh A beard that projects from the base of the chin

Pheomelanin A naturally occurring hair pigment that is yellowish or golden in colour

Pigments The natural substances, eumelanin, pheomelanin and trichosiderin, within the hair that gives us our hair colour

pincurls A technique of curling with clips instead of rollers

Pityriasis capitis The technical term for dandruff

plastic apron An item of PPE

Pleat A visual description of hair that is folded, such as a French pleat

Point cutting A cutting technique where the cutting angle is changed to remove hair bulk from the ends of each cutting section

Point-of-sale material The display and promotional materials supporting a specific advertising campaign

polypeptide chains The internal, fibrous structure of hair

polyvinyl or nitrile disposable gloves An item of PPE

Porosity test A test to indicate the condition (or damage) of the outer cuticle of the hair. This is a good indicator of the hair condition and its ability to absorb chemicals and moisture

Porosity The speed at which hair absorbs (and retains) moisture

Porous Hair that has lost surface protection and therefore has a greater absorption and less resistance to chemicals and products. This affects the hair's manageability, handling and ability to hold in a style

Porous hair Hair that has lost surface protection and therefore has a greater absorption and less resistance to chemicals and products. This affects the hair's manageability, handling and ability to hold in a style

Portable appliance testing (PAT) An system for checking the safety of portable electrical equipment

Portfolio A system for recording experiences, case studies, personal accounts, results from tests or assessments and the findings from projects and assignments

Post-damping The application of perming lotion after the winding in the curlers. This means that the time taken winding doesn't affect the overall processing time

Posture The positioning of the body. Good posture is when the body is in alignment. Correct posture enables you to work longer without becoming tired. It prevents muscle fatigue (tiredness) and stiff joints

pre-bonded hot extension systems An attachment method for hair extensions

pre-cutting A term for removing excesses of hair prior to styling

Pre-damping The application of perming lotion prior to winding in the curlers

Pre-perming treatments A product applied to the hair before perming to balance out uneven porosity

Pre-pigmentation The preparatory process of adding warm tones to pre-lightened hair when (and before) reintroducing depth. This counteracts the unwanted effects that will often appear if this process is not carried out first, e.g. green hues

Pre-soften A process to soften resistant white hair with hydrogen peroxide

Prices Act (1974) The price of products has to be displayed in order to prevent a false impression to the buyer

product build-up The residual amounts of styling products e.g. wax that can build -up on the hair

Professional advice Providing information based upon experience and knowledge

Professional standards The standards expected by industry, awarding organisations, NOS

progressive dyes Hair colours containing incompatible metallic salts (Lead acetate)

Project Private study focusing upon a set topic or object

Promotion An advertising campaign with supporting material to help sell a product or service

Proportion The comparative relationship of one thing to another

Provision and Use of Work Equipment Regulations (1998) (PUWER) Regulations laying down the ways in which work equipment must be used safely

Psoriasis Non-infectious areas of thickening skin/epidermal layers usually around the elbows and knees

Public liability insurance A compulsory insurance protecting employees, customers and visitors against the consequences of personal injury

PW Appointment abbreviation for permanent wave (perm).

Quasi-permanent (colour) A colour that is mixed with a low-strength developer to create a longer-lasting effect. This treatment does show a regrowth and does need a skin test 24–48 hours prior to the service.

Radial brush A completely round brush. The inner body of the brush is usually metal allowing the brush to heat up. It is used for blow-drying with volume, lift, wave and curl on short and long length hair

Razor A cutting tool for shaving

Record cards Confidential cards recording the personal details of each client registered at the salon. These cards also record services a client received and retail product purchases. The information may be stored electronically on the salon's computer

Reducing agent A product that releases hydrogen into the hair such as colour strippers, de-colour, perm lotion

reduction The chemical process that takes place when hydrogen (in alkaline substances) is introduced to hair

Referral (client) The situations where you need to redirect clients to other sources of treatment or service, i.e. when there are adverse hair and skin conditions, or because of other services that your salon doesn't provide

re-touch/regrowth The band of natural hair growing back at the root area (12.5mm per month) which will require some form of processing to match the mid lengths and ends

Regrowth The band of natural hair growing back at the root area (12.5mm per month) which will require some form of processing to match the mid lengths and ends

Relaxer/relaxing A chemical process (usually in two parts) which removes natural movement/curl from the hair

Resale Prices Acts (1964 and 1976) The manufacturers can supply a recommended retail price (MRRP), but the seller is not obliged to sell at the recommended price

Reshape/reshaping Cutting hair back into style. A six-weekly reshape cut will maintain a hairstyle

Resources The variety of means available to a business that can be utilized or employed within any given task or project including time, money, staff, equipment, stock, etc

Restructurant A deep acting treatment that will help to re-strengthen natural hair

Restyle Cutting hair into a new style

Reverse graduation A cutting technique that joins together shorter hair down to longer hair in one continuous cutting angle

RIDDOR Reporting of Injuries, Diseases and Dangerous Occurrences Regulations. This legislation requires the employer to report certain injuries or diseases occurring in the workplace

Ringworm A fungal disease also known as tinea capitis. It is a very contagious contra-indication and must be referred to a GP

Risk assessment A process of looking for and assessing the hazards within the workplace

Risk The likelihood of harm occurring from a potential hazard

role play A simulation of an activity or process

Rollers A variety of circular formers of differing diameters used for setting hair when dry (e.g. Velcro self-cling) or wet (e.g. 'Skelox')

Rooftop moustache A shape that extends from under the nose to form a straight 'chevron' or inverted 'V' shape

Root lift mousse A mousse that has a directional nozzle allowing you to apply foam at or near to the roots. It is used on hair that needs body

Rotary massage A quicker and firmer circular movement used during the shampooing process

Round An outline perimeter facial shape that has proportions that roughly resemble a circular or round shape

Round facial shape An outline perimeter facial shape that has proportions that roughly resemble a circular or round shape

Safety razor A hand-held razor that is fitted with disposable blades providing a more convenient, hygienic option, as the blades can be replaced for each client

Sale and Supply of Goods Act (1994) The vendor must ensure that the goods they sell are of satisfactory quality and reasonably fit. The goods must be the standard that would be regarded by a reasonable person as satisfactory having taken into account the description of the goods, the price and other relevant circumstances. The vendor must ensure that the goods can meet the purpose they are claimed to do

Salon policy The hairdressing procedures or work rules issued by the salon management

Salon services The extent and variety of all the services offered in your workplace

salt bonds Weaker bonds between polypeptide chains that are broken during shampooing

Scabies The common name of the itch mite. This animal parasite burrows beneath the surface of the skin and is very highly contagious. Referral to a GP is essential

Scalp plaits Also known as a French plait, a cane row or cornrow

Scalp The skin covering the top of the head

Scissor over comb A technique of cutting hair with scissors, using the back of the comb as a guide. This technique is usually used when the hair is at a length that cannot be held between the fingers

Scrunch drying A form of finger drying technique, where the lengths of the hair are dried (often with the aid of a diffuser) and compacted/crushed by the fingers to maximize the hair's natural movement

Sebaceous cyst A swelling of the oil gland within the hair follicle

Sebaceous glands Sack-like appendages on the sides of the follicle that secrete sebum onto the hair shaft

Seborrhea An overproduction of natural oils causing a greasy scalp and hair

Sebum A natural oil produced by the sebaceous gland

self-adhesive extension An attachment method for hair extensions

Semi-permanent colour A semi permanent colour is not mixed with hydrogen peroxide. It only penetrates to the lower cuticle and therefore lasts for a few washes

Senegalese twists A twisting technique that resembles the plaited effect created by cornrows

Serum A silicone-based product that is used as a finishing product to smooth the hair and to add shine

Shape, proportion and balance The physical and notional aspects that control hair design and hairstyling

Shaper razor A type of razor with disposable blades that is used for cutting and styling hair, but not for shaving. It therefore has uses for both women's and men's hairstyling

Sharps box A sharps box is a designated sealed container used for the safe disposal of sharp items, e.g. used razor blades

Sharps A term to describe sharp objects, e.g. razors, razor blades and scissors

Shaving cream Moisturizes the skin while providing a good lubricant for shaving. Moisturizing shaving creams can be used for all skin types, but normal to drier skins will benefit most from the creams

Shelftalkers A point of sale show card that is fixed to a shelf so that it stands out and can attract attention because it stands out from the other products

Short graduations Haircuts where the inner and upper layers of a haircut are longer than the lengths of the outline, perimeter hair

sideburns Men's facial hair that extends from the sides, in front of the ears, downwards

skin sensitivities A predisposition to certain chemicals or environments

Skin tests As with hair tests, there are a number of tests that can be carried out prior to a service to help evaluate the effects of processing upon the skin. These tests could reveal contra-indications to services by providing information on how the skin reacts under certain conditions

Slicing (colouring) Sections of colour placed in the hair to bring attention to style lines or styling features

Slicing A texturizing technique for cutting hair using the sharp blades of scissors without opening and closing them, like using a razor or shaper

Soya (shampoo ingredient) Helps to lock in moisture for the hair and scalp

Special offers See multi-buys

Sphenoid bone The bone at the base of the cranium, behind the eye sockets

Spiral wind A perming technique of winding longer hair from root to point to create cascading curls

Split ends A condition of the hair where a damaged cuticle exposes the inner cortex of the hair allowing it to split along its length (fragilitas crinium)

Square An outline perimeter facial shape that has proportions that roughly resemble a square shape

Square facial shape An outline perimeter facial shape that has proportions that roughly resemble a square shape

Steamer An item of salon equipment that is used for accelerating the development time of bleach lighteners. It produces a moist heat which stops the bleach drying out during the lightening process

Sterile Free from germs

Sterilization The complete eradication of living bacteria and germs

stock control A system for organizing the purchases, holding levels and movements of consumables within a business

storyboard A visual representation of a sequence of events

Straightener (chemical) An ammonium-based lotion similar to perms that can be used to remove wave in hair

Straightening Reducing the curl or wave in hair

Strand test A test carried out upon hair prior to chemical services to determine the effects of processing

Strengths and weaknesses The difference between personal skill areas that you excel in and those that you need to work on

Style line The directions in which the hair is positioned or appears to flow

Styling glaze A thick, glossy, water resistant styling product

Styling mousse A general styling aid for adding volume and providing hold when blow-drying or setting

Stylist Another name for a qualified hairdresser or hairstylist

Subcutaneous fatty layer/Subcutaneous tissue A fatty layer of cells at the lower dermis beneath the skin

Surface conditioner A light conditioner that works on the outside of the hair to smooth and fill areas of damaged, missing or worn cuticle until the next shampoo

surface tension The tension of the surface film of a liquid caused by the attraction of the particles in the surface layer by the bulk of the liquid

Surfactant A surface acting chemical detergent that cleanses the surface of the hair and skin

Sweat gland Small tubes in the skin of the dermis and epidermis which excrete sweat. Their function is to regulate body temperature through the evaporation of sweat from the skin's surface

Sweat A clear, salty liquid produced by glands in the skin that helps to regulate body temperature

SWOT analysis An evaluation process for identifying; strengths, weaknesses, opportunities and threats

Sycosis An inflammatory disease affecting the follicles, particularly the beard. Appearing as pustules or papules, perforated by the hair

Symmetrical Balanced by means of an even and equal distribution of hair on either side

Synthetic colour Any form of colour that is not a naturally occurring pigment. A term that is often used instead of artificial colour

T liner/outliner A type of clipper with a different blade type to standard clippers, enabling closer cut outlines around ears, necklines and facial hair shapes

T-section highlights A partial highlighting technique around the hairline and along the parting only

Tail or pin comb A comb that provides tension when combing through sections and helps to manage hair. It is used for sectioning hair into workable sizes depending on the setting, plaiting or twisting technique used

Tapered necklines Soft outlines that follow the natural hairline shape so that the nape outline appears to fade out with no harsh lines visible

Tapering Cutting a hair section by removing thickness towards the ends of the hair to form a tapered point, i.e. a point like that of a sharpened pencil

Tapotement A brisk tapping or slapping massage movement which is also known as percussion

Tea tree oil (shampoo ingredient) A natural essential oil, like an antiseptic, which will fight infections on the scalp

Telogen The period during which a hair ceases to grow before it is shed

Temporal bones Form the lower sides of the head

Temporary bonds   The hydrogen bonds within the hair that are modified and fix the style into shape

Temporary colours   Colours that do not penetrate the hair cuticle or affect the natural hair colour, but remain on the hair until washed off

Tensile strength test   A test that will determine the breaking point of a hair. This relates directly to the internal structure of the hair within the cortex

Tension   The state of being stretched

Terminal hair   The coarser type of hair that is found on the scalp and other areas of the body. There are three specific stages of terminal hair growth: anagen, telogen and catagen

Texturizing   A variety of cutting techniques that are used to achieve different effects within the cutting scheme of a hairstyle

Thinning scissors   Scissors which will remove uniform bulk from any point between the root area and ends

Thinning   A way of reducing the thickness or amount of hair without having an effect on the overall (apparent) hair length. Techniques would include razoring, texturizing or by using thinning scissors

Tinea capitis   A fungal disease commonly known as ringworm. It is a very contagious contra-indication and must be referred to a GP

tone on tone colours   Demi, or Quasi permanent colours

Tone   Refers to the tonal (the colour) properties of hair. These are grouped into reds, golds, mahogany, ash, chestnut, etc

Toner/toning   Adding pastel colours to previously, lightened hair to control the final desired effect. Toning can neutralize unwanted tones or add depth or colour to hair that is too light

Tonging   A technique of styling hair with heated equipment. The tongs are cylindrical in shape and, when heated, hair is wound around and held in place for a few seconds and then released

Total look   A term that is often used to describe a visual themed effect that incorporates hair, clothes, accessories and make-up

Traction alopecia   An area of baldness that is caused by the excessive pulling of hair at the root. It is often associated with longer hair worn in plaits, twists, hair-ups and extensions

Trade Descriptions Act (1968)   Products must not be falsely or misleadingly described in relation to their quality, fitness, price or purpose, by advertisements, orally, displays or descriptions. Since 1972 it is also a requirement to label a product clearly, so that the buyer can see where the product was made

Tramliner   A type of hair clipper

Triangular facial shape   An outline perimeter facial shape where the chin is very narrow

Trichologist   A professionally qualified person who specializes in the diagnosis and treatment of hair and scalp problems

Trichorrhexis nodosa   A condition where the hair has damaged sites of cuticle allowing the fibrous cortex to break through. This makes the hair weakened, very knotted and hard to manage

Trichosiderin   An iron-containing pigment found in human red hair

Trim/Trimming   A trim denotes a haircut where very little is taken off in order to maintain a hairstyle. Typically a six-weekly reshape is another name for a trim

Twist   A technique of styling hair, or multiple stems of hair, by twisting them together.

Ultraviolet radiation   A form of sterilization carried out in salons by putting tools and equipment into a UV cabinet

Under-processing   A state where the normal expected results are not allowed to fully develop

Uniform layer cut   This type of haircut has sections that are equal, i.e. the same length throughout

UV cabinet   A system for sterilising tools and equipment using ultra violet rays

Velcro rollers   Self-cling setting rollers for use on dry hair. They produce a softer curl effect than wet setting rollers

Vented brush   A parallel, flat brush with a double row of rigid, plastic bristles (short and long) affixed to a brush head that is not solid. It is used for general brushing and straightening of short to mid-length hair

vertical roll   A technique for dressing hair in a folded pleat

virgin hair   Untreated natural hair

Virus   The smallest micro-organisms that cause infection and disease

visual aids   Anything used to provide a visual representation e.g.. colour chart, pictures etc

VRQ   An abbreviation for Vocationally Related Qualifications. These are job ready qualifications at a range of different levels

W/C   Appointment abbreviation for wet cutting

Warmth   A reference to hair tones that appear golden, copper or red in colour

Wefts   Long continuous strands of pre-coloured, pre-bonded hair that create a 'curtain' of hair that can be used to add to, or extend, a client's own natural hair

Wetting agent   A chemical agent that allows a liquid to spread more easily across or into a surface by lowering the liquid's surface tension

Whorls   A circular hair growth pattern that will influence or limit the styling options for a client, e.g. nape whorls

Widow's peak   A distinct point in the hairline in the centre of the forehead

X readings   A sub-total of sales held within the till

Z reading   A final till reading providing summaries of all sales/petty cash etc.

Index